Molecular Therapies for Inherited Retinal Diseases

Molecular Therapies for Inherited Retinal Diseases

Editors

Rob W.J. Collin
Alejandro Garanto

MDPI • Basel • Beijing • Wuhan • Barcelona • Belgrade • Manchester • Tokyo • Cluj • Tianjin

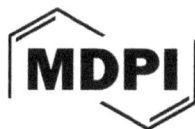

Editors
Rob W.J. Collin
Radboud University Medical Center
The Netherlands

Alejandro Garanto
Radboud University Medical Center
The Netherlands

Editorial Office
MDPI
St. Alban-Anlage 66
4052 Basel, Switzerland

This is a reprint of articles from the Special Issue published online in the open access journal *Genes* (ISSN 2073-4425) (available at: https://www.mdpi.com/journal/genes/special_issues/mol_therap_IRD).

For citation purposes, cite each article independently as indicated on the article page online and as indicated below:

LastName, A.A.; LastName, B.B.; LastName, C.C. Article Title. *Journal Name* **Year**, *Article Number*, Page Range.

ISBN 978-3-03943-176-2 (Hbk)
ISBN 978-3-03943-177-9 (PDF)

Cover image courtesy of Susanne Roosing and Alejandro Garanto.

© 2020 by the authors. Articles in this book are Open Access and distributed under the Creative Commons Attribution (CC BY) license, which allows users to download, copy and build upon published articles, as long as the author and publisher are properly credited, which ensures maximum dissemination and a wider impact of our publications.
The book as a whole is distributed by MDPI under the terms and conditions of the Creative Commons license CC BY-NC-ND.

Contents

About the Editors vii

Rob W.J. Collin and Alejandro Garanto
Preface of Special Issue "Molecular Therapies for Inherited Retinal Diseases"
Reprinted from: *Genes* **2020**, *11*, 169, doi:10.3390/genes11020169 1

Peter M.J. Quinn and Jan Wijnholds
Retinogenesis of the Human Fetal Retina: An Apical Polarity Perspective
Reprinted from: *Genes* **2019**, *10*, 987, doi:10.3390/genes10120987 3

Ivana Trapani
Adeno-Associated Viral Vectors as a Tool for Large Gene Delivery to the Retina
Reprinted from: *Genes* **2019**, *10*, 287, doi:10.3390/genes10040287 43

Jasmina Cehajic Kapetanovic, Alun R. Barnard and Robert E. MacLaren
Molecular Therapies for Choroideremia
Reprinted from: *Genes* **2019**, *10*, 738, doi:10.3390/genes10100738 55

**Jasmina Cehajic Kapetanovic, Michelle E McClements,
Cristina Martinez-Fernandez de la Camara and Robert E MacLaren**
Molecular Strategies for *RPGR* Gene Therapy
Reprinted from: *Genes* **2019**, *10*, 674, doi:10.3390/genes10090674 71

**Laura R. Bohrer, Luke A. Wiley, Erin R. Burnight, Jessica A. Cooke, Joseph C. Giacalone,
Kristin R. Anfinson, Jeaneen L. Andorf, Robert F. Mullins, Edwin M. Stone
and Budd A. Tucker**
Correction of NR2E3 Associated Enhanced S-cone Syndrome Patient-specific iPSCs
using CRISPR-Cas9
Reprinted from: *Genes* **2019**, *10*, 278, doi:10.3390/genes10040278 87

Sarah Naessens, Laurien Ruysschaert, Steve Lefever, Frauke Coppieters and Elfride De Baere
Antisense Oligonucleotide-Based Downregulation of the G56R Pathogenic Variant Causing
NR2E3-Associated Autosomal Dominant Retinitis Pigmentosa
Reprinted from: *Genes* **2019**, *10*, 363, doi:10.3390/genes10050363 101

Marta Zuzic, Jesus Eduardo Rojo Arias, Stefanie Gabriele Wohl and Volker Busskamp
Retinal miRNA Functions in Health and Disease
Reprinted from: *Genes* **2019**, *10*, 377, doi:10.3390/genes10050377 113

**Iris Barny, Isabelle Perrault, Christel Michel, Nicolas Goudin, Sabine Defoort-Dhellemmes,
Imad Ghazi, Josseline Kaplan, Jean-Michel Rozet and Xavier Gerard**
AON-Mediated Exon Skipping to Bypass Protein Truncation in Retinal Dystrophies Due to the
Recurrent *CEP290* c.4723A > T Mutation. Fact or Fiction?
Reprinted from: *Genes* **2019**, *10*, 368, doi:10.3390/genes10050368 129

Alejandro Garanto, Lonneke Duijkers, Tomasz Z. Tomkiewicz and Rob W. J. Collin
Antisense Oligonucleotide Screening to Optimize the Rescue of the Splicing Defect Caused by
the Recurrent Deep-Intronic *ABCA4* Variant c.4539+2001G>A in Stargardt Disease
Reprinted from: *Genes* **2019**, *10*, 452, doi:10.3390/genes10060452 147

Siebren Faber and Ronald Roepman
Balancing the Photoreceptor Proteome: Proteostasis Network Therapeutics for Inherited Retinal Disease
Reprinted from: *Genes* **2019**, *10*, 557, doi:10.3390/genes10080557 . . . . **161**

Arianna Tolone, Soumaya Belhadj, Andreas Rentsch, Frank Schwede and François Paquet-Durand
The cGMP Pathway and Inherited Photoreceptor Degeneration: Targets, Compounds, and Biomarkers
Reprinted from: *Genes* **2019**, *10*, 453, doi:10.3390/genes10060453 . . . . **187**

Sònia Trigueros, Elena B. Domènech, Vasileios Toulis and Gemma Marfany
In Vitro Gene Delivery in Retinal Pigment Epithelium Cells by Plasmid DNA-Wrapped Gold Nanoparticles
Reprinted from: *Genes* **2019**, *10*, 289, doi:10.3390/genes10040289 . . . . **203**

Irene Vázquez-Domínguez, Alejandro Garanto and Rob W.J. Collin
Molecular Therapies for Inherited Retinal Diseases—Current Standing, Opportunities and Challenges
Reprinted from: *Genes* **2019**, *10*, 654, doi:10.3390/genes10090654 . . . . **215**

Ben Shaberman and Todd Durham
The Foundation Fighting Blindness Plays an Essential and Expansive Role in Driving Genetic Research for Inherited Retinal Diseases
Reprinted from: *Genes* **2019**, *10*, 511, doi:10.3390/genes10070511 . . . . **245**

About the Editors

Rob W.J. Collin Following the completion of his MSc studies in Chemistry, Dr. Collin obtained his Ph.D. studying the physiological role of proteins involved in Alzheimer's disease. Thereafter, he moved to the field of Human Genetics, where he first was involved in identifying the genetic causes of inherited hearing loss and, later, visual impairment. Intrigued by the upcoming potential of genetic therapies to treat these diseases, Dr. Collin shifted gears and built his own group around the topic of developing novel therapeutic strategies for inherited retinal diseases. Dr. Collin is currently an Associate Professor on "Molecular therapies for eye diseases" at the Department of Human Genetics of the Radboudumc.

Alejandro Garanto studied Biology at the University of Barcelona. Subsequently, he enrolled in the Ph.D. program of the Department of Genetics to study the function of a frequently mutated gene associated with inherited retinal disease. After the completion of his PhD, he worked on the exciting topic of deubiquitinating enzymes and their role in the retinal fate. In 2012, he moved to Nijmegen and joined the group of Dr. Collin at the Radboudumc as a postdoc. Since then, he has focused his scientific career on the development of novel therapeutic interventions for inherited retinal disease. Currently, Dr. Garanto is an Assistant Professor leading the "DNA and RNA editing for inherited retinal diseases" group at the Department of Human Genetics of the Radboudumc.

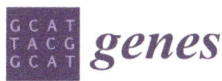

Editorial

Preface of Special Issue "Molecular Therapies for Inherited Retinal Diseases"

Rob W.J. Collin * and Alejandro Garanto *

Department of Human Genetics and Donders Institute for Brain, Cognition and Behaviour, Radboud University Medical Center, P.O. Box 9101, 6500 HB Nijmegen, The Netherlands
* Correspondence: rob.collin@radboudumc.nl (R.W.J.C.); alex.garanto@radboudumc.nl (A.G.)

Received: 29 January 2020; Accepted: 4 February 2020; Published: 5 February 2020

Inherited retinal diseases (IRDs) are a group of progressive disorders that lead to severe visual impairment or even complete blindness. IRDs display a vast heterogeneity, clinically as well as genetically, with over 250 genes identified in which mutations can cause one or more clinical subtypes of IRD. Long considered incurable diseases, intense research over the last two decades, combined with major technological advancements, have enabled the development of the first therapeutic approaches for these diseases. The approval of LuxturnaTM (voretigene neparvovec), a gene augmentation therapy vector for *RPE65*-associated IRD, by the US Food and Drug Administration and the European Medicines Agency, is considered a true milestone in the field, and has led to the development of similar, or different therapeutic strategies for many other subtypes of IRD. Despite these major achievements, there are still many aspects that can—and need to—be improved, including more insights into the relationship between genetic variation and cellular dysfunction, optimization of the vectors and sequences used, improving delivery methods, as well as understanding and modulating the (local) immune response. In addition, the extreme rarity of some genetic subtypes of IRDs poses an enormous challenge on the development of novel therapies, in terms of e.g., costs and regulatory affairs.

In this Special Issue of Genes, we focus our attention on molecular therapeutic approaches for IRD, i.e., strategies that aim to overcome the primary genetic defect, or its consequences, by using genetic material or small compounds to restore molecular and cellular function. The issue is comprised of original research articles as well as (mini-)reviews, on topics such as gene augmentation, RNA-based therapies, genome editing, proteostasis, small molecule approaches and delivery vectors. The manuscripts mainly contain preclinical research, varying from work in cellular systems to in vivo studies. Some reviews summarize the current stage of ongoing clinical trials, i.e., for *CHM*- and *RPGR*-associated IRD. We close this Special Issue with a contribution of the Foundation Fighting Blindness USA on the patient's (organizations') perspective on the current landscape, as well as a future perspective on the era that lies ahead of us. With this, we aim to provide a contemporary overview on the development and implementation of novel (personalized) therapies for IRD, and identify the tremendous possibilities as well as the key bottlenecks that currently exist.

© 2020 by the authors. Licensee MDPI, Basel, Switzerland. This article is an open access article distributed under the terms and conditions of the Creative Commons Attribution (CC BY) license (http://creativecommons.org/licenses/by/4.0/).

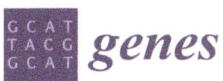

Review

Retinogenesis of the Human Fetal Retina: An Apical Polarity Perspective

Peter M.J. Quinn [1] and Jan Wijnholds [1,2,*]

[1] Department of Ophthalmology, Leiden University Medical Center, 2300 RC Leiden, The Netherlands; pq2138@cumc.columbia.edu
[2] The Netherlands Institute for Neuroscience, Royal Netherlands Academy of Arts and Sciences, 1105 BA Amsterdam, The Netherlands
* Correspondence: J.Wijnholds@lumc.nl; Tel.: +31-71-526-9269

Received: 21 August 2019; Accepted: 26 November 2019; Published: 29 November 2019

Abstract: The Crumbs complex has prominent roles in the control of apical cell polarity, in the coupling of cell density sensing to downstream cell signaling pathways, and in regulating junctional structures and cell adhesion. The Crumbs complex acts as a conductor orchestrating multiple downstream signaling pathways in epithelial and neuronal tissue development. These pathways lead to the regulation of cell size, cell fate, cell self-renewal, proliferation, differentiation, migration, mitosis, and apoptosis. In retinogenesis, these are all pivotal processes with important roles for the Crumbs complex to maintain proper spatiotemporal cell processes. Loss of Crumbs function in the retina results in loss of the stratified appearance resulting in retinal degeneration and loss of visual function. In this review, we begin by discussing the physiology of vision. We continue by outlining the processes of retinogenesis and how well this is recapitulated between the human fetal retina and human embryonic stem cell (ESC) or induced pluripotent stem cell (iPSC)-derived retinal organoids. Additionally, we discuss the functionality of in utero and preterm human fetal retina and the current level of functionality as detected in human stem cell-derived organoids. We discuss the roles of apical-basal cell polarity in retinogenesis with a focus on Leber congenital amaurosis which leads to blindness shortly after birth. Finally, we discuss Crumbs homolog (*CRB*)-based gene augmentation.

Keywords: apical polarity; crumbs complex; fetal retina; PAR complex; retinal organoids; retinogenesis; gene augmentation; adeno-associated virus (AAV); Leber congenital amaurosis

1. The Physiology of Vision

Vision is perhaps the most dominant sense in daily life and both non-correctable unilateral and bilateral vision loss severely impact the quality of life [1]. Vision begins with the processing of light, which is electromagnetic radiation that travels as waves (Figure 1A). Light waves, as with all waves, can be characterized by their wavelength (distance between wave peaks), frequency (number of wavelengths within a time period), and amplitude (the height of each peak or depth of each trough). Visible light is a narrow group of wavelengths between approximately 400 nm and 760 nm which we interpret as a spectrum of different colors (Figure 1B) [2]. Light can be reflected (bounce of a surface), absorbed (transfer of energy to a surface), or refracted (bending of light between two mediums) (Figure 1C).

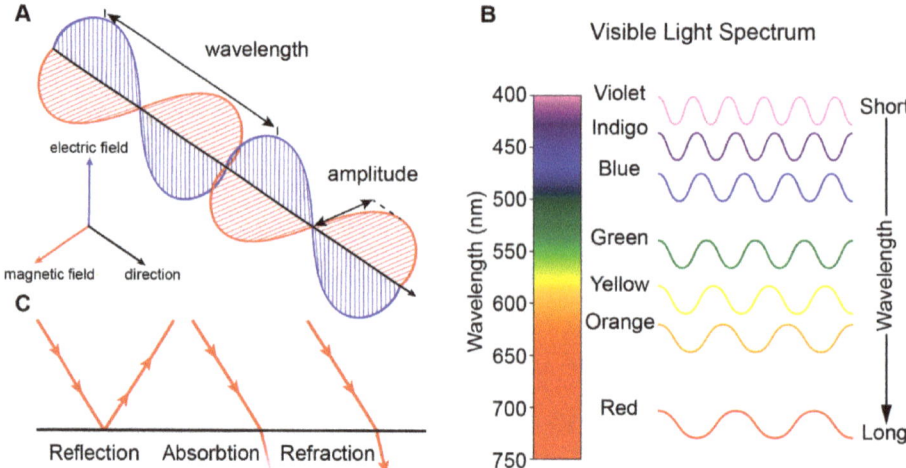

Figure 1. Transmission of light. (**A**) Light is electromagnetic radiation that travels as waves consisting of perpendicular oscillating electric and magnetic fields. (**B**) Visible light is a narrow group of wavelengths between approximately 400 nm (short wavelength) and 760 nm (long wavelength) which we interpret as a spectrum of different colors. Wavelengths outside this range are not visible to humans. (**C**) Light can be reflected, absorbed and refracted.

When light first enters the eye, it is refracted by the cornea through the pupil, whose size is controlled by the iris. The iris, the colored part of the eye, controls the amount of light entering the eye while the lens focuses the light through the vitreous humor and on to the proximal surface of the retina (Figure 2A). The adult retina consists of one glial cell type, the Müller glial cells, and six major types of neurons, the rod and cone photoreceptors, bipolar cells, amacrine cells, horizontal cells, and ganglion cells (Figure 2B). Their cell bodies are distributed across three nuclear layers, the outer nuclear layer (ONL), inner nuclear layer (INL), and ganglion cell layer (GCL). Two synaptic layers, the outer plexiform layer (OPL) and inner plexiform layer (IPL), contain the axonal and dendritic processes of the cells [3]. Whereas there is one type of rod photoreceptor, there are various subtypes of cone photoreceptor, bipolar, amacrine, horizontal, and ganglion cells that differ in their functional roles and morphology [4]. Besides Müller glial cells there are two other glial cell types that serve to maintain retinal homeostasis, the astrocytes and resident microglia [5]. Light must be channelled through the retina and absorbed by its three light responsive cells: the rod and cone photoreceptors and the intrinsically-photosensitive retinal ganglion cells (ipRGCs). The mammalian retina contains various opsin proteins involved in the photoreception synchronisation of circadian rhythms (photoentrainment). These are the cone opsins (M/LWS, red/green opsin; SWS1, blue opsin) responsible for high visual acuity, resolution, and color vision (photopic vision), and rod opsin (RH1, Rhodopsin) responsible for dim light vision (scotopic vision) and ipRGCs opsin (OPN4, Melanopsin) responsible for synchronisation of the circadian rhythms and ambient light perception [6–9]. The cones are less sensitive to light and rods are more sensitive to light and are also used together under intermediated light conditions (mesopic vision) [10]. Most forms of inherited retinal disease negatively affect the function of photoreceptors, resulting in progressive loss of rod and/or cone photoreceptors. Müller glial cells mediate the channelling of light through the retina towards the photoreceptors [11,12]. Müller glial cells can channel different wavelengths of light to specific subsets of photoreceptors to optimise day vision [13]. The visual pigments of the photoreceptors contain an opsin protein covalently linked to the chromophore 11-*cis*-retinal. Upon the absorption of a photon 11-*cis*-retinal becomes isomerised to all-*trans*-retinal, this leads to an activated opsin intermediate (metarhodopsin II, rods; Meta-II, cones). This active intermediate leads to triggering of a transduction cascade resulting in hyperpolarisation of the photoreceptors, due to the closure of cyclic guanosine 3′,5′-monophosphate (cGMP)-gated channels, and a reduction in glutamate release [14]. This electrophysiological signal is then further propagated to the inner retina and can be propagated through many different pathways to the ganglion cells. Prototypically these signals can be direct, from photoreceptor (PRC) to bipolar cells to ganglion cells. However, it can also be indirect with lateral modulation of the electrophysiological signals being made by horizontal cell processes in the OPL or by amacrine cell processes in the IPL [10,15,16]. Thus, creating radially aligned "functional units" of photoreceptors, bipolar cells, amacrine cells, horizontal cells, and ganglion cells. The fovea contains a specialised pathway, termed the midget pathway, which helps account for its ability to provide high visual acuity [17–19].

The visual system, however, is not solely comprised of the eye but also the topographically mapped ganglion cell axonal projections connecting the retina to the superior colliculus (SC) and lateral geniculate nucleus (LGN) in the brain [20]. The ganglion cell axonal projections exit the left and right eyes as bundles, the optic nerves, and they extend to below the hypothalamus to the optic chiasm. The optic chiasm is the crossover point for the nasal axons of each eye which combine with the opposing eyes temporal axons. The two optic tracts extend from the optic chiasm to the SC and the LGN, with the optic radiations further extending from the LGN to the primary visual cortex (Figure 2C) [21]. The SC, LGN, and pulvinar nuclei are all involved in the process of relaying and refining visual information to the primary visual cortex [22,23]. Interestingly, despite the severe retinal dysfunction of Leber congenital amaurosis-2 (LCA2) patients, recovery of both retinal function, but also reorganization and maturation of synaptic connectivity in the visual pathway, is found upon administration of a gene therapy treatment [24]. Such recovery highlights the relative plasticity of the human visual system.

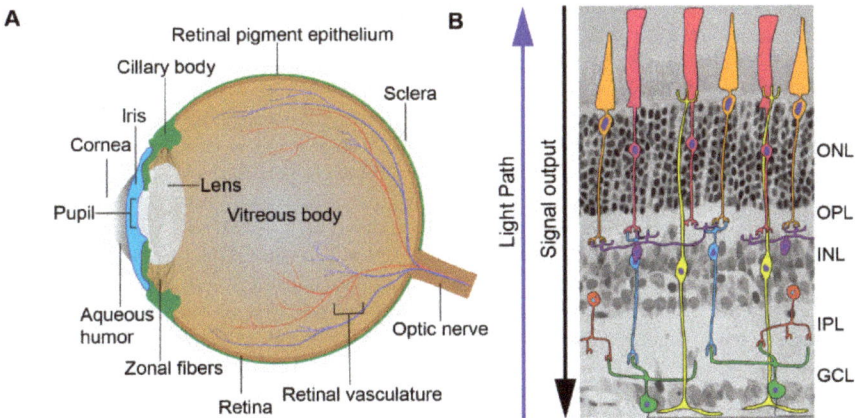

Figure 2. *Cont.*

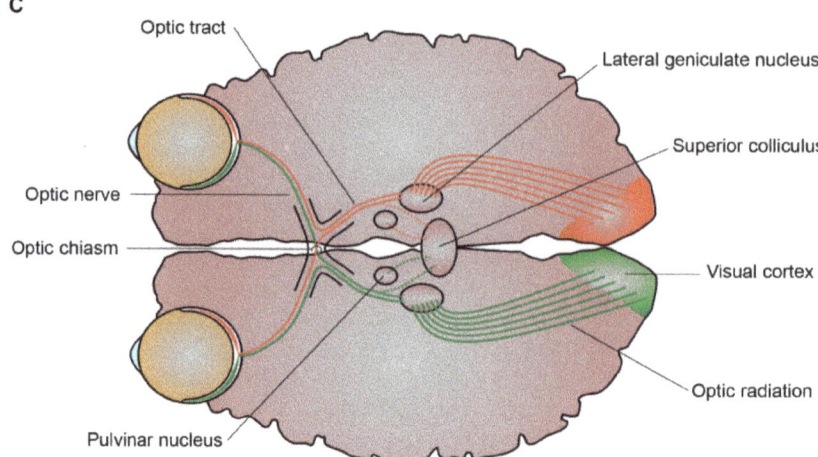

Figure 2. Processing of light. (**A**) Schematic picture of the eye. The eye is comprised of the aqueous humor, ciliary body, cornea, iris, lens, optic nerve, pupil, retina, retinal pigment epithelium, retinal vasculature, sclera, vitreous body, and zonal fibers. When light first enters the eye, it is refracted by the cornea through the pupil, whose size is controlled by the iris. The iris, the colored part of the eye, controls the amount of light entering the eye while the lens focuses the light through the vitreous humor and on to the proximal surface of the retina. (**B**) Schematic picture of the retina. The retina is composed of seven cell types: amacrine cells (red), bipolar cells (blue), cones (orange), ganglion cells (green), horizontal cells (purple), Müller glial cells (yellow), and rods (pink). When light first enters the retina, it goes through the ganglion cell layer (GCL), then the inner plexiform layer (IPL), inner nuclear layer (INL), outer plexiform layer (OPL), and outer nuclear layer (ONL). As light is passing through the retina it is absorbed by its light responsive cells: rod and cone photoreceptors and the intrinsically-photosensitive retinal ganglion cells (ipRGCs). This creates electrophysiological signals that then are further propagated to the inner retina and can be propagated through many different cell to cell pathways to the ganglion cells. (**C**) Schematic picture of the visual pathway. The axons of the retinal ganglion cells exit the eyes as bundles, the optic nerve, and extend to the optic chiasm were the nasal axons of each eye crossover and combine with the contralateral eyes temporal axons and subsequently via the optic tract travel to the lateral geniculate nucleus (LGN) and superior colliculus (SC). The LGN, SC, and pulvinar nucleus are all involved in the process of relaying and refining visual information to the visual cortex. Visual information is relayed to the visual cortex via optic radiations which extend from the LGN.

2. Retinogenesis

The retina, part of the central nervous system, offers an extremely accessible and relatively immune-privileged model system for investigating the mechanisms of neural development and vision [25]. A high conservation of the genes involved in retinal development exists across species allowing us to gain an in-depth fundamental knowledge of these mechanisms. Retinal development is both a pre- and postnatal process. The development of the retina begins when the anterior neural plate subdivides into a number of domains, with the medial region specifying as the eye field (Figure 3). The formation of the eye field is coordinated by expression of the eye field transcription factors (EFTFs), shortly after gastrulation. There are a number of EFTFs in mammals including Pax6, Rax, Lhx2, Six3, and Six6. The eye field consists of all the progenitors which go on to form all the neural-derived cell types and structures of the eye [26–30]. The progenitors of the eye field begin to specialize very early in development, hence the large number of bilateral diseases of eye morphogenesis [28]. From the eye field, bilateral optic sulci form and evaginate from the diencephalon at human fetal embryonic day 22

(E22) forming optic vesicles at E24 (Figure 3). The optic vesicles extend towards the surface ectoderm remaining connected to the forebrain through the optic stalk, which eventually develops into the optic nerve. The hyaloid artery, running from the optic stalk and into the retinal neuroepithelium through the optic fissure, provides the basis for the vascularisation of the retina and developing eye. As the optic vesicles invaginate forming the two-layered optic cups by E32, the surface ectoderm thickens forming the lens placode and further develops into lens vesicle, sitting behind the surface ectoderm (Figure 3). The anterior rim of the optic cup will become the iris and ciliary body, while the posterior rim will become the pigmented and neural retina. The outer layer of the posterior optic cup remains as a single cuboidal layer becoming the retinal pigment epithelium (RPE). The single inner layer of the posterior optic cup proliferates and differentiates, beginning in the 7th fetal week (Fwk), developing into the multilayered neural retina [28,31].

The processes of the newborn progenitors of the inner optic cup, the retinal neuroepithelium, extend and attach both apically through adherens junctions (AJs) at the outer limiting membrane (OLM), and basally through integrin- and proteoglycan-based focal adhesions at the inner limiting membrane (ILM) [32,33]. Retinal progenitors undergo interkinetic nuclear migration in which their nuclei move in an apical-basal manner in phase with the cell cycle, this occurs in mainly a stochastic manner but becomes briefly directed at cell division (Figure 4A) [33–35]. Progenitors initially undergo symmetric cell division leading to an increase in the pool of progenitors and thus thickening of the neuroepithelium. After that the progenitors go through asymmetric divisions, and produce one daughter cell to maintain the stem cell pool and one terminally differentiated postmitotic cell. Later in development depletion of the retinal progenitor pool occurs through symmetric divisions leading to two postmitotic terminally differentiated daughter cells (Figure 4B) [34,36]. Cell intrinsic and extrinsic factors govern cell fate choice and thus tissue architecture and function. The retinal cells governed by these factors progress from multipotent retinal progenitors to competent postmitotic precursors, which undergo further specification before becoming the final differentiated adult cell type [4,37–39].

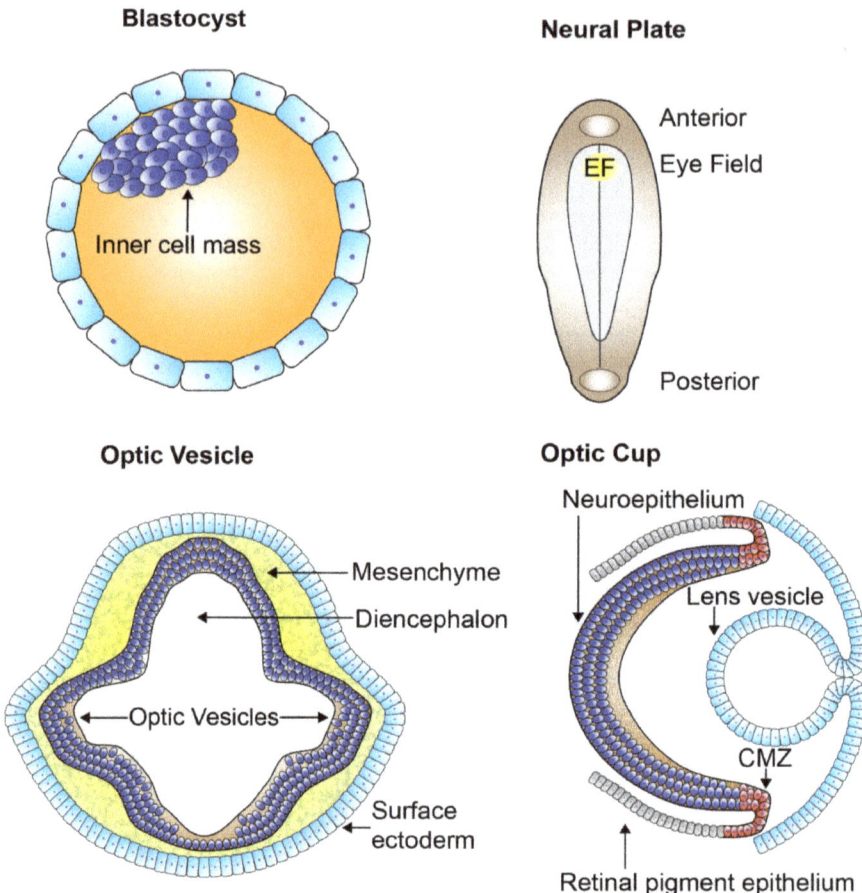

Figure 3. The organization of the developing retina. Schematic picture of early retinal development. From the blastocyst which contains the pluripotent cell mass gastrulation and neurulation occur forming the neural plate. The eye field specifies at the medial region of the anterior neural plate and contains all the progenitors which go on to form all the neural-derived cell types and structures of the eye. Bilateral optic sulci develop from the eye field forming the optic vesicles which extend towards the surface ectoderm. The optic vesicles invaginate forming the two-layered optic cups and the lens vesicle forms and sits behind the surface ectoderm. The outer layer of the optic cup remains as a single cuboidal layer becoming the retinal pigment epithelium. The single inner layer of the optic cup proliferates and differentiates forming the multilayered neural retina. EF: eye field; CMZ: ciliary marginal zone.

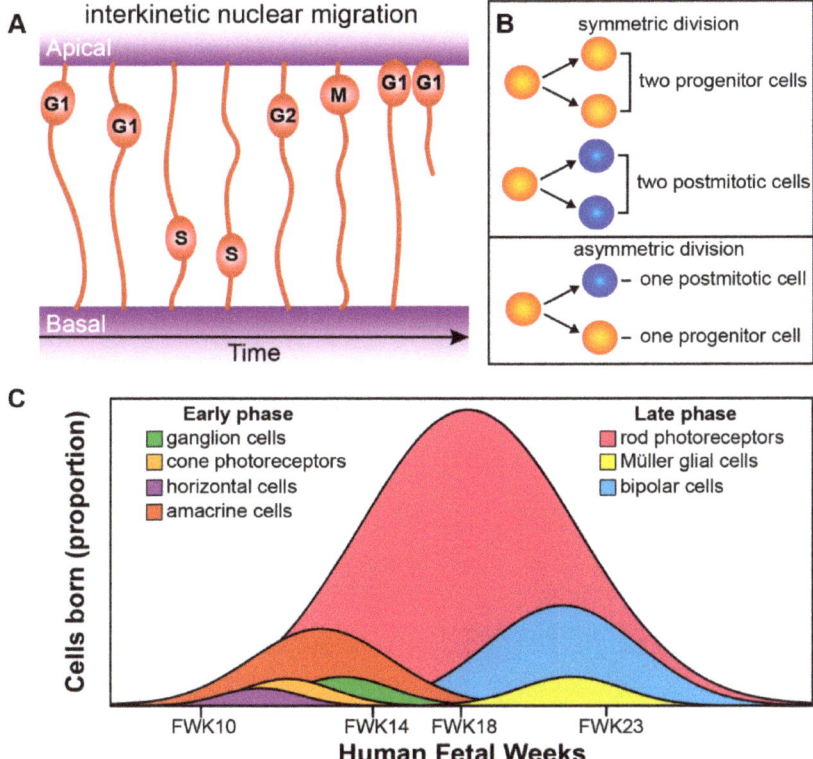

Figure 4. Retinogenesis. (**A**) Radial progenitor cells undergoing interkinetic nuclear migration during cell cycle phases G1, S, G2, and M. The mitosis (M) phase takes place at the apical side, whereas the DNA synthesis (S) phase takes place more basally. (**B**) Symmetric versus asymmetric cell division. (**C**) Genesis of retinal cells born during the development of the human eye can be divided into an early phase (ganglion cells, cone photoreceptors, horizontal cells, and amacrine cells) and an overlapping late phase (rod photoreceptors, Müller glial cells, and bipolar cells; see Aldiri et al. 2017 [40]). FWK—fetal week.

The birth of the seven major cell types of retina occur from the early multipotent retinal progenitor cells and happens in an orderly and overlapping manner [39]. The genesis of the major cell types group into an early phase and a late phase. The early phase consists of the birth of the first ganglion cells, cone photoreceptors, horizontal cells, and amacrine cells. The overlapping late phase consists of the birth of the first rod photoreceptors, Müller glial cells and bipolar cells (Figure 4C) [39]. Recently, both Aldiri et al. (2017) and Hoshino et al. (2017) described similar retinal time courses for the developing human retina based on RNA-Seq analysis [40,41]. The newborn postmitotic cell types must become positioned correctly within the retina; this occurs through migration of cells along the radial axis (apical-basal) of the retina or by tangential migration of cells perpendicular to the radial axis of the retina. Interestingly, only the early born cell types (ganglion cells, cone photoreceptors, horizontal cells, and amacrine cells) exhibit tangential migration (Figure 5A) [42,43].

There are a number of modes of radial migration for newborn neurons including: glial cell-guided, the migration of neurons along radial glial progenitors (Figure 5B); Somal translocation, the movement of nuclei across inherited apical or basal processes (Figure 5C); Multipolar migratory mode, nuclei movement due to multiple cell processes with no retention of apical or basal attachment to facilitate nuclei movement (Figure 5D); No translocation, inefficient migration due to retention of the apical or basal process and slow release of opposing process (Figure 5E). These various modes of migration are cell type-specific [44–47]. Tangential dispersion is driven by a mix of diffusible signals and/or contact-mediated interactions that drive a local spacing rule to keep a minimum distance between neighboring cells of the same cell type [48].

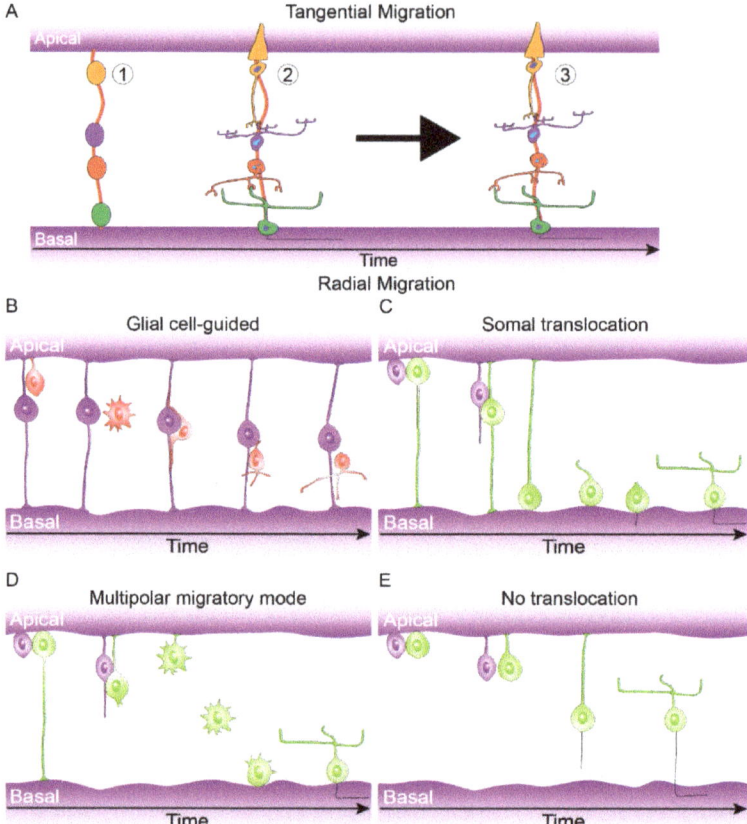

Figure 5. Tangential and Radial migration. (**A**) Tangential migration can be described in three steps: (1) Early born cell type progenitors localize to their correct laminar position (Cones: orange, Bipolar cells: purple, amacrine cells: red, ganglion cells: green), (2) they undergo morphological differentiation, (3) tangential migration coincides with morphological differentiation allowing subsets of early born cell types to move a short distance within their laminar position (see Reese et al. 1999 [43]). (**B**) Glial cell-guided, apically born neurons become initially detached and subsequently attach to radial glial progenitor cells. They then migrate along the radial glial progenitor cells to the target laminar location where they fully integrate. (**C**) Somal translocation, apically born nuclei can move along there inherited basally attached process from. Once they move to their final laminar location they fully integrate (This process can also occur with only apically inherited processes). (**D**) Multipolar migratory mode, in rare case apically born neurons can loses both apical and basal attachments but can move to their final laminar position and integrate due to a multipolar mode. (**E**) No translocation, inefficient migration due to retention of the apical or basal process and slow release of opposing process. For further details see Icha et al. 2016 and Amini et al. 2018 [45,47].

Retinal mosaic is the term used for the distribution of a neuronal cell type orthogonal to the apical-basal axis in a particular retinal layer. There is a highly ordered mosaic architecture in the mammalian retina leading to the non-random distribution of its cell bodies and dendritic process. This mosaic patterning is essential for retinal functionality, tying information together in a regularly patterned/ordered way from radially aligned "functional units" such that complete sampling and coverage of an image is achieved. Development of mosaics may be due to a combination of tangential dispersion (for early born cell types), programmed cell death, and lateral inhibition [45,48,49]. Interestingly, mosaic patterning can apply to a group of cells that have yet to reach their final developmental position, suggesting a pre-orchestrated cell intrinsic process [45].

Thus, retinogenesis is a precise orchestration of spatiotemporal processes such as symmetric and asymmetric cell division, cell fate choice (determination, competence, specification, and differentiation), cell migration (interkinetic nuclear migration, radial migration, and tangential migration), and maturation (integration and specialization of retinal spatiotemporal processes to provide adult functionality). The developing retinal neuroepithelium has a large amount of plasticity to accommodate these spatiotemporal process while maintaining its tissue integrity and architecture.

3. The Genetics of Retinal Development

As briefly highlighted in the previous section a number of genes are responsible for forming the early eye field. In this section we will shortly expand on some of the important gene regulatory networks (GRNs) essential for retinal development. GRNs can establish precise spatial, temporal, and cellular context specific controlled changes in gene expression patterns through the synergistic relationship of sets of transcription factors (TF) and their action on cis-regulatory modules (CRMs). The CRMS typically are a collection of TF-binding sites on the same strand of DNA as they affect [50–53]. GRNs are important as they can provide us with mechanistic insight into what is need to acquire and maintain a particular cell type identity. We will discuss the GRNs responsible for retinal progenitors and subsequent competent postmitotic precursors and their cell type specification. Mutations in, or misregulation of, several of these early developmental genes can lead to inherited retinal diseases. A number of recent papers have focused on retinal development using bulk transcriptomic [40,41,54,55] and single-cell transcriptomic approaches [54,56–61] to study human fetal retina and retinal organoids. These works add too many of the findings from work on mammalian animal models which have defined developmental or cell specific gene clusters and networks [62–70].

Several genes have been attributed to neuroretinal specification as well as the proliferative and multipotent ability of retinal progenitor cells, including *Vsx2* (also known as *Chx10*), *Pax6*, *Lhx2*, *Rax*, *Six3*, and *Six6* [71–79]. Many of the genes are also implicated in retinal abnormalities; for instance, *Pax6* mutations can lead to foveal hypoplasia, while *Rax* mutations can cause microphthalmia leading to retinal dysplasia [80,81]. Two genes, *Ikzf1* and *Casz1*, are required for the temporal regulation of retinal progenitor cell fate, with dysregulation of these genes leading to changes in the production of early versus late-born retinal cell types [82,83]. Interestingly, many retinal progenitor cell transcription factors are also important in Müller glia cell specification [68]. This includes the Hippo effector Yap, which is essential for retinal progenitor cell cycle progression. Additionally, Yap is required for Müller glial cell reprogramming and cell cycle re-entry and is misregulated in retinal disease [84–87]. Other factors related to retinal progenitors and Müller glial cells include Notch factors Hes1 and Hes5 as well as Lhx2, Rax, and Sox9 [88–91].

Several retinal TFs including Otx2, Crx, Nrl, and Nr2e3 control rod and cone-specific photoreceptor specification. Mutations in *Crx* can cause Leber congenital amaurosis (LCA), cone-rod dystrophy (CRD), and Retinitis pigmentosa (RP), while *Nrl* and *Nr2e3* mutations can cause RP and enhanced S-cone syndrome [92–98]. Otx2 can determine both rod and cone photoreceptor cell fate, while Crx acts with Nrl and Rorβ for terminal photoreceptor gene expression controlling the cone/rod ratio [99–102]. Activation of *Nrl* expression leads to the subsequent activation of the *Nr2e3* rod-specific factor; both Nrl and Nr2e3 can suppress cone cell fate genes [101,103,104]. Prdm1 (also known as Blimp1) also promotes rod specification while repressing bipolar fate [105,106]. Thrβ2 and RXRgamma are required for cone generation and subtype specification [107–109]. A CRM of the *Thrb* gene is regulated by Otx2 and Onecut1 transcription factors for the production of cones and horizontal cells, with Onecut1 found to be critical in specifying cone versus rod fate [110]. Recently, the Emerson Lab further confirmed that ThrbCRM1 progenitor cells preferentially form cone photoreceptors as well as subtypes of horizontal and ganglion cells [111].

Bipolar cells are also specified from Otx2 component postmitotic precursors in which expression with Vsx2 leads to their cell specification [105,106]. Vsx1 and Bhlhb5 are required for bipolar cell subtype fate [112,113]. The other interneurons, amacrine cells, and horizontal cells arise from Pax6, Ptf1a and Foxn4 expressing retinal progenitor cells [76,114,115]. Prox1 lies further downstream of Foxn4 and Ptf1a and specifies horizontal cell fate [116]. While, Onecut1 acts downstream of Foxn4, in parallel with Ptf1a, but upstream of Prox1 to specify horizontal cell fate [117]. Additionally, Lim1, Isl1 and Lhx1 also specify horizontal cell fate [118–120]. Tfap2a and 2b, Barhl2, Bhlhb5, NeuroD factors, and Isl1 act downstream of Ptf1a to specify an amacrine cell fate [113,121–124]. Lastly, Pou4f2 and Isl1 are essential in the acquisition of ganglion cell fate being downstream of retinal progenitor cell factor Atoh7 [125,126]. Additionally, genes promoting ganglion cell specification include *Neurod1*, *Sox4*, and *Sox11* [127,128].

Nevertheless, what has been found out about *CRB1* transcript expression in early retinal development? Recently, Hu et al. found using single-cell RNA-seq that *CRB1* transcripts were particularly enriched during human retinal development in retinal progenitor and Müller glial cells from human fetal retina [56]. In human retinal organoids, *CRB1* transcripts were found to be lowly expressed in very early organoids with moderate expression in later organoids [57]. In a study by Clark et al. they found using single-cell RNA-seq that transcripts for *Crb1* in mouse retina increased from embryonic to postnatal stages. Interestingly, they found the opposite for *Crb2* transcripts, being more abundant early embryonically and decreasing postnatally [63]. This pattern is in agreement with studies of human fetal retina and retinal organoids that show initial low protein levels of CRB1 and higher levels of CRB2 in early development [129]. Redundancy of function for CRB1 and CRB2 has been identified in the mouse retina. With knockout of either *Crb1* or *Crb2* in mouse Müller glial cells leading to mild retinal morphological phenotypes, while ablation of both *Crb1* and *Crb2* concomitantly from mouse Müller glial cells leads to a severe Leber congenital amaurosis phenotype [130–132]. However, while *Crb1* knockout mice are viable, *Crb2* ablation causes lethality in mice and genetic variants of the *CRB2* gene cause a syndromic phenotype in humans [133,134]. CRB3 is more widely expressed in epithelial tissues than either CRB1 or CRB2 and does not share their large extracellular domains. Ablation of *Crb3* leads to lethality shortly after birth with defects in (lung and intestinal) epithelial tissue morphogenesis [135,136].

4. Morphological and Molecular Recapitulation of the Human Fetal Retina

Studying retinal development in animal models is useful to understand the underlying cellular processes, but some of these processes are remarkably different in the human retina. There are molecular and morphological similarities between mammalian retina, but subtle differences highlight caution when applying information from other species to the human retina and its diseases, even between non-human primate and human retina [137–140]. Additionally, limited access to human fetal and adult cadaveric donor retina limited the studies in human retina at a tissue or single cell type level in regards to pathobiology, signaling dynamics, and physiology. Retinal organoids derived from human embryonic stem cells or induced pluripotent stem cells mimic the three-dimensional laminated structure of the retina allowing us to study basic eye development, disease modelling, drug potency assays, gene augmentation, and cell therapeutic strategies [141–146].

Multiple recent studies have directly compared human fetal retina with human stem cell-derived retinal organoids, analyzing their morphology or transcriptome, or both [54,147–149]. Additionally, a large body of research exists regarding the morphology and transcriptome of either human fetal retina [8,40,41,150–160] or human stem cell-derived retinal organoids [58,141,142,161–170]. Together, these studies provide a unique insight into human retinogenesis and allow us to have a reference point between in vivo human retinal development and in vitro models of it. Do human stem cell-derived retinal organoids sufficiently recapture the cell type diversity including all sub-types, morphological cues, synaptic wiring, and light sensitivity of the human fetal retina and subsequent adult retina?

Human retinal organoids have been found to recapitulate the main temporal and spatial cues of the in vivo human retina producing all the retinal layers and containing the 7 major cell types [142,145,171]. The spatiotemporal birth and maturation of retinal cell types differ depending on their location within the retina. In the human fetal retina, photoreceptors are born and remain located in the apical retina. However, in human stem cell-derived retinal organoids, photoreceptors reside mostly apically but are also seen in more basal positions particularly in early developmental stages, suggesting incomplete positional cues. Interestingly, Kaewkhaw et al. (2015) were able to track basally located photoreceptors from DD42 to DD44 with live cell imaging, finding that they translocated their soma apically [168]. The mammalian retina matures in a centroperipheral manner with the peripheral retina organizing its adult like lamination later than the central retina [155]. This delayed peripheral maturation is also detected in gene expression profiles comparing these regions. Cell type expression patterns, analyzed by immunohistochemistry, can be delayed by at least 50 days in the peripheral compared to more central retina. Differences are also found between nasal and temporal retina [41]. Additionally, sustained differences in gene expression profiles of peripheral and macula of the human adult retina is found, but this has been attributed to the anatomical differences between these two regions [172]. Mammals are known to contain a peripherally located ciliary marginal zone (CMZ), a stem cell-like niche able to contribute postmitotic cells to the retina in addition to radial glial progenitor cells [173,174]. However, little data is available on the CMZ of the human fetal retina, but studies on human and mouse stem cell-derived retinal organoids have highlighted its presence [164,165].

The human retina contains a central region termed the macula in which the 1.5 mm fovea centralis resides. The fovea, required for high visual acuity and color vision, in particular, was found to develop and mature much earlier than the rest of the retina [41,175]. The developing fovea, already free of mitotic cells at Fwk 8.4, initially consists of a single row of cone photoreceptors. The rapidly maturing foveal inner retina already consists of the main components of the midget ganglion pathway as well as of presynaptic markers present in the OPL and IPL by Fwk 13.7 [41]. However, a small depression called the foveal pit develops from Fwk 25 which leads to a gradual receding of all retinal layers except for the outer nuclear layer which begins to thicken. Foveal development continues in early childhood with elongation of cone outer segments and is considered adult-like in early- to mid-adolescence [152,153,160,176,177]. Newborns still have underdeveloped outer segments at the cone-rich fovea after birth. Therefore, suggesting that human newborns rely on extrafoveal vision initially [138]. Immature cones are present from Fwk 8 and immature rods from Fwk 10. Cone S opsin expresses from Fwk 12 while cone L and M opsin and rhodopsin express at Fwk 15 [8,151,153,155,159]. Rod photoreceptor maturation defined as the development of both inner and outer segments, occurs quicker in the mid-peripheral human retina than the parafoveal region [150]. Full maturation of the human retina does not occur until early adolescence. The average adult human retina contains 4.6 million cones, decreasing sharply in density outward from the fovea. However, the average number of rods in the adult human retina, 92 million, far exceeds the number of cones. The density of rods is highest around the optic nerve and decrease in density towards the peripheral retina and are absent from the central fovea [156].

Retinal organoids do not yet form a separate specialized fovea. However, they do form all of the main photoreceptor subtypes including photoreceptors with Rhodopsin, L/M-opsin and S-opsin [146,178,179]. Retinal organoid photoreceptors form both inner and outer segments and contain many of the prototypic morphological structures including: mitochondria, basal body, centriole, connecting cilium, and outer segment discs. Additionally, adjacent structures, such as the adherens junctions of the OLM, the microvilli of radial glial progenitors, and subsequently Müller glial cells are also found [142,162,163,169–171,179]. The quality of these structures greatly varied between studies and in particularly outer segments had very few or disorganized disk stacks. Recently, Eldred et al. (2018) found that the DD200 retinal organoids can recreate the temporal generation of cones having a similar distribution, gene expression profile, and morphology as adult human retina. They also identified a temporal switch which promotes the differentiation of S cones towards L/M cones through thyroid hormone signaling. Going one step further they also found that the two thyroid hormone states, T3 and T4, were modulated by different deiodinase enzymes in early or late organoids to specify the change from S to L/M cone subtypes and found that temporal gene expression of these enzymes correlated with data from Hoshino et al. (2017) on the human developing retina [41,146]. Interestingly, preterm human infants that have low T3/T4 are more likely to have defects in color vision [180]. Local modulation of thyroid signaling in retinal organoids may specify a more cone-rich, fovea-like region, making them a step closer to the in vivo human retina. Such modulation of thyroid signaling in retinal organoids might be achieved through optogenetically controlled protein expression. Recently, Kim et al. were able to make more cone-rich retinal organoids by using an improved differentiation protocol [57].

5. Light Responsiveness and Synaptic Transmission of the Fetal Retina and Stem Cell-Derived Retinal Organoids

Light responsiveness and synaptic transmission are critical milestones for a functioning retina. As previously mentioned, the fetal retina does have both rods and cones with developing inner and outer segments as early as Fwk 15. The fetal retina is however considered not fully mature until post birth. The eyelids open by approximately Fwk 25, a milestone that suggests that the fine tuning of the retina to visual stimulation can begin from this point [181]. In utero visual stimulation is considered very limited. However, fetal responses to visual stimulus as measured by heart rate, physical movement and brain activity have been reported. Transabdominal illumination has been reported to increase fetal heart rate at Fwk 36 (Smyth et al. 1965: Fwk not reported, Kiuchi et al. 2000: Fwk 36–40) and fetal movement at Fwk 26 [182,183]. Fetal heart rate increase has also been shown during amnioscopy in which a cold light source was exposed to the amnion and fetus for 30 s at Fwk 38 [184]. An increase in fetal heart rate in response to light with increasing gestational age as analyzed by actocardiogram is seen from Fwk 18 to 41 [185]. However, fetuses have only been reported to reliably respond to light stimulation from Fwk 37; this is likely due to differences in abdominal and uterine wall thicknesses, light sources used, the distance of light source, and its focus on the fetus eyes [185–187]. Magnetoencephalography (MEG) studies have recorded visually evoked brain activity from as early as Fwk 28 [188–191]. Functional magnetic resonance imaging (fMRI) has also been successfully used to measure fetal response to transabdominal illumination, finding activity in the frontal lobes but not the visual cortex from Fwk 36 [192].

Two main techniques have been utilized to measure preterm neonatal vision, the electroretinogram (ERG) for retinal activity and visual evoked potentials (VEP) for brain activity. VEP studies suggest that extrauterine age accelerates the development of the fetal visual system once a maturational threshold has been reached at post Fwk 25 [193–196]. Interestingly, this coincides with the approximate age of eyelid opening. Similarly, from as early as Fwk 31, ERG studies on preterm neonates suggest that improvements in retinal activity are correlated with postconception age and extrauterine age [196–198]. Improvements in retinal activity can be recorded by a decrease in a- and b-wave latency with an increase in amplitude. Preterm ERG studies cannot be used to assess if in vivo retinal activity also has a maturational threshold because the eyelids are yet closed before Fwk 25. Other features of preterm ERG include decreasing rod threshold with increasing postconception age, adult-like b-wave sensitivity is reached at six months after normal birth [199,200]. Rod functional maturation occurs peripherally and then parafoveally [201]. Preterm birth, however, has been consistently linked with reduced rod and cone function when compared to usual term infants [202–204]. This suggests that premature exposure of the retina to light is harmful. It is unknown if premature light exposure harms cultured stem cell-derived retinal organoids.

As previously mentioned, human retinal organoids develop photoreceptor outer segments of different quality between week (Wk) 16-28 [142,146,162,163,167,169–171,179,205]. Retinal as well as brain organoids have been shown to respond to light [142,162,206]. Zhong et al. (2014) found that 2 out of 13 rod cells with putative outer segments in Wk 25–27 hiPSC-derived retinal organoids responded to light as measured by perforated-patch recordings in the voltage-clamp mode. The sensitivity of these immature human rod cells was less than found in adult non-human primate photoreceptors. Multiple responses could not be elicited in these retinal organoids, likely due to a depletion in components required for phototransduction [142]. Hallam et al. (2018) used a 4096 channel multielectrode array (MEA) on which they flattened longitudinally opened Wk 21.4 (DD150) hiPSC-derived retinal organoids ganglion side down and detected changing spike activity from pulses of white light. They also used puffs of cGMP, which depolarizes photoreceptors leading to an unstimulated condition (Dark Current), to show that the light responses found were driven by phototransduction in photoreceptors and not the potential activity of ipRGCs [162]. Quadrato et al. (2017) found that eight month hiPSC-derived brain organoids exhibited spontaneously-active neuronal networks, using high-density silicon microelectrodes. Additionally, subpopulations of neurons were identified which were responsive to 530 nm light in 4 out of 10 organoids. However, they were unable to attribute the responses directly to the photosensitive cells or the downstream neuronal networks [206].

Human stem cell-derived retinal organoids can develop some synaptic maturity. Electron microscopy data showed the presence of electron-dense ribbons surrounded by synaptic vesicles. Immunohistochemistry markers such as PSD-95, vGlut1, PNA, Synaptophysin, and Syntaxin 3, confirm synapses in human stem cell-derived retinal organoids. Markers such as RIBEYE (as detected by CtBP2) and Bassoon confirm the presence of ribbon synapses. These markers roughly aligned at the outer plexiform layer of retinal organoids. However, this varied between protocols and degeneration of the inner retina in ageing organoids may also play a factor [148,162,167,170,171,178]. Interestingly, Dorgau et al. (2018) showed that blocking of the extracellular matrix protein Laminin γ3 in late-stage retinal organoids led to the disruption of ribbon synapse marker Bassoon. This may be due to the significant disruption of Müller glial cell end feet at the inner limiting membrane [148]. Wahlin et al. (2017) showed that both excitatory (L-aspartate, glutamate) and inhibitory (GABA, glycine) neurotransmitters of the retina were present in Wk 43 (DD300) hiPSC-derived retinal organoids. L-aspartate was found in the ONL, glutamate and GABA throughout the retina and glycine in the INL [170]. Hallam et al. (2018) used puffs of GABA to highlight the emerging functional neural networks in Wk 21 (DD150) human stem cell-derived retinal organoids [162]. Wahlin et al. (2017) used whole-cell patch clamp recordings to elicit membrane capacitance changes as an index of voltage-dependent synaptic vesicle release in retinal organoid photoreceptors [170]. Similarly, Deng et al. (2018) were able to show the electrophysiological response from whole-cell patch clamp recorded rod photoreceptors from hiPSC-derived retinal organoids [178].

Together, these data highlight the potential for producing light responsive human stem cell-derived retinal organoids with maturing synapses that are capable of transferring information from the photoreceptors to the inner retina. At the least, retinal organoids have "functional units" of photoreceptors, bipolar cells, and ganglion cells. Work needs to be carried out to assess the quality of these neural networks and how well all cell types contribute. More emphasis needs to be put on comparing the early in vivo and in vitro retinal response to light and how that ties in with the maturational stage. Unsurprisingly, retinal organoids represent an immature/incomplete development stage, and thus functional responses reflect this. Improved culturing methods and better control of the microenvironment might help in further maturation of the retinal organoids.

6. Improved Retinal Organoid Modelling

Despite ongoing issues with batch to batch variations, many of the current differentiation protocols lead to the generation of well laminated retinal organoids that contain all the primary retinal cell types but have putative photoreceptor segments or show in long-term cultures degeneration of the inner retina. This may be due to the lack of correct microenvironmental cues and structural support. Degeneration of the inner retina is likely due to the lack of access by medium components, particularly as the retina thickens during development. Furthermore, misregulation of ECM components in human stem cell-derived retinal organoids may significantly affect their correct lamination [148]. Reproducibility and staging of human retinal organoids is also an important consideration particular as we further explore their use in developmental studies and disease modelling [207]. Many teams are focusing on new methodologies to improve the quality of retinal organoids by tweaking protocols, using bioreactors, or microfluidic systems, [163,167,169,170]. Recently, Mellough et al. (also with slight modification performed by Cowan et al.) showed that mechanical dissociation at the embryoid body formation stage lead to improved formation of human retinal organoids [208,209]. The use of bioreactor setups, instead of static culture setups, may help solve a number of these problems as they allow for improved aeration and distribution of nutrients as well as allow for scaling up of organoid production. Bioreactor setups report stem cell-derived retinal organoids with better lamination and enhanced differentiation, an increased yield of photoreceptors with outer segment structures, improved cone formation and a better recapitulation of the spatiotemporal development of in vivo retina [167]. While the initial stages of differentiation require hypoxic conditions, improved oxygen diffusion at later stages is essential for greater cell proliferation and ganglion cell survival. In the absence of vascularized stem cell-derived retinal organoids, bioreactors help facilitate this mechanism. A number of teams have also very recently come up with methods that lead to better cone and rod specification in human retinal organoids [57,210–213].

Many of the differentiation procedures used to derive human retinal organoids lead to the concomitant production of RPE. However, it produces RPE that is consistently not directly adjacent to the photoreceptor segments when using a 2D to 3D differentiation protocol. It does allow however medium that is conditioned by both the retinal organoids and RPE, which may provide some essential diffusible factors for both structures. Production of full-length photoreceptor segments by Wahlin et al. (2017) suggested that contact of RPE is non-essential for their development/maturation [170]. However, correctly located RPE may provide essential structural support and may help to facilitate a number of the physiological roles of photoreceptor segments such as phototransduction. Microfluidic systems for retinal organoids may help to promote improved cell to cell interaction and additionally provide tighter control of the microenvironment [214,215]. One of the future uses of human stem cell-derived retinal organoid technology is potentially as a source of transplantable tissue and in particularly photoreceptor cells to treat retinal diseases [171,216–218]. Integration and functionality of transplanted photoreceptors into host retina has been shown to be much more limited than initially thought, with predominant cytoplasmic material transfer including fluorescent reporter proteins [219–221]. Transplanted photoreceptors may not facilitate their physiological roles fully due to lack of interaction with the host RPE. One way to enhance the photosensitivity of transplanted photoreceptors from human stem cell-derived retinal organoids is to use optogenetically transformed photoreceptors [222]. Material transfer is found as well from conjugates formed from transplanted NTPDase2-positive CellTracker Green labelled Müller Glial Cells [223,224]. Material transfer represents a novel route to develop cell-based therapeutics which may be able to transfer "healthy components" to diseased retinal cells [225].

7. The Apical CRB and PAR Complexes

Apical-basal cell polarity is pivotal for the formation and functionality of epithelial tissues being governed by conserved canonical factors that define the apical domains. Apical polarity factors are for example the Crumbs-homologues (CRB1 and CRB2), Protein associated with Lin Seven 1 (PALS1 also called MAGUK p55 subfamily member 5 or MPP5), Partitioning defective-6 homolog (PAR6), atypical protein kinase C (aPKC), and PAR3. Basolateral polarity factors are for example Protein scribble homolog (SCRIB), Discs large homolog (DLG), and Lethal giant larvae protein homolog (LGL). However, recent work in the fruit fly *Drosophila* mid gut indicates that there are alternative apical polarizing factors other than the canonical epithelia polarity factors and that this may also extend to some types of vertebrate epithelia [226]. Additionally, there also exists planar cell polarity (PCP) in tissue epithelia, which is orthogonal to the apical-basal axis (Figure 6A) [227]. The retinal sub-apically localized CRB and PAR complexes (Figure 6B) are pivotal in maintaining the spatiotemporal processes of retinogenesis. The CRB complex has a prominent role in the control of apical-basal polarity acting as a sensor for cell density and upon polarization leading to regulation of Adherens Junctions (AJs) to promote maintenance of cell adhesion [228,229]. Disruption of the CRB complex leads to loss of polarity and can lead to subsequent loss of adhesion, ectopic localization of progenitors and postmitotic cells due to disrupted apically anchored process and coordinated cell migration, increase in cycling progenitor cells and late-born cell types, increase in early retinal apoptosis, and disruption of lamination. A long-term consequence of loss of retinal apical polarity is mild to severe retinal degeneration with a concurrent loss of retinal function in line with morphological deficit [130,131,230–233]. The complex acts in the role of conductor coordinating multiple downstream signaling pathways which have essential roles in development, such as the Notch and Hippo pathways [228,234,235]. Thus, leading to the regulation of cell size, cell fate determination, cell self-renewal, proliferation, differentiation, mitosis, and apoptosis. However, how these intertwined cellular responses are mediated collectively by the core complex remains ambiguous.

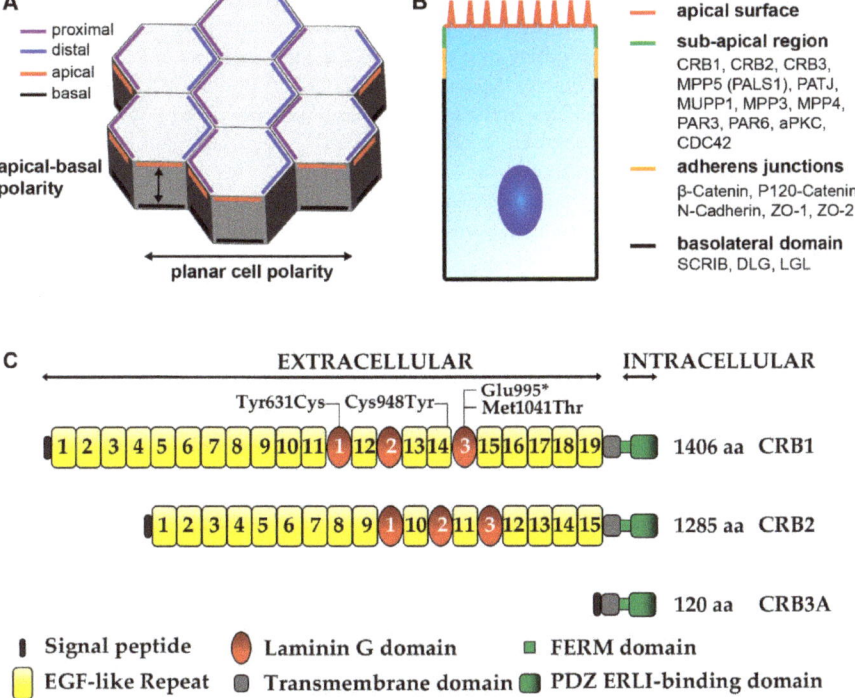

Figure 6. Schematic picture of Epithelial polarity. (A) Epithelial cell polarity consist of apical-cell polarity and orthogonal to this axis planar cell polarity (PCP). PCP is the collective alignment of cell polarity across the tissue plane and involves asymmetric segregation of proximal (purple) and distal (blue) PCP components. Apical-basal polarity involves the antagonistic, functional, and spatial segregation of apical (red) and basal (black) components. (B) In the retina the CRB and PAR complexes are located at the sub-apical region (green), below the apical surface (red) and adjacent to the adherens junctions (yellow). Scribbled (SCRIB), discs large (DLG), and lethal giant larvae (LGL) form a basolateral domain (black) extending below the adherens junctions. (C) Schematic overview of the prototypic CRB1, CRB2, and CRB3 proteins. Mutations from the three iPSC CRB1 RP patients lines recently derived to retinal organoids are mapped to their protein location in CRB1. Adapted from Quinn et al. 2017 [144].

The mammalian retinal CRB complex comprises of at least one of the three CRB family members, CRB1, CRB2, and CRB3 (isoform CRB3A which has a conserved C-terminus, isoform CRB3B which lacks the conserved C-terminus), in addition to PALS1 (also called MPP5), PATJ, MUPP1, MPP3, and MPP4. Both CRB1 and CRB2 have a large extracellular domain with epidermal growth factor (EGF) and laminin-globular domains. As discovered in *Drosophila* epithelia cells CRB1, CRB2, and CRB3A have a single transmembrane domain juxtaposing a short intracellular C-terminus of 37 amino acids which contains a FERM-binding motif (4.1, ezrin, radixin, moesin) and PSD-95/Discs-large/ZO-1 (PDZ)-binding motif ERLI (Glu-Arg-Leu-Ile) [144,229,235,236]. The three prototypic CRB proteins are shown in Figure 6C, for further details also on other isoforms details can be found in Quinn et al. 2017 [144]. Alternatively, the non-prototypic CRB3B isoform, which has a role in ciliogenesis and cell division, contains a C-terminal PDZ-binding motif CLPI (Cys- Leu-Pro-Ile) that does not interact with the PAR complex as found in Madin-Darby canine kidney epithelial cells (MDCK) [237,238]. The FERM motif can bind to proteins such as EPB4.1L5 which plays a role in epithelial-to-mesenchymal transition during gastrulation in mice and similar proteins are negative regulators of photoreceptor size in *Drosophila* and zebrafish [239–243]. EPB4.1L5 oligomerization is essential for its binding to CRB and is mediated through its FERM and FERM adjacent (FA) domains, as found in *Drosophila* and in MDCK cells [244]. EPB4.1L5 controls the actomyosin cytoskeleton at both apical junctions and basal focal adhesions, as found in the mouse kidney and during mouse development [239,245]. EPB4.1L5 is predominantly located basolaterally in early development, repressing CRB, but is recruited by CRB apically at later stages of differentiation. In the adult mammalian retina EPB4.1L5 has been found to localize to the OLM [242,243]. PAR complex member aPKC can bind and phosphorylate the FA domain of EPB4.1L5 leading to the dismantling of the EPB4.1L5 oligomer. This phosphorylation by aPKC prevents the premature apical localization of EPB4.1L5, in turn EPB4.1L5 restrains aPKC signaling thus antagonizing each other, leading to tightly controlled segregation of apical/basal membrane domains, as found in *Drosophila* and in MDCK cells [244,246]. The 4 amino acid PDZ-binding motif ERLI of CRB allows for interaction with adaptor proteins such as PALS1 and PAR6, as found in *Drosophila* and in MDCK cells [247,248]. Binding of PALS1 to the C-terminal PDZ domain of CRB leads to recruitment of PATJ or MUPP1 through binding of the PALS1 N-terminal L27 domain to the L27 domain of PATJ or MUPP1, as found in *Drosophila* and in MDCK cells [249,250]. Additionally, PALS1 can recruit MPP3 and MPP4 to the apical complex, in the mouse retina [251,252]. PALS1 is abundantly expressed at the OLM and tight junction of the RPE. Ablation of PALS1 in the mouse neural retina resulted in late onset retinal degeneration suggestion redundancy of MPPs in the neural retina, whereas ablation of PALS1 in the mouse RPE and neural retina results in early onset retinal degeneration suggesting specific roles for PALS1 in RPE [231].

Binding of PAR6 to the C-terminal PDZ binding domain of CRB leads to the recruitment of the other PAR complex members PAR3, aPKC, and cell division control 42 (CDC42). PAR6 can interact with PAR3 through their PDZ domains, with aPKC through their N-terminal Phox and Bem1 (PB1) domains, and with CDC42 through their semi-CDC42- and Rac-interactive binding (CRIB) domains, as found in *Caenorhabditis elegans* and mammalian tissue lysates and cos1 cells [253–256]. The activity of aPKC is suppressed by PAR6 binding, but this suppression is partially relieved when GTP bound CDC42 interacts with the complex, as found in *Drosophila* and in MDCK cells [257,258]. However, the activity of aPKC has also been shown to be promoted by PAR6 [259]. PAR3 is both an inhibitor of aPKC activity but also its substrate, found in mammalian tissue lysates [256]. At adherens junctions, PAR3 can also bind to the scaffolding proteins FERM domain containing 4A (FRMD4A) and FRMD4B (also known as GRSP-1) leading to the recruitment of cytohesin-1 (CYTH)1 and causing subsequent activation of ARF6, this complex being essential for epithelial polarity [260]. FRMD4B and CYTH3 (also known as GRP1) also exist in a complex, found in COS1 cells [261]. Recently, in the mouse retina a variant of FRMD4B, $Frmd4b^{Tvrm222}$, led to the suppression of OLM fragmentation and photoreceptor dysplasia in $Nr2e3^{rd7}$ and $Nrl^{-/-}$ mice. Whole exome sequencing revealed that the $Frmd4b^{Tvrm222}$ variant had a substitution of serine residue 938 by proline (S938P). Transfection of COS7 cells with either

S938P or wild-type FRMD4B and the addition of insulin, an agonist of the phosphoinositide 3-kinase (PI3K)-AKT pathway, revealed that the FRMD4B variant does not translocate to the plasma membrane as occurs with wildtype FRMD4B. The $Frmd4b^{Tvrm222}$ mice showed reduced AKT phosphorylation and an increase in cell junction proteins, activated AKT leads to loss of apical-basal polarity. Therefore, the interactions of the FRMD4B variant and cytohesin-3 may modulate both the PAR3 activated ARF6 pathway and/or PI3K-AKT pathway to prevent retinal dysplasia in $Nr2e3^{rd7}$ and $Nrl^{-/-}$ mice [262]. CDC42 in addition to its role in regulating aPKC has recently been shown to regulate another kinase to the apical domain, p21-activated kinase-1 (PAK1), as found in *Drosophila* and mammalian epithelial cells [258,263]. Loss of PAK1 or aPKC leads to a moderate polarity phenotype however a dramatic loss of epithelial polarity was detected when PAK1 as well as aPKC are inactive. Both aPKC and PAK1 act redundantly downstream of CDC42. PAK1 is expressed throughout the mouse retina [263,264]. The CRB and PAR complexes may interact additionally through direct interaction of the amino terminus of PALS1 and the PDZ domain of PAR6, the interaction being regulated by GTP bound CDC42, as investigated in mammalian cell lines [265]. PAR6, PAR3 and aPKC are located at the OLM in the embryonic mouse retina while CDC42 is located throughout the retina [266–268].

8. The Localization of the Mammalian Retinal CRB Complex

The developing mammalian retina expresses both CRB1 and CRB2. In mouse retina, both CRB1 and CRB2 are expressed at the subapical region adjacent to adherens junctions of progenitor cells at embryonic day 12.5 (Figure 7A), which is equivalent to the early 1st trimester human fetal retinal development, transcriptionally [40,41,232,242,269]. However, in 1st trimester human fetal retina, while CRB2 labelling is found at the subapical region adjacent to adherens junctions in putative photoreceptor inner segments and the apical villi of radial glial progenitor cells, CRB1 is almost below detection level (Figure 7B). Subsequently, in mid 2nd trimester human fetal retina CRB1 and CRB2 labelling could be clearly detected at the subapical region adjacent to adherens junctions between putative photoreceptor inner segments and in the apical villi of radial glial progenitor cells/ Müller glial cells. In addition to CRB1 and CRB2 expression other CRB complex members PALS1, MUPP1, and PAR3 were found to be expressed in 1st and 2nd trimester human fetal retina. In 1st trimester human fetal retina we also found PATJ expression this was not analyzed in 2nd trimester retina. The onset of CRB1 and CRB2 expression and other members of the CRB complex in the human fetal retina was found to be recapitulated in early versus late differentiated human induced-pluripotent stem cell (iPSC)-derived retinal organoids [129].

In the adult mammalian retina CRB1, CRB2, and CRB3 proteins localize at the subapical region in the Müller glial cells of mice, non-human primates and humans (Figure 7C–E). However, while CRB3 is present at the subapical region of photoreceptors in all three species, the expression patterns of CRB1 and CRB2 at the subapical region of photoreceptors differs between the three species (Figure 7C–E). CRB2 is present at the subapical region of mouse photoreceptors, whereas CRB1 is not (Figure 7C). In non-human primates both CRB1 and CRB2 are present in photoreceptors (Figure 7D). In cadaveric human retinas collected 2-days after death CRB1 is present at the subapical region whereas CRB2 is present at vesicles in the photoreceptor inner segments but at some distance from the subapical region (Figure 7E) [130,132,270,271]. Interestingly, all 3 CRB proteins in the adult human retina are detected in the photoreceptor inner segments at a distance from the outer limiting membrane [272]. Additionally, CRB3 is also detected in the inner retina of mice, non-human primates and humans [132,270,273]. All of the ultrastructural immuno-electron microscopy studies using anti-CRB on adult human cadaveric retina were carried out using two-days-old tissue samples, and might for that reason differ with the results obtained when using freshly collected non-human-primate retinas. In other studies, a negative correlation between protein abundance and post-mortem time has been found in the human retina [274,275].

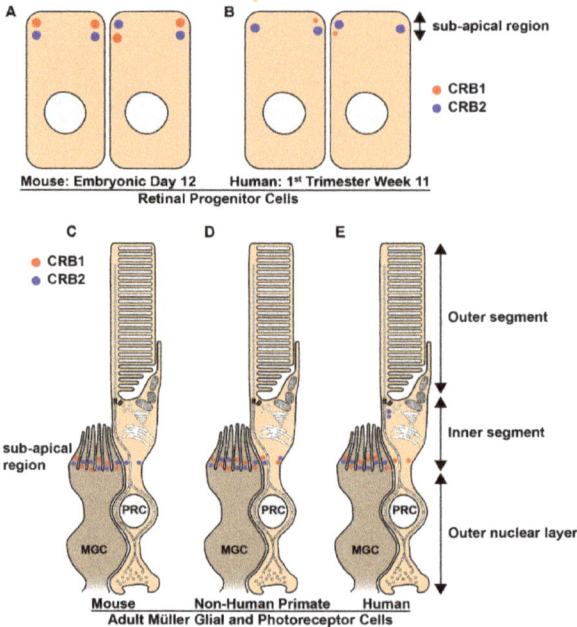

Figure 7. Schematic picture of the localization of the CRB proteins in mammalian adult retinal Müller glial and photoreceptor cells. (**A**–**E**) CRB1 (red) and CRB2 (blue) proteins localize at the subapical region in mouse (**A**) and human (**B**) retinal progenitors cells and adult Müller glial cells of mice (**C**), non-human primates (**D**) and humans (**E**). However, the expression of CRB1 in the early developing human retina is low and sporadic. Additionally, the expression patterns of CRB1 and CRB2 at the subapical region of adult photoreceptors differs between the three species. CRB2 is present at the subapical region of mouse photoreceptors, whereas CRB1 is not (**C**). In non-human primates both CRB1 and CRB2 are present in photoreceptors (**D**). In cadaveric human retinas collected 2-days after death CRB1 is present at the subapical region whereas CRB2 is present in the photoreceptor inner segments but at some distance from the subapical region (**E**). PRC: Photoreceptor; MGC: Müller glial cells.

In the adult mouse RPE, 1st and 2nd trimester human fetal RPE, and human iPSC-derived RPE CRB2 has been found to be expressed [129,276]. In the both human fetal and iPSC-derived RPE CRB2 immuno-EM labeling was found above adherens junctions and tight junctions in the apical membrane and microvilli [129].

9. CRB1 and Leber Congenital Amaurosis

Leber congenital amaurosis (LCA) is an early-onset disease leading to blindness from near birth with *CRB1* mutations accounting for 7–17% of cases and affecting approximately 10,000 patients worldwide [235,277–279]. Currently, there is no treatment available for *CRB1*-LCA patients, but proof-of-concept gene supplementation studies have shown functional rescue in *CRB1* retinitis pigmentosa (RP) mouse models which sets a ground work for proof-of-concept in *CRB1*-LCA-like mouse models [272]. *CRB1* gene mutations cause LCA8 with patients having severely attenuated or non-recordable ERG, abnormal pupillary reflex and nystagmus and their retinas have abnormal layering with reports of the retina being thickened, thinned or unchanged [280–289]. Mutations in CRB1 also lead to the development of RP with patients developing night blindness and a progressive loss of visual field due to rod degeneration [92]. *CRB1* mutations are associated with RP type 12 and are characterized by preservation of the para-arteriolar retinal pigment epithelium (PPRPE) and, due to macular involvement, a progressive loss of visual field. Disease onset can be from early childhood, however, some patients do not exhibit symptoms until after the first decade of life [290–292]. Additional CRB1 clinically relevant features include macular atrophy, keratoconus, Coats-like exudative vasculopathy, RP without PPRPE, pigmented paravenous chorioretinal atrophy, and nanophthalmos [288,293–297].

Human stem cell-derived retinal organoids which mimic retinal disease are an excellent tool for understanding disease mechanisms as well as a platform for testing therapeutic strategies. Other teams, including our own, are investigating pathobiology and disease mechanism of stem cell-derived retinal organoids from *CRB1* patients. We, have recently shown for the first time that three hiPSC lines (LUMC0116iCRB; LUMC0117iCRB; LUMC0128iCRB) from *CRB1* RP patients showed a phenotype similar as previously found in 3 month-old $Crb1^{KO}$ RP mice when differentiated into retinal organoids [129,130]. LUMC0116iCRB has c.3122T>C p.(Met1041Thr) homozygote missense mutations. LUMC0117iCRB has 2983G>T p.(Glu995*) and c.1892A>G p.(Tyr631Cys) mutations. LUMC0128iCRB has c.2843G>A p.(Cys948Tyr) and c.3122T>C p.(Met1041Thr) missense mutations. Mutations are mapped to their protein location in Figure 6C. Compared to control retinal organoids (Figure 8A), *CRB1* patient derived retinal organoids at DD180 showed disruptions at the OLM demonstrated by ectopic photoreceptor nuclei above the OLM and altered localization of CRB complex members at the OLM (Figure 8B,D). Furthermore, the CRB1 variant proteins localized to the subapical region above the adherens junctions, as in controls, but additionally showed a curved and broadened expression pattern (Figure 8C,E). Mislocalization of the CRB1 variant protein was also found mislocalized in the apical area of the NBL [129]. However, these studies are in their early stages with the underlying effects of the variant CRB1 proteins on protein-protein interactions and downstream cell signaling pathways still to be elucidated. Many rodent models of CRB retinal degeneration exist and have provided us with a deep insight into the pathobiology and mechanisms underlying CRB disease [130,144,232,235]. *CRB1*-LCA-like models have further built on our previous data [132,298,299].

One of the main working hypothesis that we draw from our four *CRB1*-LCA-like models is that CRB2 protein levels may be lower or that a less functional variant is of CRB2 is expressed in *CRB1* LCA patients compared to less severe *CRB1* retinal diseases [132,298,299]. Clinical reports of *CRB1* LCA patients have shown that degeneration can affect all quadrants of the retina while other reports show restriction to the inferior retina [285,288,300,301]. This is highly suggestive of the presence of a modifying factor. Variants of *CRB2* have been associated with retinal aberrations and more recently a missense mutation of *CRB2* has been found to cause retinitis pigmentosa [134,302]. Additionally, CRB2 is present in the fetal human retina in the first-trimester, whereas CRB1 expression starts from the second trimester [129]. In the mouse, both CRB1 and CRB2 are found in the early embryonic retina [232,242,269]. Therefore, missense variants of *CRB2* in humans are likely to have small but important effects on retinal diseases. A number of transcript variants have been reported for CRB1, and new novel isoforms of CRB1 are reported in the mouse and human retina and may also lead to the phenotypic variability in *CRB1* patients [144,303]. Currently there has been no link between *CRB3* mutations and retinal disease.

The four *CRB1*-LCA-like models had both alleles of *Crb2* disrupted in either retinal progenitor cells (ΔRPC), immature photoreceptors ($\Delta imPRC$), or Müller glial cells (ΔMG) on genetic backgrounds with either reduced levels of ($Crb1^{KO/WT}Crb2^{\Delta RPC}$) or complete knockout of Crb1 ($Crb1^{KO}Crb2^{\Delta RPC}$, $Crb1^{KO}Crb2^{\Delta imPRC}$, $Crb1^{KO}Crb2^{\Delta MG}$). All of these models had abnormally layered and transiently thickened retina, disruptions of the outer limiting membrane and ectopic localization of mitotic progenitors, cycling cells, and immature photoreceptors. The thickened retinas observed were in part due to the ectopic birth or displacement of early progenitors which we found increased in the $Crb1^{KO}Crb2^{\Delta RPC}$ and $Crb1^{KO}Crb2^{\Delta imPRC}$ mouse retinas, but not in the $Crb1^{KO}Crb2^{\Delta MG}$. This led to adult retinas in which we detected ectopic cells in the ganglion cell layer either sporadically ($Crb1^{KO}Crb2^{\Delta RPC}$), at the peripheral retina ($Crb1^{KO}Crb2^{\Delta MG}$), or within most of the retina ($Crb1^{KO}Crb2^{\Delta imPRC}$), or throughout the retina ($Crb1^{KO}Crb2^{\Delta RPC}$). We hypothesize that *CRB1* LCA patients which exhibit a thickened retina and abnormal layering do so due to similar mechanisms as found in our *CRB1*-LCA-like mouse models, displacement or the ectopic birth of progenitor cells, cycling cells, and immature photoreceptor cells [132,285,298,299]. Additionally, the reported thinned or unchanged retinal thickness of *CRB1* LCA patients is likely due to measurements made when significant retinal degeneration had already occurred. In our *CRB1*-LCA-like mouse models we detected transient changes in retinal thickness [288,289].

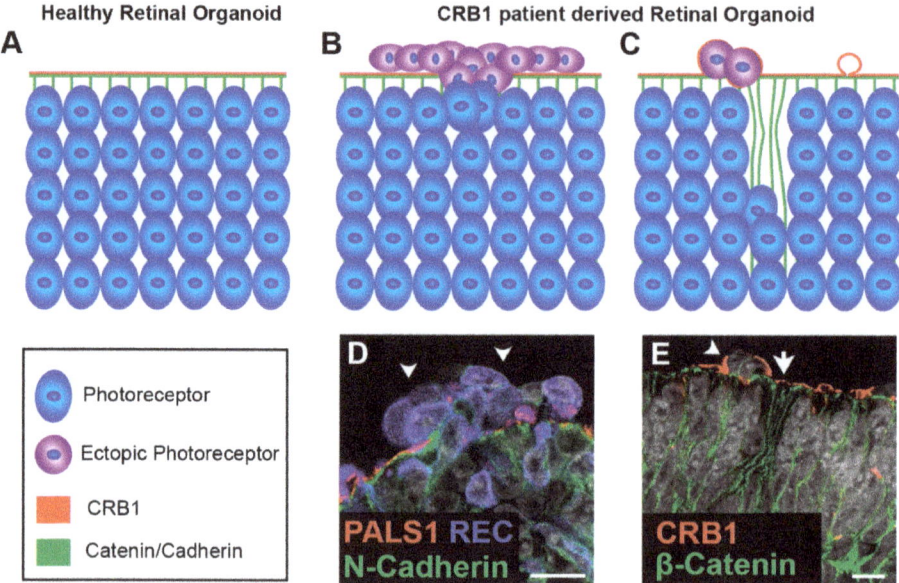

Figure 8. Disruptions at the outer limiting membrane in retinal organoids from *CRB1* retinitis pigmentosa (RP) patients. Schematic depiction of healthy (**A**) and *CRB1* patient (**B,C**) derived retinal organoids. (**A**) In healthy organoids CRB1 is located at the subapical region adjacent to the adherens junctions. (**B,D**) In retinal organoids from *CRB1* retinitis pigmentosa patient (LUMC0116iCRB) disruptions of the outer limiting membrane (OLM) and ectopic photoreceptors have been found. (**C,E**) Additionally, budding of the apical membrane and mislocalization of the CRB1 variant in the NBL also occurs. Scale bars (**D,E**), 20 µm. Panels (**C,D**) are modified from [178] under a Creative Commons license.

While in the $Crb1^{KO/WT}Crb2^{\Delta RPC}$ and $Crb1^{KO}Crb2^{\Delta RPC}$ mouse models no differences in retinal degenerations were reported between superior/inferior or central/peripheral retina, the $Crb1^{KO}Crb2^{\Delta imPRC}$ and $Crb1^{KO}Crb2^{\Delta MG}$ retina showed superior/inferior or central/peripheral phenotypes, respectively [132,298,299]. Interestingly, a new *Crb1Crb2* double knockout mouse model which disrupted both alleles of *Crb2* in rods (Δrods) on a genetic background lacking *Crb1* ($Crb1^{KO}Crb2^{\Delta rods}$) does not have an LCA-like but RP-like phenotype. The $Crb1^{KO}Crb2^{\Delta rods}$ retinas have a phenotype that mainly affects the peripheral and central superior retina [304]. These differences may be attributed to opposing gradients of mouse CRB1 and CRB2 at the subapical region between the superior and inferior retina as well as the contribution of CRB1 and CRB2 to either photoreceptors (CRB2) or Müller glial cells (CRB1 and CRB2) [130,270,271]. Another common feature of the *CRB1*-LCA-like mouse models is the early formation of retinal rosettes [132,298,299]. A comparison of the *Crb1Crb2* double knockout mouse models can be found in Table 1.

Table 1. Comparison of Crb1Crb2 double knockout mouse models.

	Crb1KOCrb2ΔRPC	Crb1KOCrb2ΔimPRC	Crb1KO/WTCrb2ΔRPC	Crb1KOCrb2ΔMG	Crb1KOCrb2Δrods
Severity	++++	+++	++	++	+
CRB1 + CRB2 in MGC/PRC/RPC Cre Mosaicism	0/0/0 50%	60/0/60 95%	20/0/20 50%	0/100/60 95%	60/03/60 99–100%
Phenotype onset	E13 whole retina	E15 whole retina	E15 periphery	E17 periphery	3M periphery
OLM disruption	++++	++++	++	+++ centrally ++++ at periphery	+ whole retina
Abnormal retinal lamination	YES	YES	YES	YES	NO
Ectopic localization retinal cells	YES (of all neurons)	YES of PRC and RPC	YES of PRC, BC, AC and GC	YES of PRC, MGC, BC, AC and RPC	YES of PRC
Transiently thickened retina	YES	YES	YES	YES	NO
Intermingling of nuclei of the ONL and INL	YES	YES	YES But moderately	YES at peripheral retina	YES Sporadic
Ectopic retinal cells in GCL	++++	+++	(+) sporadic ectopic cells	+ periphery	NO
ERG max b-waves 1M/3M	25%/0%	*/*	25%/10%	50%/0%	100%/90%
IS/OS at P14	NO	NO	NO	NO	YES
ONL at P14	NO	NO	YES	YES but not at periphery	YES
OPL at P14	NO	NO	At foci	YES but not at periphery	YES
INL at P14	NO	NO	YES	YES	YES
IPL at P14	YES	YES	YES	YES	YES
GCL at P14	Thickened in all of retina	Thickened in majority of retina	Thickened in part of retina	Thickened at peripheral retina	YES
Increase number of RPC	YES	YES	YES	NO	NA
Severity retinal phenotype	Throughout retina	Superior > inferior	Peripheral > central	Peripheral > central	Peripheral and Central Superior
Neovascularization	YES	YES	YES	YES	NA
Photoreceptors lost at 3M	YES (some sparse nuclei)	NA	thin ONL	YES (some sparse nuclei)	Minimal
Retinal overgrowth by late-born cells	YES	NO	NO	NO	NA
Apoptosis increased	YES	YES	YES	NA	NA

MGC—Müller glial cell; PRC—rod and cone photoreceptors; RPC—retinal progenitor cell; E—embryonic day; M—month; OLM—outer limiting membrane; BC—bipolar cell; AC—amacrine cell; GC—ganglion cell; ONL—outer nuclear layer; INL—inner nuclear layer; GCL—ganglion cell layer; ERG—electroretinography; *, mice not analyzed by ERG due to severe hydrocephalous; IS—inner segment; OS—outer segment; OPL—outer plexiform layer; IPL—inner plexiform layer; NA—not analyzed. Percentages distribution: CRB1 estimated 40% and CRB2 60% weight in MGC and RPC. CRB2 estimated 100% weight in PRC. # Rods estimated at 97% and cones at 3%. Adapted from [132].

Rosette formation has been extensively described in many retinal conditions including retinitis pigmentosa, diabetic retinopathy, and retinoblastoma [305–307]. The formation of rosettes has been attributed to the disruption of the OLM both chemically and genetically [130,231,233,266,308–312]. A defining hallmark of CRB mouse models is the formation of photoreceptor rosettes which may be concurrent with the loss of polarity in a CRB dependent manner. The more severe CRB models have a low level of total CRB, less stable AJs and thus an earlier phenotype onset and rosette formation. The less severe CRB models have a higher level of total CRB, more stable AJs and thus a later phenotype onset and rosette formation [144]. Rosette formation is preceded by aberrant localization of retinal cells into the subretinal space at foci where loss of adhesion is found. In the developing retina, this is usually seen as "volcanic-like" cell eruptions, while in the mature retina this is seen as a loss of complete rows of photoreceptors [130–132,232,270,298,299]. The $Crb1^{KO}Crb2^{\Delta MG}$ retina has a peripheral to central degenerative phenotype. At P1 in the $Crb1^{KO}Crb2^{\Delta MG}$, retina rosettes can be detected peripherally while only protrusions into the subretinal space are found in the central retina. By P14 the peripheral rosettes are gone due to advancement of the phenotype, but rosettes can now be found in the central retina [132]. Differences in the number of aberrant cells in early- versus late-disrupted OLM phenotypes likely arise from both the extent of OLM disruption as well as the developmental stage of the retina. Earlier cells are less mature/competent and are still undergoing division and migration changes. Rosette formation is likely independent of any increased cell proliferation seen in early-onset RP-like and LCA-like CRB models as rosettes are also present in later onset CRB, CRB-related, and non-CRB mouse models that do not exhibit changes in proliferation [130–132,232,298,299,310,311,313].

Although the mechanism by which rosettes are formed in retinal disease is not fully alluded to, it has been related to changes in the extracellular matrix, adhesion molecules, and the cytoskeleton, all of which can be affected by an imbalance between apical and basal polarity domains [314–317]. Loss of CRB in mutant mouse models may not be uniform due to opposing gradients of CRB1 and CRB2 proteins in the superior versus inferior retina as well as the non-uniform localization of CRB between photoreceptors (CRB2) and Müller glial cells (CRB1 and CRB2), leading to imbalance of CRB levels at the OLM in the mutant models [130,270,271]. Differences in adjacent apical levels of CRB are well studied as this is part of the process for tube invagination, similar mechanisms in opposing CRB levels between adjacent cells may lead to rosette formation, which are in fact invaginations of the apical retinal surface [318–320].

10. Gene Augmentation for Hereditary Retinopathies

Gene augmentation, via recombinant adeno-associated virus (rAAV) delivery, is currently the "go to" therapeutic strategy for targeting hereditary retinal diseases. Luxturna (voretigene neparvovec-rzyl) has led the way for eye gene therapeutics by becoming the first FDA- and EMA-approved AAV gene therapy for patients with biallelic *RPE65* gene mutations [321,322]. As such a large number of AAV mediated gene therapeutics are currently going under clinical trials focused on the treatment of achromatopsia, autosomal recessive retinitis pigmentosa, choroideremia, Leber hereditary optic neuropathy, retinitis pigmentosa, X-linked retinitis pigmentosa, X-linked Retinoschisis, and wet age-related macular degeneration (summarized in Table 1, Alves and Wijnholds 2018 [323]). The clinical success of rAAV mediated eye gene therapeutics is in part due to its low toxicity; the small amount of rAAV required to infect the retinal pigment epithelium or retina; the surgical accessibility of the eye; the large number of non-invasive techniques for monitoring disease progression, such as ERG, scanning laser ophthalmoscopy (SLO) and spectral domain optical coherence tomography (SD-OCT); and the immune-privileged status of the eye, having a good safety profile with low immunogenicity. Additionally, rAAV vectors can transduce both dividing but also non-dividing cells such as photoreceptors and display varied cell tropisms due to a plethora of capsid variants [323,324].

Wild type AAVs are small non-enveloped single stranded DNA viruses that belong to the parvovirus family in the genus Dependovirus and as such require assistance for replication. Cell surface receptors such as heparin sulfate and sialic acid mediate AAV endocytosis. AAV is then processed through the cytosol too the nucleus where it is uncoated and processed into nuclear episomal structures. The AAV genome includes three open reading frames which express the Replication (*rep*), Capsid (*cap*) and assembly activating protein (*aap*) genes. Two T-shaped 145 nucleotide-long inverted terminal repeats (ITRs) flank the genome. The ITRs and the four proteins encoded by the *rep* gene, Rep78, Rep68, Rep52, and Rep40, are needed for genome replication and packaging. Virion proteins (VP1), VP2, and VP3 from *cap* gene transcripts form an icosahedral symmetry shell ~26 nm in diameter defined by 60 subunits in a molar ratio of 1:1:10 (VP1:VP2:VP3). The assembly of the virions is promoted by the scaffolding function of AAP. However, in rAAV the *rep* and *cap* genes and the element required for site-specific integration into the genomic locus *AAVS1* are deleted. This means for replication a helper plasmid containing the *rep* and *cap* genes along with helper genes from adenovirus (*E4*, *E2a*, and *VA*) must be supplied [324].

Development of a *CRB*-based gene therapy approach was particularly challenging due to the cDNA size of 4.2 kb for human *CRB1*. With the addition of promoter, polyadenylation, and ITR sequences this is at the very edge of the approximate 4.7 kb packaging space of rAAV. Additionally, human *CRB1* cDNA required codon optimization to achieve sufficient levels of expression. However, alternative strategies employing the use of the 3.85 kb human *CRB2* cDNA and the development of minimal promoters for the expression of CRB proteins in photoreceptors and Müller glial cells has led to proof-of-concept for a *CRB*-based gene therapeutic [272,325]. These proof-of-concept pre-clinical studies found both morphological and functional rescue in two *CRB1*-RP-like mouse models when using an AAV-*CRB2*-based gene therapy vector. We found that expression of *CRB1* was deleterious in *CRB1* RP-like mouse models but not in wild-type mice. The *CRB2*-based gene therapy used a combination of AAV9 and the ubiquitous CMV promoter to target both photoreceptors (cone and rods) and Müller glial cells to achieve rescue. No rescue was achieved if either photoreceptors or Müller glial cells were targeted independently. We hypothesize that physiological relevant levels of CRB proteins are required at the subapical regions in neighboring photoreceptors and Müller glial cells [272]. There are a large number of transcript variants for CRB1 [144]. The Kay lab has identified a number of novel CRB1 isoforms in both mouse and human retina [303].

Cultured human iPSC-derived retinal organoids recapitulate well the human fetal retina, and might therefore be good models to test gene therapy vectors [143]. Recently we used transgene expression assays in human iPSC-derived retinal organoids and adult cadaveric human retinal explants to assess the tropism of three AAV serotypes: AAV9, AAV5, and ShH10Y using the ubiquitous CMV promoter. We found a preference of AAV5 and ShH10Y445F over AAV9 to infect Müller glial cells in hiPSC-derived retinal organoids. We observed as well a higher efficacy of AAV5 than ShH10Y445F or AAV9 serotypes for infection of photoreceptors and Müller glial cells in cultured human donor retinal explants. Together, our data indicate that AAV5 serotype in combination with the CMV promoter may be a viable strategy to express the *CRB* gene in human photoreceptors (rods and cones) and Müller glial cells [129]. An additional clinically relevant finding we discovered was the higher efficacy of AAV5-CMV-*GFP*, ShH10Y445F-CMV-*GFP*, and AAV9-CMV-*GFP* to express in Müller glial cells than photoreceptors in human retinal explants lacking photoreceptor segments. This indicated (1) that in the absence of photoreceptor segments there is an increased bioavailability of AAV vectors, allowing targeting of less-abundant/preferred receptors for AAV uptake; (2) that there may be a common mechanism of active AAV uptake to photoreceptors through there segments, e.g., putative sites of receptor-dependent or -independent clathrin- and caveolae-mediated endocytosis; (3) that intact photoreceptor segments allow for efficient AAV5 gene therapy vector transduction of human photoreceptors, whereas loss of intact photoreceptor segments allows for efficient AAV5 gene therapy vector transduction of Müller glial cells [129].

11. Concluding Remarks

Human stem cell-derived retinal organoids faithfully recapture in part many of the facets of the human fetal retina, including retinal cell type diversity, morphological cues, synaptic wiring, and light sensitivity. Improved retinal organoid culturing methods using bioreactors or microfluidic organ-on-a-chip technology, which also allows for tight control of the physiological microenvironment, bring us a further step towards an in vivo like retina [167,215,326]. Furthermore, retinal organoid models derived from patients may be used in conjunction with two-photon imaging and light sheet microscopy as well as tissue clearing methods such as DISCO and PACT [47,169,327–329]. This will allow unparalleled analysis of live and fixed cellular events including spatiotemporal process such as proliferation, differentiation and migration. Additionally, new methods such as ferrofluid droplets as mechanical actuators allow analysis of the mechanics of 3D developing tissues. This tool in combination with optogenetics or calcium imaging would provide insight into how neuronal and mechanical responses may influence each other in retinal development and disease [330,331]. Together, these are all valuable tools to further evaluate the mechanisms by which the misregulation of the apical CRB and PAR complexes affects retinogenesis leading to the severe retinal degeneration seen in LCA patients. Additionally, *CRB*-based gene augmentation is a viable option for *CRB1*-related retinitis pigmentosa and needs to be further evaluated for *CRB1*-related LCA.

Author Contributions: Conceptualization, P.M.J.Q. and J.W.; writing—original draft preparation, P.M.J.Q.; writing—review and editing, P.M.J.Q. and J.W.; visualization, P.M.J.Q.; funding acquisition, J.W.

Funding: This research was funded by Foundation Fighting Blindness [TA-GT-0715-0665-LUMC], The Netherlands Organisation for Health Research and Development [43200004], Curing Retinal Blindness Foundation, Stichting Retina Nederland Fonds, Landelijke St. Blinden en Slechtzienden, Rotterdamse Stichting, Blindenbelangen, St. Blindenhulp, St. Blinden- Penning and MaculaFonds.

Acknowledgments: We would like to thank members of the Wijnholds Lab for their input.

Conflicts of Interest: The authors declare no conflict of interest. The LUMC is the holder of patent number PCT/NL2014/050549, which describes the potential clinical use of CRB2; J.W. is listed as inventor on this patent and is an employee of the LUMC. The authors declare that the research was conducted without any commercial or financial relationships that could be construed as a potential conflict of interest.

References

1. Vu, H.T.V.; Keeffe, J.E.; McCarty, C.A.; Taylor, H.R. Impact of unilateral and bilateral vision loss on quality of life. *Br. J. Ophthalmol.* **2005**, *89*, 360–363. [CrossRef] [PubMed]
2. Youssef, P.N.; Sheibani, N.; Albert, D.M. Retinal light toxicity. *Eye* **2011**, *25*, 1–14. [CrossRef] [PubMed]
3. Marquardt, T.; Gruss, P. Generating neuronal diversity in the retina: One for nearly all. *Trends Neurosci.* **2002**, *25*, 32–38. [CrossRef]
4. Xiang, M. Intrinsic control of mammalian retinogenesis. *Cell. Mol. Life Sci.* **2013**, *70*, 2519–2532. [CrossRef] [PubMed]
5. Vecino, E.; Rodriguez, F.D.; Ruzafa, N.; Pereiro, X.; Sharma, S.C. Glia-neuron interactions in the mammalian retina. *Prog. Retin. Eye Res.* **2016**, *51*, 1–40. [CrossRef] [PubMed]
6. Foster, R.G.; Hankins, M.W. Non-rod, non-cone photoreception in the vertebrates. *Prog. Retin. Eye Res.* **2002**, *21*, 507–527. [CrossRef]
7. Ebrey, T.; Koutalos, Y. Vertebrate photoreceptors. *Prog. Retin. Eye Res.* **2001**, *20*, 49–94. [CrossRef]
8. Xiao, M.; Hendrickson, A. Spatial and Temporal Expression of Short, Long/Medium, or Both Opsins in Human Fetal Cones. *J. Comp. Neurol.* **2000**, *559*, 545–559. [CrossRef]
9. Roorda, A.; Williams, D.R. The arrangement of the three cone classes in the living human eye. *Nature* **1999**, *397*, 520–522. [CrossRef]
10. Grimes, W.N.; Songco-Aguas, A.; Rieke, F. Parallel Processing of Rod and Cone Signals: Retinal Function and Human Perception. *Annu. Rev. Vis. Sci* **2018**, *4*, 123–141. [CrossRef]
11. Franze, K.; Grosche, J.; Skatchkov, S.N.; Schinkinger, S.; Foja, C.; Schild, D.; Uckermann, O.; Travis, K.; Reichenbach, A.; Guck, J. Muller cells are living optical fibers in the vertebrate retina. *Proc. Natl. Acad. Sci. USA* **2007**, *104*, 8287–8292. [CrossRef] [PubMed]
12. Labin, A.M.; Ribak, E.N. Retinal glial cells enhance human vision acuity. *Phys. Rev. Lett.* **2010**, *104*, 1–4. [CrossRef] [PubMed]

13. Labin, A.M.; Safuri, S.K.; Ribak, E.N.; Perlman, I. Muller cells separate between wavelengths to improve day vision with minimal effect upon night vision. *Nat. Commun.* **2014**, *5*, 4319. [CrossRef] [PubMed]
14. Kefalov, V.J. Rod and cone visual pigments and phototransduction through pharmacological, genetic, and physiological approaches. *J. Biol. Chem.* **2012**, *287*, 1635–1641. [CrossRef]
15. Lee, B.B.; Martin, P.R.; Grünert, U. Retinal connectivity and primate vision. *Prog. Retin. Eye Res.* **2010**, *29*, 622–639. [CrossRef]
16. Rivlin-Etzion, M.; Grimes, W.N.; Rieke, F. Flexible Neural Hardware Supports Dynamic Computations in Retina. *Trends Neurosci.* **2018**, *41*, 224–237. [CrossRef]
17. Kolb, H.; Marshak, D. The midget pathways of the primate retina. *Doc. Ophthalmol.* **2003**, *106*, 67–81. [CrossRef]
18. Dacey, D.M. The mosaic of midget ganglion cells in the human retina. *J. Neurosci.* **1993**, *13*, 5334–5355. [CrossRef]
19. Provis, J.M.; Penfold, P.L.; Cornish, E.E.; Sandercoe, T.M.; Madigan, M.C. Anatomy and development of the macula: Specialisation and the vulnerability to macular degeneration. *Clin. Exp. Optom.* **2005**, *88*, 269–281. [CrossRef]
20. Ellis, E.M.; Gauvain, G.; Sivyer, B.; Murphy, G.J. Shared and distinct retinal input to the mouse superior colliculus and dorsal lateral geniculate nucleus. *J. Neurophysiol.* **2016**, *116*, 602–610. [CrossRef]
21. Erskine, L.; Herreral, E. Connecting the retina to the brain. *ASN Neuro* **2015**, *6*. [CrossRef]
22. Ahmadlou, M.; Zweifel, L.S.; Heimel, J.A. Functional modulation of primary visual cortex by the superior colliculus in the mouse. *Nat. Commun.* **2018**, *9*, 3895. [CrossRef] [PubMed]
23. Warner, C.E.; Kwan, W.C.; Wright, D.; Johnston, L.A.; Egan, G.F.; Bourne, J.A. Preservation of vision by the pulvinar following early-life primary visual cortex lesions. *Curr. Biol.* **2015**, *25*, 424–434. [CrossRef]
24. Ashtari, M.; Zhang, H.; Cook, P.A.; Cyckowski, L.L.; Shindler, K.S.; Marshall, K.A.; Aravand, P.; Vossough, A.; Gee, J.C.; Maguire, A.M.; et al. Plasticity of the human visual system after retinal gene therapy in patients with Leber's congenital amaurosis. *Sci. Transl. Med.* **2015**, *7*, 1–13. [CrossRef]
25. Benhar, I.; London, A.; Schwartz, M. The privileged immunity of immune privileged organs: The case of the eye. *Front. Immunol.* **2012**, *3*, 1–6. [CrossRef]
26. Kenyon, K.L.; Zaghloul, N.; Moody, S.A. Transcription factors of the anterior neural plate alter cell movements of epidermal progenitors to specify a retinal fate. *Dev. Biol.* **2001**, *240*, 77–91. [CrossRef]
27. Li, H.; Tierney, C.; Wen, L.; Wu, J.Y.; Rao, Y. A single morphogenetic field gives rise to two retina primordia under the influence of the prechordal plate. *Development* **1997**, *124*, 603–615.
28. Heavner, W.; Pevny, L. Eye development and retinogenesis. *Cold Spring Harb. Perspect. Biol.* **2012**, *4*. [CrossRef]
29. Zaghloul, N.A.; Yan, B.; Moody, S.A. Step-wise specification of retinal stem cells during normal embryogenesis. *Biol. Cell* **2005**, *97*, 321–337. [CrossRef]
30. Graw, J. Eye development. *Curr. Top. Dev. Biol.* **2010**, *90*, 343–386.
31. O'Rahilly, R. The prenatal development of the human eye. *Exp. Eye Res.* **1975**, *21*, 93–112. [CrossRef]
32. Randlett, O.; Norden, C.; Harris, W.A. The vertebrate retina: A model for neuronal polarization in vivo. *Dev. Neurobiol.* **2011**, *71*, 567–583. [CrossRef]
33. Baye, L.M.; Link, B.A. Nuclear migration during retinal development. *Brain Res.* **2008**, *1192*, 29–36. [CrossRef]
34. Baye, L.M.; Link, B.A. Interkinetic Nuclear Migration and the Selection of Neurogenic Cell Divisions during Vertebrate Retinogenesis. *J. Neurosci.* **2007**, *27*, 10143–10152. [CrossRef]
35. Norden, C.; Young, S.; Link, B.A.; Harris, W.A. Actomyosin Is the Main Driver of Interkinetic Nuclear Migration in the Retina. *Cell* **2009**, *138*, 1195–1208. [CrossRef]
36. Cayouette, M. The orientation of cell division influences cell-fate choice in the developing mammalian retina. *Development* **2003**, *130*, 2329–2339. [CrossRef]
37. Yang, X.J. Roles of cell-extrinsic growth factors in vertebrate eye pattern formation and retinogenesis. *Semin. Cell Dev. Biol.* **2004**, *15*, 91–103. [CrossRef]
38. Jin, K. Transitional Progenitors during Vertebrate Retinogenesis. *Mol. Neurobiol.* **2017**, *54*, 3565–3576. [CrossRef]
39. Cepko, C.L.; Austin, C.P.; Yang, X.; Alexiades, M.; Ezzeddine, D. Cell fate determination in the vertebrate retina. *Proc. Natl. Acad. Sci. USA* **1996**, *93*, 589–595. [CrossRef]

40. Aldiri, I.; Xu, B.; Wang, L.; Chen, X.; Hiler, D.; Griffiths, L.; Valentine, M.; Shirinifard, A.; Thiagarajan, S.; Sablauer, A.; et al. The Dynamic Epigenetic Landscape of the Retina During Development, Reprogramming, and Tumorigenesis. *Neuron* **2017**, *94*, 550–568.e10. [CrossRef]
41. Hoshino, A.; Ratnapriya, R.; Brooks, M.J.; Chaitankar, V.; Wilken, M.S.; Zhang, C.; Starostik, M.R.; Gieser, L.; La Torre, A.; Nishio, M.; et al. Molecular Anatomy of the Developing Human Retina. *Dev. Cell* **2017**, *43*, 763–779.e4. [CrossRef]
42. Reese, B.E.; Harvey, A.R.; Tan, S.S. Radial and tangential dispersion patterns in the mouse retina are cell-class specific. *Proc. Natl. Acad. Sci. USA* **1995**, *92*, 2494–2498. [CrossRef]
43. Reese, B.E.; Necessary, B.D.; Tam, P.P.; Faulkner-Jones, B.; Tan, S.S. Clonal expansion and cell dispersion in the developing mouse retina. *Eur. J. Neurosci.* **1999**, *11*, 2965–2978. [CrossRef]
44. Pearson, R.A.; Lüneborg, N.L.; Becker, D.L.; Mobbs, P. Gap junctions modulate interkinetic nuclear movement in retinal progenitor cells. *J. Neurosci.* **2005**, *25*, 10803–10814. [CrossRef]
45. Amini, R.; Rocha-martins, M.; Norden, C. Neuronal Migration and Lamination in the Vertebrate Retina. **2018**, *11*, 1–16. [CrossRef]
46. Kay, J.N. Radial migration: Retinal neurons hold on for the ride. *J. Cell Biol.* **2016**, *215*, 147–149. [CrossRef]
47. Icha, J.; Kunath, C.; Martins, M.R.; Norden, C. Independent modes of ganglion cell translocation ensure correct lamination of the zebrafish retina. *J. Cell Biol.* **2016**, *215*, 259–275. [CrossRef]
48. Reese, B.E.; Galli-Resta, L. The role of tangential dispersion in retinal mosaic formation. *Prog. Retin. Eye Res.* **2002**, *21*, 153–168. [CrossRef]
49. Reese, B.E.; Keeley, P.W. Design principles and developmental mechanisms underlying retinal mosaics. *Biol. Rev. Camb. Philos. Soc.* **2015**, *90*, 854–876. [CrossRef]
50. Davidson, E.H. cis -Regulatory Modules, and the Structure/Function Basis. In *The Regulatory Genome Gene Regulatory Networks In Development And Evolution*; Academic Press: Cambridge, MA, USA, 2006; pp. 31–86.
51. Peter, I.S.; Davidson, E.H. Evolution of gene regulatory networks controlling body plan development. *Cell* **2011**, *144*, 970–985. [CrossRef]
52. Allan, D.W.; Thor, S. Transcriptional selectors, masters, and combinatorial codes: Regulatory principles of neural subtype specification. *Wiley Interdiscip. Rev. Dev. Biol.* **2015**, *4*, 505–528. [CrossRef] [PubMed]
53. Suryamohan, K.; Halfon, M.S. Identifying transcriptional cis-regulatory modules in animal genomes. *Wiley Interdiscip. Rev. Dev. Biol.* **2015**, *4*, 59–84. [CrossRef]
54. Welby, E.; Lakowski, J.; Di Foggia, V.; Budinger, D.; Gonzalez-Cordero, A.; Lun, A.T.L.; Epstein, M.; Patel, A.; Cuevas, E.; Kruczek, K.; et al. Isolation and Comparative Transcriptome Analysis of Human Fetal and iPSC-Derived Cone Photoreceptor Cells. *Stem Cell Rep.* **2017**, *9*, 1898–1915. [CrossRef]
55. Mellough, C.B.; Bauer, R.; Collin, J.; Dorgau, B.; Zerti, D.; Dolan, D.W.P.; Jones, C.M.; Izuogu, O.G.; Yu, M.; Hallam, D.; et al. An integrated transcriptional analysis of the developing human retina. *Development* **2019**, *146*. [CrossRef]
56. Hu, Y.; Wang, X.; Hu, B.; Mao, Y.; Chen, Y.; Yan, L.; Yong, J.; Dong, J.; Wei, Y.; Wang, W.; et al. Dissecting the transcriptome landscape of the human fetal neural retina and retinal pigment epithelium by single-cell RNA-seq analysis. *PLOS Biol.* **2019**, *17*, e3000365. [CrossRef]
57. Kim, S.; Lowe, A.; Dharmat, R.; Lee, S.; Owen, L.A.; Wang, J.; Shakoor, A.; Li, Y.; Morgan, D.J.; Hejazi, A.A.; et al. Generation, transcriptome profiling, and functional validation of cone-rich human retinal organoids. *Proc. Natl. Acad. Sci. USA* **2019**, *116*, 10824–10833. [CrossRef]
58. Phillips, M.J.; Jiang, P.; Howden, S.; Barney, P.; Min, J.; York, N.W.; Chu, L.-F.; Capowski, E.E.; Cash, A.; Jain, S.; et al. A Novel Approach to Single Cell RNA-Sequence Analysis Facilitates In Silico Gene Reporting of Human Pluripotent Stem Cell-Derived Retinal Cell Types. *Stem Cells* **2018**, *36*, 313–324. [CrossRef]
59. Collin, J.; Queen, R.; Zerti, D.; Dorgau, B.; Hussain, R.; Coxhead, J.; Cockell, S.; Lako, M. Deconstructing Retinal Organoids: Single Cell RNA-Seq Reveals the Cellular Components of Human Pluripotent Stem Cell-Derived Retina. *Stem Cells* **2019**, *37*, 593–598. [CrossRef]
60. Langer, K.B.; Ohlemacher, S.K.; Phillips, M.J.; Fligor, C.M.; Jiang, P.; Gamm, D.M.; Meyer, J.S. Retinal Ganglion Cell Diversity and Subtype Specification from Human Pluripotent Stem Cells. *Stem Cell Rep.* **2018**, *10*, 1282–1293. [CrossRef]
61. Mao, X.; An, Q.; Xi, H.; Yang, X.-J.; Zhang, X.; Yuan, S.; Wang, J.; Hu, Y.; Liu, Q.; Fan, G. Single-Cell RNA Sequencing of hESC-Derived 3D Retinal Organoids Reveals Novel Genes Regulating RPC Commitment in Early Human Retinogenesis. *Stem Cell Rep.* **2019**, *13*, 747–760. [CrossRef]

62. Kim, J.W.; Yang, H.J.; Brooks, M.J.; Zelinger, L.; Karakülah, G.; Gotoh, N.; Boleda, A.; Gieser, L.; Giuste, F.; Whitaker, D.T.; et al. NRL-Regulated Transcriptome Dynamics of Developing Rod Photoreceptors. *Cell Rep.* **2016**, *17*, 2460–2473. [CrossRef]
63. Clark, B.S.; Stein-O'Brien, G.L.; Shiau, F.; Cannon, G.H.; Davis-Marcisak, E.; Sherman, T.; Santiago, C.P.; Hoang, T.V.; Rajaii, F.; James-Esposito, R.E.; et al. Single-Cell RNA-Seq Analysis of Retinal Development Identifies NFI Factors as Regulating Mitotic Exit and Late-Born Cell Specification. *Neuron* **2019**, *102*, 1111–1126.e5. [CrossRef]
64. Kim, J.W.; Yang, H.J.; Oel, A.P.; Brooks, M.J.; Jia, L.; Plachetzki, D.C.; Li, W.; Allison, W.T.; Swaroop, A. Recruitment of Rod Photoreceptors from Short-Wavelength-Sensitive Cones during the Evolution of Nocturnal Vision in Mammals. *Dev. Cell* **2016**, *37*, 520–532. [CrossRef]
65. Mo, A.; Luo, C.; Davis, F.P.; Mukamel, E.A.; Henry, G.L.; Nery, J.R.; Urich, M.A.; Picard, S.; Lister, R.; Eddy, S.R.; et al. Epigenomic landscapes of retinal rods and cones. *Elife* **2016**, *5*, 1–29. [CrossRef]
66. Hughes, A.E.O.; Enright, J.M.; Myers, C.A.; Shen, S.Q.; Corbo, J.C. Cell Type-Specific Epigenomic Analysis Reveals a Uniquely Closed Chromatin Architecture in Mouse Rod Photoreceptors. *Sci. Rep.* **2017**, *7*, 1–16. [CrossRef]
67. Norrie, J.L.; Lupo, M.S.; Xu, B.; Al Diri, I.; Valentine, M.; Putnam, D.; Griffiths, L.; Zhang, J.; Johnson, D.; Easton, J.; et al. Nucleome Dynamics during Retinal Development. *Neuron* **2019**, *104*, 521–528.e11. [CrossRef]
68. Blackshaw, S.; Harpavat, S.; Trimarchi, J.; Cai, L.; Huang, H.; Kuo, W.P.; Weber, G.; Lee, K.; Fraioli, R.E.; Cho, S.-H.; et al. Genomic Analysis of Mouse Retinal Development. *PLoS Biol.* **2004**, *2*, e247. [CrossRef]
69. Lo Giudice, Q.; Leleu, M.; La Manno, G.; Fabre, P.J. Single-cell transcriptional logic of cell-fate specification and axon guidance in early-born retinal neurons. *Development* **2019**, *146*, dev178103. [CrossRef]
70. Rheaume, B.A.; Jereen, A.; Bolisetty, M.; Sajid, M.S.; Yang, Y.; Renna, K.; Sun, L.; Robson, P.; Trakhtenberg, E.F. Single cell transcriptome profiling of retinal ganglion cells identifies cellular subtypes. *Nat. Commun.* **2018**, *9*. [CrossRef]
71. Diacou, R.; Zhao, Y.; Zheng, D.; Cvekl, A.; Liu, W. Six3 and Six6 Are Jointly Required for the Maintenance of Multipotent Retinal Progenitors through Both Positive and Negative Regulation. *Cell Rep.* **2018**, *25*, 2510–2523.e4. [CrossRef]
72. Liu, W.; Cvekl, A. Six3 in a small population of progenitors at E8.5 is required for neuroretinal specification via regulating cell signaling and survival in mice. *Dev. Biol.* **2017**, *428*, 164–175. [CrossRef] [PubMed]
73. Liu, W.; Lagutin, O.; Swindell, E.; Jamrich, M.; Oliver, G. Neuroretina specification in mouse embryos requires Six3-mediated suppression of Wnt8b in the anterior neural plate. *J. Clin. Investig.* **2010**, *120*, 3568–3577. [CrossRef] [PubMed]
74. Burmeister, M.; Novak, J.; Liang, M.Y.; Basu, S.; Ploder, L.; Hawes, N.L.; Vidgen, D.; Hoover, F.; Goldman, D.; Kalnins, V.I.; et al. Ocular retardation mouse caused by Chx10 homeobox null allele: Impaired retinal progenitor proliferation and bipolar cell differentiation. *Nat. Genet.* **1996**, *12*, 376–384. [CrossRef]
75. Li, X.; Perissi, V.; Liu, F.; Rose, D.W.; Rosenfeld, M.G. Tissue-specific regulation of retinal and pituitary precursor cell proliferation. *Science* **2002**, *297*, 1180–1183. [CrossRef]
76. Marquardt, T.; Ashery-Padan, R.; Andrejewski, N.; Scardigli, R.; Guillemot, F.; Gruss, P. Pax6 is required for the multipotent state of retinal progenitor cells. *Cell* **2001**, *105*, 43–55. [CrossRef]
77. Gordon, P.J.; Yun, S.; Clark, A.M.; Monuki, E.S.; Murtaugh, L.C.; Levine, E.M. Lhx2 balances progenitor maintenance with neurogenic output and promotes competence state progression in the developing retina. *J. Neurosci.* **2013**, *33*, 12197–12207. [CrossRef]
78. Zibetti, C.; Liu, S.; Wan, J.; Qian, J.; Blackshaw, S. Epigenomic profiling of retinal progenitors reveals LHX2 is required for developmental regulation of open chromatin. *Commun. Biol.* **2019**, *2*, 1–13. [CrossRef]
79. Tétreault, N.; Champagne, M.-P.; Bernier, G. The LIM homeobox transcription factor Lhx2 is required to specify the retina field and synergistically cooperates with Pax6 for Six6 trans-activation. *Dev. Biol.* **2009**, *327*, 541–550. [CrossRef]
80. Azuma, N.; Nishina, S.; Yanagisawa, H.; Okuyama, T.; Yamada, M. PAX6 missense mutation in isolated foveal hypoplasia. *Nat. Genet.* **1996**, *13*, 141–142. [CrossRef]
81. Voronina, V.A.; Kozhemyakina, E.A.; O'Kernick, C.M.; Kahn, N.D.; Wenger, S.L.; Linberg, J.V.; Schneider, A.S.; Mathers, P.H. Mutations in the human RAX homeobox gene in a patient with anophthalmia and sclerocornea. *Hum. Mol. Genet.* **2004**, *13*, 315–322. [CrossRef]

82. Mattar, P.; Ericson, J.; Blackshaw, S.; Cayouette, M. A conserved regulatory logic controls temporal identity in mouse neural progenitors. *Neuron* **2015**, *85*, 497–504. [CrossRef] [PubMed]
83. Elliott, J.; Jolicoeur, C.; Ramamurthy, V.; Cayouette, M. Ikaros Confers Early Temporal Competence to Mouse Retinal Progenitor Cells. *Neuron* **2008**, *60*, 26–39. [CrossRef] [PubMed]
84. Hamon, A.; Masson, C.; Bitard, J.; Gieser, L.; Roger, J.E.; Perron, M. Retinal Degeneration Triggers the Activation of YAP/TEAD in Reactive Müller Cells. *Investig. Opthalmol. Vis. Sci.* **2017**, *58*, 1941. [CrossRef] [PubMed]
85. Kim, J.Y.; Park, R.; Lee, J.H.J.; Shin, J.; Nickas, J.; Kim, S.; Cho, S.H. Yap is essential for retinal progenitor cell cycle progression and RPE cell fate acquisition in the developing mouse eye. *Dev. Biol.* **2016**, *419*, 336–347. [CrossRef] [PubMed]
86. Rueda, E.M.; Hall, B.M.; Hill, M.C.; Swinton, P.G.; Tong, X.; Martin, J.F.; Poché, R.A. The Hippo Pathway Blocks Mammalian Retinal Müller Glial Cell Reprogramming. *Cell Rep.* **2019**, *27*, 1637–1649.e6. [CrossRef]
87. Hamon, A.; García-García, D.; Ail, D.; Bitard, J.; Chesneau, A.; Dalkara, D.; Locker, M.; Roger, J.E.; Perron, M. Linking YAP to Müller Glia Quiescence Exit in the Degenerative Retina. *Cell Rep.* **2019**, *27*, 1712–1725.e6. [CrossRef]
88. Furukawa, T.; Mukherjee, S.; Bao, Z.Z.; Morrow, E.M.; Cepko, C.L. rax, Hes1, and notch1 promote the formation of Muller glia by postnatal retinal progenitor cells. *Neuron* **2000**, *26*, 383–394. [CrossRef]
89. Hojo, M.; Ohtsuka, T.; Hashimoto, N.; Gradwohl, G.; Guillemot, F.; Kageyama, R. Glial cell fate specification modulated by the bHLH gene Hes5 in mouse retina. *Development* **2000**, *127*, 2515–2522.
90. Poché, R.A.; Furuta, Y.; Chaboissier, M.-C.; Schedl, A.; Behringer, R.R. Sox9 is expressed in mouse multipotent retinal progenitor cells and functions in Müller glial cell development. *J. Comp. Neurol.* **2008**, *510*, 237–250. [CrossRef]
91. de Melo, J.; Zibetti, C.; Clark, B.S.; Hwang, W.; Miranda-Angulo, A.L.; Qian, J.; Blackshaw, S. Lhx2 Is an Essential Factor for Retinal Gliogenesis and Notch Signaling. *J. Neurosci.* **2016**, *36*, 2391–2405. [CrossRef]
92. Verbakel, S.K.; van Huet, R.A.C.; Boon, C.J.F.; den Hollander, A.I.; Collin, R.W.J.; Klaver, C.C.W.; Hoyng, C.B.; Roepman, R.; Klevering, B.J. Non-syndromic retinitis pigmentosa. *Prog. Retin. Eye Res.* **2018**, 1–30. [CrossRef] [PubMed]
93. Haider, N.B.; Jacobson, S.G.; Cideciyan, A.V.; Swiderski, R.; Streb, L.M.; Searby, C.; Beck, G.; Hockey, R.; Hanna, D.B.; Gorman, S.; et al. Mutation of a nuclear receptor gene, NR2E3, causes enhanced S cone syndrome, a disorder of retinal cell fate. *Nat. Genet.* **2000**, *24*, 127–131. [CrossRef] [PubMed]
94. Sohocki, M.M.; Sullivan, L.S.; Mintz-Hittner, H.A.; Birch, D.; Heckenlively, J.R.; Freund, C.L.; Mclnnes, R.R.; Daiger, S.P. A range of clinical phenotypes associated with mutations in CRX, a photoreceptor transcription-factor gene. *Am. J. Hum. Genet.* **1998**, *63*, 1307–1315. [CrossRef] [PubMed]
95. Swain, P.K.; Chen, S.; Wang, Q.L.; Affatigato, L.M.; Coats, C.L.; Brady, K.D.; Fishman, G.A.; Jacobson, S.G.; Swaroop, A.; Stone, E.; et al. Mutations in the cone-rod homeobox gene are associated with the cone-rod dystrophy photoreceptor degeneration. *Neuron* **1997**, *19*, 1329–1336. [CrossRef]
96. Newman, H.; Blumen, S.C.; Braverman, I.; Hanna, R.; Tiosano, B.; Perlman, I.; Ben-Yosef, T. Homozygosity for a recessive loss-of-function mutation of the NRL gene is associated with a variant of enhanced S-cone syndrome. *Investig. Ophthalmol. Vis. Sci.* **2016**, *57*, 5361–5371. [CrossRef]
97. DeAngelis, M.M.; Grimsby, J.L.; Sandberg, M.A.; Berson, E.L.; Dryja, T.P. Novel mutations in the NRL gene and associated clinical findings in patients with dominant retinitis pigmentosa. *Arch. Ophthalmol.* **2002**, *120*, 369–375. [CrossRef]
98. Gire, A.I.; Sullivan, L.S.; Bowne, S.J.; Birch, D.G.; Hughbanks-Wheaton, D.; Heckenlively, J.R.; Daiger, S.P. The Gly56Arg mutation in NR2E3 accounts for 1-2% of autosomal dominant retinitis pigmentosa. *Mol. Vis.* **2007**, *13*, 1970–1975.
99. Nishida, A.; Furukawa, A.; Koike, C.; Tano, Y.; Aizawa, S.; Matsuo, I.; Furukawa, T. Otx2 homeobox gene controls retinal photoreceptor cell fate and pineal gland development. *Nat. Neurosci.* **2003**, *6*, 1255–1263. [CrossRef]
100. Furukawa, T.; Morrow, E.M.; Cepko, C.L. Crx, a novel otx-like homeobox gene, shows photoreceptor-specific expression and regulates photoreceptor differentiation. *Cell* **1997**, *91*, 531–541. [CrossRef]
101. Mears, A.J.; Kondo, M.; Swain, P.K.; Takada, Y.; Bush, R.A.; Saunders, T.L.; Sieving, P.A.; Swaroop, A. Nrl is required for rod photoreceptor development. *Nat. Genet.* **2001**, *29*, 447–452. [CrossRef]

102. Fu, Y.; Liu, H.; Ng, L.; Kim, J.W.; Hao, H.; Swaroop, A.; Forrest, D. Feedback induction of a photoreceptor-specific isoform of retinoid-related orphan nuclear receptor β by the rod transcription factor NRL. *J. Biol. Chem.* **2014**, *289*, 32469–32480. [CrossRef] [PubMed]
103. Chen, J.; Rattner, A.; Nathans, J. The rod photoreceptor-specific nuclear receptor Nr2e3 represses transcription of multiple cone-specific genes. *J. Neurosci.* **2005**, *25*, 118–129. [CrossRef]
104. Oh, E.C.T.; Khan, N.; Novelli, E.; Khanna, H.; Strettoi, E.; Swaroop, A. Transformation of cone precursors to functional rod photoreceptors by bZIP transcription factor NRL. *Proc. Natl. Acad. Sci. USA* **2007**, *104*, 1679–1684. [CrossRef]
105. Wang, S.; Sengel, C.; Emerson, M.M.; Cepko, C.L. A gene regulatory network controls the binary fate decision of rod and bipolar cells in the vertebrate retina. *Dev. Cell* **2014**, *30*, 513–527. [CrossRef]
106. Brzezinski, J.A.; Lamba, D.A.; Reh, T.A. Blimp1 controls photoreceptor versus bipolar cell fate choice during retinal development. *Development* **2010**, *137*, 619–629. [CrossRef]
107. Ng, L.; Hurley, J.B.; Dierks, B.; Srinivas, M.; Saltó, C.; Vennström, B.; Reh, T.A.; Forrest, D. A thyroid hormone receptor that is required for the development of green cone photoreceptors. *Nat. Genet.* **2001**, *27*, 94–98. [CrossRef]
108. Roberts, M.R.; Hendrickson, A.; McGuire, C.R.; Reh, T.A. Retinoid X receptor γ is necessary to establish the S-opsin gradient in cone photoreceptors of the developing mouse retina. *Investig. Ophthalmol. Vis. Sci.* **2005**, *46*, 2897–2904. [CrossRef]
109. Roberts, M.R.; Srinivas, M.; Forrest, D.; De Escobar, G.M.; Reh, T.A. Making the gradient: Thyroid hormone regulates cone opsin expression in the develoninn mouse retina. *Proc. Natl. Acad. Sci. USA* **2006**, *103*, 6218–6223. [CrossRef]
110. Emerson, M.M.; Surzenko, N.; Goetz, J.J.; Trimarchi, J.; Cepko, C.L. Otx2 and Onecut1 promote the fates of cone photoreceptors and horizontal cells and repress rod photoreceptors. *Dev. Cell* **2013**, *26*, 59–72. [CrossRef]
111. Schick, E.; McCaffery, S.D.; Keblish, E.E.; Thakurdin, C.; Emerson, M.M. Lineage tracing analysis of cone photoreceptor associated cis-regulatory elements in the developing chicken retina. *Sci. Rep.* **2019**, *9*, 1–14. [CrossRef]
112. Chow, R.L.; Volgyi, B.; Szilard, R.K.; Ng, D.; McKerlie, C.; Bloomfield, S.A.; Birch, D.G.; McInnes, R.R. Control of late off-center cone bipolar cell differentiation and visual signaling by the homeobox gene Vsx1. *Proc. Natl. Acad. Sci. USA* **2004**, *101*, 1754–1759. [CrossRef] [PubMed]
113. Huang, L.; Hu, F.; Feng, L.; Luo, X.-J.; Liang, G.; Zeng, X.-Y.; Yi, J.-L.; Gan, L. Bhlhb5 is required for the subtype development of retinal amacrine and bipolar cells in mice. *Dev. Dyn.* **2014**, *243*, 279–289. [CrossRef] [PubMed]
114. Fujitani, Y.; Fujitani, S.; Luo, H.; Qiu, F.; Burlison, J.; Long, Q.; Kawaguchi, Y.; Edlund, H.; MacDonald, R.J.; Furukawa, T.; et al. Ptf1a determines horizontal and amacrine cell fates during mouse retinal development. *Development* **2006**, *133*, 4439–4450. [CrossRef]
115. Li, S.; Mo, Z.; Yang, X.; Price, S.M.; Shen, M.M.; Xiang, M. Foxn4 controls the genesis of amacrine and horizontal cells by retinal progenitors. *Neuron* **2004**, *43*, 795–807. [CrossRef] [PubMed]
116. Dyer, M.A.; Livesey, F.J.; Cepko, C.L.; Oliver, G. Prox1 function controls progenitor cell proliferation and horizontal cell genesis in the mammalian retina. *Nat. Genet.* **2003**, *34*, 53–58. [CrossRef]
117. Wu, F.; Li, R.; Umino, Y.; Kaczynski, T.J.; Sapkota, D.; Li, S.; Xiang, M.; Fliesler, S.J.; Sherry, D.M.; Gannon, M.; et al. Onecut1 is essential for horizontal cell genesis and retinal integrity. *J. Neurosci.* **2013**, *33*, 13053–13065. [CrossRef]
118. Liu, W.; Wang, J.H.; Xiang, M. Specific expression of the LIM/homeodomain protein Lim-1 in horizontal cells during retinogenesis. *Dev. Dyn.* **2000**, *217*, 320–325. [CrossRef]
119. Edqvist, P.H.; Myers, S.M.; Hallböök, F. Early identification of retinal subtypes in the developing, pre-laminated chick retina using the transcription factors Prox1, Lim1, Ap2α, Pax6, Isl1, Isl2, Lim3 and Chx10. *Eur. J. Histochem.* **2006**, *50*, 147–154.
120. Poché, R.A.; Kin, M.K.; Raven, M.A.; Furuta, Y.; Reese, B.E.; Behringer, R.R. Lim1 is essential for the correct laminar positioning of retinal horizontal cells. *J. Neurosci.* **2007**, *27*, 14099–14107. [CrossRef]
121. Jin, K.; Jiang, H.; Xiao, D.; Zou, M.; Zhu, J.; Xiang, M. Tfap2a and 2b act downstream of Ptf1a to promote amacrine cell differentiation during retinogenesis. *Mol. Brain* **2015**, *8*, 1–14. [CrossRef]
122. Elshatory, Y.; Everhart, D.; Deng, M.; Xie, X.; Barlow, R.B.; Gan, L. Islet-1 controls the differentiation of retinal bipolar and cholinergic amacrine cells. *J. Neurosci.* **2007**, *27*, 12707–12720. [CrossRef]

123. Cherry, T.J.; Wang, S.; Bormuth, I.; Schwab, M.; Olson, J.; Cepko, C.L. NeuroD factors regulate cell fate and neurite stratification in the developing retina. *J. Neurosci.* **2011**, *31*, 7365–7379. [CrossRef]
124. Ding, Q.; Chen, H.; Xie, X.; Libby, R.T.; Tian, N.; Gan, L. BARHL2 differentially regulates the development of retinal amacrine and ganglion neurons. *J. Neurosci.* **2009**, *29*, 3992–4003. [CrossRef] [PubMed]
125. Wu, F.; Kaczynski, T.J.; Sethuramanujam, S.; Li, R.; Jain, V.; Slaughter, M.; Mu, X. Two transcription factors, Pou4f2 and Isl1, are sufficient to specify the retinal ganglion cell fate. *Proc. Natl. Acad. Sci. USA* **2015**, *112*, E1559–E1568. [CrossRef]
126. Mu, X.; Fu, X.; Beremand, P.D.; Thomas, T.L.; Klein, W.H. Gene-regulation logic in retinal ganglion cell development: Isl1 defines a critical branch distinct from but overlapping with Pou4f2. *Proc. Natl. Acad. Sci. USA* **2008**, *105*, 6942–6947. [CrossRef]
127. Mao, C.A.; Wang, S.W.; Pan, P.; Klein, W.H. Rewiring the retinal ganglion cell gene regulatory network: Neurod1 promotes retinal ganglion cell fate in the absence of Math5. *Development* **2008**, *135*, 3379–3388. [CrossRef]
128. Jiang, Y.; Ding, Q.; Xie, X.; Libby, R.T.; Lefebvre, V.; Gan, L. Transcription factors SOX4 and SOX11 function redundantly to regulate the development of mouse retinal ganglion cells. *J. Biol. Chem.* **2013**, *288*, 18429–18438. [CrossRef]
129. Quinn, P.M.; Buck, T.M.; Mulder, A.A.; Ohonin, C.; Alves, C.H.; Vos, R.M.; Bialecka, M.; van Herwaarden, T.; van Dijk, E.H.C.; Talib, M.; et al. Human iPSC-Derived Retinas Recapitulate the Fetal CRB1 CRB2 Complex Formation and Demonstrate that Photoreceptors and Müller Glia Are Targets of AAV5. *Stem Cell Rep.* **2019**, *12*, 906–919. [CrossRef]
130. van de Pavert, S.A.; Kantardzhieva, A.; Malysheva, A.; Meuleman, J.; Versteeg, I.; Levelt, C.; Klooster, J.; Geiger, S.; Seeliger, M.W.; Rashbass, P.; et al. Crumbs homologue 1 is required for maintenance of photoreceptor cell polarization and adhesion during light exposure. *J. Cell Sci.* **2004**, *117*, 4169–4177. [CrossRef]
131. Alves, C.H.; Pellissier, L.P.; Vos, R.M.; Garcia Garrido, M.; Sothilingam, V.; Seide, C.; Beck, S.C.; Klooster, J.; Furukawa, T.; Flannery, J.G.; et al. Targeted ablation of Crb2 in photoreceptor cells induces retinitis pigmentosa. *Hum. Mol. Genet.* **2014**, *23*, 3384–3401. [CrossRef]
132. Quinn, P.M.; Mulder, A.A.; Henrique Alves, C.; Desrosiers, M.; de Vries, S.I.; Klooster, J.; Dalkara, D.; Koster, A.J.; Jost, C.R.; Wijnholds, J. Loss of CRB2 in Müller glial cells modifies a CRB1-associated retinitis pigmentosa phenotype into a Leber congenital amaurosis phenotype. *Hum. Mol. Genet.* **2019**, *28*, 105–123. [CrossRef] [PubMed]
133. Xiao, Z.; Patrakka, J.; Nukui, M.; Chi, L.; Niu, D.; Betsholtz, C.; Pikkarainen, T.; Pikkarainan, T.; Vainio, S.; Tryggvason, K. Deficiency in Crumbs homolog 2 (Crb2) affects gastrulation and results in embryonic lethality in mice. *Dev. Dyn.* **2011**, *240*, 2646–2656. [CrossRef]
134. Lamont, R.E.; Tan, W.-H.; Innes, A.M.; Parboosingh, J.S.; Schneidman-Duhovny, D.; Rajkovic, A.; Pappas, J.; Altschwager, P.; DeWard, S.; Fulton, A.; et al. Expansion of phenotype and genotypic data in CRB2-related syndrome. *Eur. J. Hum. Genet.* **2016**, *24*, 1436–1444. [CrossRef]
135. Charrier, L.E.; Loie, E.; Laprise, P. Mouse Crumbs3 sustains epithelial tissue morphogenesis in vivo. *Sci. Rep.* **2015**, *5*, 1–16. [CrossRef]
136. Whiteman, E.L.; Fan, S.; Harder, J.L.; Walton, K.D.; Liu, C.-J.; Soofi, A.; Fogg, V.C.; Hershenson, M.B.; Dressler, G.R.; Deutsch, G.H.; et al. Crumbs3 Is Essential for Proper Epithelial Development and Viability. *Mol. Cell. Biol.* **2014**, *34*, 43–56. [CrossRef]
137. Haverkamp, S.; Haeseleer, F.; Hendrickson, A. A comparison of immunocytochemical markers to identify bipolar cell types in human and monkey retina. *Vis. Neurosci.* **2003**, *20*, 589–600. [CrossRef]
138. Abramov, I.; Gordon, J.; Hendrickson, A.; Hainline, L.; Dobson, V.; Labossiere, E. The retina of the newborn human infant. *Science* **1982**, *217*, 265–267. [CrossRef]
139. Bibb, L.C.; Holt, J.K.; Tarttelin, E.E.; Hodges, M.D.; Gregory-Evans, K.; Rutherford, A.; Lucas, R.J.; Sowden, J.C.; Gregory-Evans, C.Y. Temporal and spatial expression patterns of the CRX transcription factor and its downstream targets. Critical differences during human and mouse eye development. *Hum. Mol. Genet.* **2001**, *10*, 1571–1579. [CrossRef]
140. Hendrickson, A. A morphological comparison of foveal development in man and monkey. *Eye* **1992**, *6*, 136–144. [CrossRef]

141. Reichman, S.; Terray, A.; Slembrouck, A.; Nanteau, C.; Orieux, G.; Habeler, W.; Nandrot, E.F.; Sahel, J.-A.; Monville, C.; Goureau, O. From confluent human iPS cells to self-forming neural retina and retinal pigmented epithelium. *Proc. Natl. Acad. Sci. USA* **2014**, *111*, 8518–8523. [CrossRef]
142. Zhong, X.; Gutierrez, C.; Xue, T.; Hampton, C.; Vergara, M.N.; Cao, L.-H.; Peters, A.; Park, T.S.; Zambidis, E.T.; Meyer, J.S.; et al. Generation of three-dimensional retinal tissue with functional photoreceptors from human iPSCs. *Nat. Commun.* **2014**, *5*, 4047. [CrossRef] [PubMed]
143. Quinn, P.M.; Buck, T.M.; Ohonin, C.; Mikkers, H.M.M.; Wijnholds, J. Production of iPS-Derived Human Retinal Organoids for Use in Transgene Expression Assays. *Methods Mol. Biol.* **2018**, *1715*, 261–273.
144. Quinn, P.M.; Pellissier, L.P.; Wijnholds, J. The CRB1 complex: Following the trail of Crumbs to a feasible gene therapy strategy. *Front. Neurosci.* **2017**, *11*, 175. [CrossRef] [PubMed]
145. Nakano, T.; Ando, S.; Takata, N.; Kawada, M.; Muguruma, K.; Sekiguchi, K.; Saito, K.; Yonemura, S.; Eiraku, M.; Sasai, Y. Self-formation of optic cups and storable stratified neural retina from human ESCs. *Cell Stem Cell* **2012**, *10*, 771–785. [CrossRef] [PubMed]
146. Eldred, K.C.; Hadyniak, S.E.; Hussey, K.A.; Brenerman, B.; Zhang, P.; Chamling, X.; Sluch, V.M.; Welsbie, D.S.; Hattar, S.; Taylor, J.; et al. Thyroid hormone signaling specifies cone subtypes in human retinal organoids. *Science* **2018**, *362*, 359950. [CrossRef]
147. Lakowski, J.; Welby, E.; Budinger, D.; Di Marco, F.; Di Foggia, V.; Bainbridge, J.W.B.; Wallace, K.; Gamm, D.M.; Ali, R.R.; Sowden, J.C. Isolation of Human Photoreceptor Precursors via a Cell Surface Marker Panel from Stem Cell-Derived Retinal Organoids and Fetal Retinae. *Stem Cells* **2018**, *36*, 709–722. [CrossRef]
148. Dorgau, B.; Felemban, M.; Sharpe, A.; Bauer, R.; Hallam, D.; Steel, D.H.; Lindsay, S.; Mellough, C.; Lako, M. Laminin γ3 plays an important role in retinal lamination, photoreceptor organisation and ganglion cell differentiation. *Cell Death Dis.* **2018**, *9*, 615. [CrossRef]
149. Felemban, M.; Dorgau, B.; Hunt, N.C.; Hallam, D.; Zerti, D.; Bauer, R.; Ding, Y.; Collin, J.; Steel, D.; Krasnogor, N.; et al. Extracellular matrix components expression in human pluripotent stem cell-derived retinal organoids recapitulates retinogenesis in vivo and reveals an important role for IMPG1 and CD44 in the development of photoreceptors and interphotoreceptor matrix. *Acta Biomater.* **2018**, *74*, 207–221. [CrossRef]
150. Hendrickson, A.; Drucker, D. The development of parafoveal and mid-peripheral human retina. *Behav. Brain Res.* **1992**, *49*, 21–31. [CrossRef]
151. Hendrickson, A.; Bumsted-O'Brien, K.; Natoli, R.; Ramamurthy, V.; Possin, D.; Provis, J. Rod photoreceptor differentiation in fetal and infant human retina. *Exp. Eye Res.* **2008**, *87*, 415–426. [CrossRef]
152. Hendrickson, A.; Possin, D.; Vajzovic, L.; Toth, C.A. Histologic Development of the Human Fovea From Midgestation to Maturity. *Am. J. Ophthalmol.* **2012**, *154*, 767–778.e2. [CrossRef] [PubMed]
153. Hendrickson, A. Development of Retinal Layers in Prenatal Human Retina. *Am. J. Ophthalmol.* **2016**, *161*, 29–35.e1. [CrossRef] [PubMed]
154. Kozulin, P.; Natoli, R.; O'Brien, K.M.B.; Madigan, M.C.; Provis, J.M. Differential expression of anti-angiogenic factors and guidance genes in the developing macula. *Mol. Vis.* **2009**, *15*, 45–59. [PubMed]
155. O'Brien, K.M.B.; Schulte, D.; Hendrickson, A.E. Expression of photoreceptor-associated molecules during human fetal eye development. *Mol. Vis.* **2003**, *9*, 401–409.
156. Curcio, C.A.; Sloan, K.R.; Kalina, R.E.; Hendrickson, A.E. Human photoreceptor topography. *J. Comp. Neurol.* **1990**, *292*, 497–523. [CrossRef]
157. Narayanan, K.; Wadhwa, S. Photoreceptor morphogenesis in the human retina: A scanning electron microscopic study. *Anat. Rec.* **1998**, *252*, 133–139. [CrossRef]
158. Cornish, E.E.; Xiao, M.; Yang, Z.; Provis, J.M.; Hendrickson, A.E. The role of opsin expression and apoptosis in determination of cone types in human retina. *Exp. Eye Res.* **2004**, *78*, 1143–1154. [CrossRef]
159. Cornish, E.E.; Hendrickson, A.E.; Provis, J.M. Distribution of short-wavelength-sensitive cones in human fetal and postnatal retina: Early development of spatial order and density profiles. *Vision Res.* **2004**, *44*, 2019–2026. [CrossRef]
160. Hendrickson, A.E.; Yuodelis, C. The Morphological Development of the Human Fovea. *Ophthalmology* **1984**, *91*, 603–612. [CrossRef]

161. Fligor, C.M.; Langer, K.B.; Sridhar, A.; Ren, Y.; Shields, P.K.; Edler, M.C.; Ohlemacher, S.K.; Sluch, V.M.; Zack, D.J.; Zhang, C.; et al. Three-Dimensional Retinal Organoids Facilitate the Investigation of Retinal Ganglion Cell Development, Organization and Neurite Outgrowth from Human Pluripotent Stem Cells. *Sci. Rep.* **2018**, *8*, 1–14. [CrossRef]
162. Hallam, D.; Hilgen, G.; Dorgau, B.; Zhu, L.; Yu, M.; Bojic, S.; Hewitt, P.; Schmitt, M.; Uteng, M.; Kustermann, S.; et al. Human induced pluripotent stem cells generate light responsive retinal organoids with variable and nutrient dependent efficiency. *Stem Cells* **2018**, *36*, 1535–1551. [CrossRef] [PubMed]
163. Luo, Z.; Zhong, X.; Li, K.; Xie, B.; Liu, Y.; Ye, M.; Li, K.; Xu, C.; Ge, J. An Optimized System for Effective Derivation of Three-dimensional Retinal Tissue via Wnt Signaling Regulation. *Stem Cells* **2018**, *36*, 1709–1722. [CrossRef] [PubMed]
164. Kuwahara, A.; Ozone, C.; Nakano, T.; Saito, K.; Eiraku, M.; Sasai, Y. Generation of a ciliary margin-like stem cell niche from self-organizing human retinal tissue. *Nat. Commun.* **2015**, *6*, 6286. [CrossRef] [PubMed]
165. Fernández-Nogales, M.; Murcia-Belmonte, V.; Chen, H.Y.; Herrera, E. The peripheral eye: A neurogenic area with potential to treat retinal pathologies? *Prog. Retin. Eye Res.* **2018**, *68*, 110–123. [CrossRef]
166. DiStefano, T.; Chen, H.Y.; Panebianco, C.; Kaya, K.D.; Brooks, M.J.; Gieser, L.; Morgan, N.Y.; Pohida, T.; Swaroop, A. Accelerated and Improved Differentiation of Retinal Organoids from Pluripotent Stem Cells in Rotating-Wall Vessel Bioreactors. *Stem Cell Rep.* **2018**, *10*, 300–313. [CrossRef]
167. Ovando-Roche, P.; West, E.L.; Branch, M.J.; Sampson, R.D.; Fernando, M.; Munro, P.; Georgiadis, A.; Rizzi, M.; Kloc, M.; Naeem, A.; et al. Use of bioreactors for culturing human retinal organoids improves photoreceptor yields. *Stem Cell Res. Ther.* **2018**, *9*, 1–14. [CrossRef]
168. Kaewkhaw, R.; Kaya, K.D.; Brooks, M.; Homma, K.; Zou, J.; Chaitankar, V.; Rao, M.; Swaroop, A. Transcriptome Dynamics of Developing Photoreceptors in Three-Dimensional Retina Cultures Recapitulates Temporal Sequence of Human Cone and Rod Differentiation Revealing Cell Surface Markers and Gene Networks. *Stem Cells* **2015**, *33*, 3504–3518. [CrossRef]
169. Reichman, S.; Slembrouck, A.; Gagliardi, G.; Chaffiol, A.; Terray, A.; Nanteau, C.; Potey, A.; Belle, M.; Rabesandratana, O.; Duebel, J.; et al. Generation of Storable Retinal Organoids and Retinal Pigmented Epithelium from Adherent Human iPS Cells in Xeno-Free and Feeder-Free Conditions. *Stem Cells* **2017**, *35*, 1176–1188. [CrossRef]
170. Wahlin, K.J.; Maruotti, J.A.; Sripathi, S.R.; Ball, J.; Angueyra, J.M.; Kim, C.; Grebe, R.; Li, W.; Jones, B.W.; Zack, D.J. Photoreceptor Outer Segment-like Structures in Long-Term 3D Retinas from Human Pluripotent Stem Cells. *Sci. Rep.* **2017**, *7*, 766. [CrossRef]
171. Gonzalez-Cordero, A.; Kruczek, K.; Naeem, A.; Fernando, M.; Kloc, M.; Ribeiro, J.; Goh, D.; Duran, Y.; Blackford, S.J.I.; Abelleira-Hervas, L.; et al. Recapitulation of Human Retinal Development from Human Pluripotent Stem Cells Generates Transplantable Populations of Cone Photoreceptors. *Stem Cell Rep.* **2017**, *9*, 820–837. [CrossRef]
172. Li, M.; Jia, C.; Kazmierkiewicz, K.L.; Bowman, A.S.; Tian, L.; Liu, Y.; Gupta, N.A.; Gudiseva, H.V.; Yee, S.S.; Kim, M.; et al. Comprehensive analysis of gene expression in human retina and supporting tissues. *Hum. Mol. Genet.* **2014**, *23*, 4001–4014. [CrossRef] [PubMed]
173. Marcucci, F.; Murcia-Belmonte, V.; Wang, Q.; Coca, Y.; Ferreiro-Galve, S.; Kuwajima, T.; Khalid, S.; Ross, M.E.; Mason, C.; Herrera, E. The Ciliary Margin Zone of the Mammalian Retina Generates Retinal Ganglion Cells. *Cell Rep.* **2016**, *17*, 3153–3164. [CrossRef] [PubMed]
174. Bélanger, M.-C.; Robert, B.; Cayouette, M. Msx1-Positive Progenitors in the Retinal Ciliary Margin Give Rise to Both Neural and Non-neural Progenies in Mammals. *Dev. Cell* **2017**, *40*, 137–150. [CrossRef]
175. Provis, J.M.; Hendrickson, A.E. The foveal avascular region of developing human retina. *Arch. Ophthalmol.* **2008**, *126*, 507–511. [CrossRef]
176. Yuodelis, C.; Hendrickson, A. A qualitative and quantitative analysis of the human fovea during development. *Vision Res.* **1986**, *26*, 847–855. [CrossRef]
177. Vajzovic, L.; Hendrickson, A.E.; O'Connell, R.V.; Clark, L.A.; Tran-Viet, D.; Possin, D.; Chiu, S.J.; Farsiu, S.; Toth, C.A. Maturation of the human fovea: Correlation of spectral-domain optical coherence tomography findings with histology. *Am. J. Ophthalmol.* **2012**, *154*, 779–789.e2. [CrossRef]
178. Deng, W.L.; Gao, M.L.; Lei, X.L.; Lv, J.N.; Zhao, H.; He, K.W.; Xia, X.X.; Li, L.Y.; Chen, Y.C.; Li, Y.P.; et al. Gene Correction Reverses Ciliopathy and Photoreceptor Loss in iPSC-Derived Retinal Organoids from Retinitis Pigmentosa Patients. *Stem Cell Rep.* **2018**, *10*, 1267–1281. [CrossRef]

179. Parfitt, D.A.; Lane, A.; Ramsden, C.M.; Carr, A.J.F.; Munro, P.M.; Jovanovic, K.; Schwarz, N.; Kanuga, N.; Muthiah, M.N.; Hull, S.; et al. Identification and Correction of Mechanisms Underlying Inherited Blindness in Human iPSC-Derived Optic Cups. *Cell Stem Cell* **2016**, *18*, 769–781. [CrossRef]
180. Simic, N.; Westall, C.; Astzalos, E.V.; Rovet, J. Visual abilities at 6 months in preterm infants: Impact of thyroid hormone deficiency and neonatal medical morbidity. *Thyroid* **2010**, *20*, 309–315. [CrossRef]
181. Duerksen, K.; Barlow, W.E.; Stasior, O.G. Fused eyelids in premature infants. *Ophthal. Plast. Reconstr. Surg.* **1994**, *10*, 234–240. [CrossRef]
182. Smyth, C.N. Exploratory methods for testing the integrity of the foetus and neonate. *BJOG Int. J. Obstet. Gynaecol.* **1965**, *72*, 920–925. [CrossRef]
183. Polishuk, W.Z.; Laufer, N.; Sadovsky, E. Fetal reaction to external light. *Harefuah* **1975**, *89*, 395–396. [PubMed]
184. Peleg, D.; Goldman, J.A. Fetal heart rate acceleration in response to light stimulation as a clinical measure of fetal well-being. A preliminary report. *J. Perinat. Med.* **1980**, *8*, 38–41. [PubMed]
185. Tatsumura, M. Studies on features of fetal movement and development of human fetus with use of fetal actogram. *Nihon Sanka Fujinka Gakkai Zasshi* **1991**, *43*, 864–873. [PubMed]
186. Kiuchi, M.; Nagata, N.; Ikeno, S.; Terakawa, N. The relationship between the response to external light stimulation and behavioral states in the human fetus: How it differs from vibroacoustic stimulation. *Early Hum. Dev.* **2000**, *58*, 153–165. [CrossRef]
187. Thanaboonyawat, I.; Wataganara, T.; Boriboonhiransarn, D.; Viboonchart, S.; Tontisirin, P. Effect of halogen light in fetal stimulation for fetal well-being assessment. *J. Med. Assoc. Thailand* **2006**, *89*, 1376–1380.
188. Eswaran, H.; Wilson, J.; Preissl, H.; Robinson, S.; Vrba, J.; Murphy, P.; Rose, D.; Lowery, C. Magnetoencephalographic recordings of visual evoked brain activity in the human fetus. *Lancet* **2002**, *360*, 779–780. [CrossRef]
189. Eswaran, H.; Lowery, C.L.; Wilson, J.D.; Murphy, P.; Preissl, H. Functional development of the visual system in human fetus using magnetoencephalography. *Exp. Neurol.* **2004**, *190*, S52–S58. [CrossRef]
190. McCubbin, J.; Murphy, P.; Eswaran, H.; Preissl, H.; Yee, T.; Robinson, S.E.; Vrba, J. Validation of the flash-evoked response from fetal MEG. *Phys. Med. Biol.* **2007**, *52*, 5803–5813. [CrossRef]
191. Matuz, T.; Govindan, R.B.; Preissl, H.; Siegel, E.R.; Muenssinger, J.; Murphy, P.; Ware, M.; Lowery, C.L.; Eswaran, H. Habituation of visual evoked responses in neonates and fetuses: A MEG study. *Dev. Cogn. Neurosci.* **2012**, *2*, 303–316. [CrossRef]
192. Fulford, J.; Vadeyar, S.H.; Dodampahala, S.H.; Moore, R.J.; Young, P.; Baker, P.N.; James, D.K.; Gowland, P.A. Fetal brain activity in response to a visual stimulus. *Hum. Brain Mapp.* **2003**, *20*, 239–245. [CrossRef] [PubMed]
193. Schwindt, E.; Giordano, V.; Rona, Z.; Czaba-Hnizdo, C.; Olischar, M.; Waldhoer, T.; Werther, T.; Fuiko, R.; Berger, A.; Klebermass-Schrehof, K. The impact of extrauterine life on visual maturation in extremely preterm born infants. *Pediatr. Res.* **2018**, *84*, 403–410. [CrossRef] [PubMed]
194. Taylor, M.J.; Menzies, R.; MacMillan, L.J.; Whyte, H.E. VEPs in normal full-term and premature neonates: Longitudinal versus cross-sectional data. *Electroencephalogr. Clin. Neurophysiol.* **1987**, *68*, 20–27. [CrossRef]
195. Tsuneishi, S.; Casaer, P. Effects of preterm extrauterine visual experience on the development of the human visual system: A flash VEP study. *Dev. Med. Child Neurol.* **2000**, *42*, 663–668. [CrossRef]
196. Leaf, A.A.; Green, C.R.; Escwk, A.; Costeloe, K.L.; Prior, P.F. Maturation of Electroretinograms and Visual Evoked Potentials in Preterm Infants. *Dev. Med. Child Neurol.* **1995**, *37*, 814–826. [CrossRef]
197. Mactier, H.; Dexter, J.D.; Hewett, J.E.; Latham, C.B.; Woodruff, C.W. The electroretinogram in preterm infants. *J. Pediatr.* **1988**, *113*, 607–612. [CrossRef]
198. Mets, M.B.; Smith, V.C.; Pokorny, J.; Pass, A. Postnatal retinal development as measured by the electroretinogram in premature infants. *Doc. Ophthalmol.* **1995**, *90*, 111–127. [CrossRef]
199. Mactier, H.; Hamilton, R.; Bradnam, M.S.; Turner, T.L.; Dudgeon, J. Contact lens electroretinography in preterm infants from 32 weeks after conception: A development in current methodology. *Arch. Dis. Child. Fetal Neonatal Ed.* **2000**, *82*, F233–F236. [CrossRef]
200. Fulton, A.B. The development of scotopic retinal function in human infants. *Doc. Ophthalmol.* **1988**, *69*, 101–109. [CrossRef]
201. Fulton, A.B.; Hansen, R.M. The development of scotopic sensitivity. *Investig. Ophthalmol. Vis. Sci.* **2000**, *41*, 1588–1596.

202. Altschwager, P.; Moskowitz, A.; Fulton, A.B.; Hansen, R.M. Multifocal erg responses in subjects with a history of preterm birth. *Investig. Ophthalmol. Vis. Sci.* **2017**, *58*, 2603–2608. [CrossRef] [PubMed]
203. Åkerblom, H.; Andreasson, S.; Larsson, E.; Holmström, G. Photoreceptor Function in School-Aged Children is Affected by Preterm Birth. *Transl. Vis. Sci. Technol.* **2014**, *3*, 7. [CrossRef] [PubMed]
204. Hansen, R.M.; Moskowitz, A.; Akula, J.D.; Fulton, A.B. The neural retina in retinopathy of prematurity. *Prog. Retin. Eye Res.* **2017**, *56*, 32–57. [CrossRef] [PubMed]
205. Lowe, A.; Harris, R.; Bhansali, P.; Cvekl, A.; Liu, W. Intercellular Adhesion-Dependent Cell Survival and ROCK-Regulated Actomyosin-Driven Forces Mediate Self-Formation of a Retinal Organoid. *Stem Cell Rep.* **2016**, *6*, 743–756. [CrossRef]
206. Quadrato, G.; Nguyen, T.; Macosko, E.Z.; Sherwood, J.L.; Min Yang, S.; Berger, D.R.; Maria, N.; Scholvin, J.; Goldman, M.; Kinney, J.P.; et al. Cell diversity and network dynamics in photosensitive human brain organoids. *Nature* **2017**, *545*, 48–53. [CrossRef]
207. Capowski, E.E.; Samimi, K.; Mayerl, S.J.; Phillips, M.J.; Pinilla, I.; Howden, S.E.; Saha, J.; Jansen, A.D.; Edwards, K.L.; Jager, L.D.; et al. Reproducibility and staging of 3D human retinal organoids across multiple pluripotent stem cell lines. *Development* **2019**, *146*, dev171686. [CrossRef]
208. Cowan, C.S.; Renner, M.; Gross-Scherf, B.; Goldblum, D.; Munz, M.; Krol, J.; Szikra, T.; Papasaikas, P.; Cuttat, R.; Waldt, A.; et al. Cell types of the human retina and its organoids at single-cell resolution: Developmental convergence, transcriptomic identity, and disease map. *bioRxiv* **2019**, 703348. [CrossRef]
209. Mellough, C.B.; Collin, J.; Queen, R.; Hilgen, G.; Dorgau, B.; Zerti, D.; Felemban, M.; White, K.; Sernagor, E.; Lako, M. Systematic Comparison of Retinal Organoid Differentiation from Human Pluripotent Stem Cells Reveals Stage Specific, Cell Line, and Methodological Differences. *Stem Cells Transl. Med.* **2019**, *8*, 694–706. [CrossRef]
210. Chichagova, V.; Hilgen, G.; Ghareeb, A.; Georgiou, M.; Carter, M.; Sernagor, E.; Lako, M.; Armstrong, L. Human iPSC differentiation to retinal organoids in response to IGF1 and BMP4 activation is line- and method-dependent. *Stem Cells* **2019**. [CrossRef]
211. Zerti, D.; Dorgau, B.; Felemban, M.; Ghareeb, A.E.; Yu, M.; Ding, Y.; Krasnogor, N.; Lako, M. Developing a simple method to enhance the generation of cone and rod photoreceptors in pluripotent stem cell-derived retinal organoids. *Stem Cells* **2019**, *50*, e95. [CrossRef]
212. Brooks, M.J.; Chen, H.Y.; Kelley, R.A.; Mondal, A.K.; Nagashima, K.; De Val, N.; Li, T.; Chaitankar, V.; Swaroop, A. Improved Retinal Organoid Differentiation by Modulating Signaling Pathways Revealed by Comparative Transcriptome Analyses with Development In Vivo. *Stem Cell Rep.* **2019**, *10*, 1–15. [CrossRef] [PubMed]
213. Kaya, K.D.; Chen, H.Y.; Brooks, M.J.; Kelley, R.A.; Shimada, H.; Nagashima, K.; de Val, N.; Drinnan, C.T.; Gieser, L.; Kruczek, K.; et al. Transcriptome-based molecular staging of human stem cell-derived retinal organoids uncovers accelerated photoreceptor differentiation by 9-cis retinal. *bioRxiv* **2019**, 733071. [CrossRef]
214. Achberger, K.; Haderspeck, J.C.; Kleger, A.; Liebau, S. Stem cell-based retina models. *Adv. Drug Deliv. Rev.* **2018**, *140*, 33–50. [CrossRef] [PubMed]
215. Achberger, K.; Probst, C.; Haderspeck, J.; Bolz, S.; Rogal, J.; Chuchuy, J.; Nikolova, M.; Cora, V.; Antkowiak, L.; Haq, W.; et al. Merging organoid and organ-on-a-chip technology to generate complex multi-layer tissue models in a human Retina-on-a-Chip platform. *Elife* **2019**, *8*. [CrossRef] [PubMed]
216. Iraha, S.; Tu, H.Y.; Yamasaki, S.; Kagawa, T.; Goto, M.; Takahashi, R.; Watanabe, T.; Sugita, S.; Yonemura, S.; Sunagawa, G.A.; et al. Establishment of Immunodeficient Retinal Degeneration Model Mice and Functional Maturation of Human ESC-Derived Retinal Sheets after Transplantation. *Stem Cell Rep.* **2018**, *10*, 1059–1074. [CrossRef]
217. Gagliardi, G.; Ben M'Barek, K.; Chaffiol, A.; Slembrouck-Brec, A.; Conart, J.B.; Nanteau, C.; Rabesandratana, O.; Sahel, J.A.; Duebel, J.; Orieux, G.; et al. Characterization and Transplantation of CD73-Positive Photoreceptors Isolated from Human iPSC-Derived Retinal Organoids. *Stem Cell Rep.* **2018**, *11*, 665–680. [CrossRef]
218. McLelland, B.T.; Lin, B.; Mathur, A.; Aramant, R.B.; Thomas, B.B.; Nistor, G.; Keirstead, H.S.; Seiler, M.J. Transplanted hESC-derived retina organoid sheets differentiate, integrate, and improve visual function in retinal degenerate rats. *Investig. Ophthalmol. Vis. Sci.* **2018**, *59*, 2586–2603. [CrossRef]
219. Pearson, R.A.; Gonzalez-Cordero, A.; West, E.L.; Ribeiro, J.R.; Aghaizu, N.; Goh, D.; Sampson, R.D.; Georgiadis, A.; Waldron, P.V.; Duran, Y.; et al. Donor and host photoreceptors engage in material transfer following transplantation of post-mitotic photoreceptor precursors. *Nat. Commun.* **2016**, *7*, 13029. [CrossRef]

220. Singh, M.S.; Balmer, J.; Barnard, A.R.; Aslam, S.A.; Moralli, D.; Green, C.M.; Barnea-Cramer, A.; Duncan, I.; MacLaren, R.E. Transplanted photoreceptor precursors transfer proteins to host photoreceptors by a mechanism of cytoplasmic fusion. *Nat. Commun.* **2016**, *7*, 13537. [CrossRef]
221. Santos-Ferreira, T.; Llonch, S.; Borsch, O.; Postel, K.; Haas, J.; Ader, M. Retinal transplantation of photoreceptors results in donor-host cytoplasmic exchange. *Nat. Commun.* **2016**, *7*, 13028. [CrossRef]
222. Garita-Hernandez, M.; Lampic, M.; Chaffiol, A.; Guibbal, L.; Routet, F.; Santos-Ferreira, T.; Gagliardi, G.; Reichman, S.; Picaud, S.; Sahel, J.-A.; et al. Restoration of visual function by transplantation of optogenetically engineered photoreceptors. *bioRxiv* **2018**, 399725. [CrossRef] [PubMed]
223. Hoek, R.M.; Quinn, P.M.; Hooibrink, B.; Wijnholds, J. Transplantation of NTPDase2-positive Sorted Müller Glial Cells into the Mouse Retina. *J. Neurosci. Neurosurg.* **2018**, *1*. [CrossRef]
224. Hoek, R.M.; Quinn, P.M.; Alves, C.H.; Hooibrink, B.; Wijnholds, J. NTPDase2 as a Surface Marker to Isolate Flow Cytometrically a Müller Glial Cell Enriched Population from Dissociated Neural Retinae. *J. Neurosci. Neurosurg.* **2018**, *1*. [CrossRef]
225. Santos-Ferreira, T.F.; Borsch, O.; Ader, M. Rebuilding the Missing Part—A Review on Photoreceptor Transplantation. *Front. Syst. Neurosci.* **2017**, *10*, 1–14. [CrossRef] [PubMed]
226. Chen, J.; Sayadian, A.-C.; Lowe, N.; Lovegrove, H.E.; St Johnston, D. An alternative mode of epithelial polarity in the Drosophila midgut. *PLoS Biol.* **2018**, *16*, e3000041. [CrossRef] [PubMed]
227. Tree, D.R.P.; Ma, D.; Axelrod, J.D. A three-tiered mechanism for regulation of planar cell polarity. *Semin. Cell Dev. Biol.* **2002**, *13*, 217–224. [CrossRef]
228. Varelas, X.; Samavarchi-Tehrani, P.; Narimatsu, M.; Weiss, A.; Cockburn, K.; Larsen, B.G.; Rossant, J.; Wrana, J.L. The Crumbs complex couples cell density sensing to Hippo-dependent control of the TGF-β-SMAD pathway. *Dev. Cell* **2010**, *19*, 831–844. [CrossRef] [PubMed]
229. Tepass, U.; Theres, C.; Knust, E. crumbs Encodes an EGFlike Protein Expressed on Apical Membranes of Drosophila Epithelial Cells and Required for Organization of Epithelia. *Cell* **1990**, *61*, 787–799. [CrossRef]
230. Alves, C.H.; Bossers, K.; Vos, R.M.; Essing, A.H.W.; Swagemakers, S.; van der Spek, P.J.; Verhaagen, J.; Wijnholds, J. Microarray and Morphological Analysis of Early Postnatal CRB2 Mutant Retinas on a Pure C57BL/6J Genetic Background. *PLoS ONE* **2013**, *8*, e82532. [CrossRef]
231. Park, B.; Alves, C.H.; Lundvig, D.M.; Tanimoto, N.; Beck, S.C.; Huber, G.; Richard, F.; Klooster, J.; Andlauer, T.F.M.; Swindell, E.C.; et al. PALS1 is essential for retinal pigment epithelium structure and neural retina stratification. *J. Neurosci.* **2011**, *31*, 17230–17241. [CrossRef]
232. Alves, C.H.; Sanz, A.S.; Park, B.; Pellissier, L.P.; Tanimoto, N.; Beck, S.C.; Huber, G.; Murtaza, M.; Richard, F.; Sridevi Gurubaran, I.; et al. Loss of CRB2 in the mouse retina mimics human retinitis pigmentosa due to mutations in the CRB1 gene. *Hum. Mol. Genet.* **2013**, *22*, 35–50. [CrossRef]
233. Dudok, J.J.; Sanz, A.S.; Lundvig, D.M.S.; Sothilingam, V.; Garrido, M.G.; Klooster, J.; Seeliger, M.W.; Wijnholds, J. MPP3 regulates levels of PALS1 and adhesion between photoreceptors and Müller cells. *Glia* **2013**, *61*, 1629–1644. [CrossRef] [PubMed]
234. Richardson, E.C.N.; Pichaud, F. Crumbs is required to achieve proper organ size control during Drosophila head development. *Development* **2010**, *137*, 641–650. [CrossRef]
235. Alves, C.H.; Pellissier, L.P.; Wijnholds, J. The CRB1 and adherens junction complex proteins in retinal development and maintenance. *Prog. Retin. Eye Res.* **2014**, *40*, 35–52. [CrossRef]
236. Bulgakova, N.A.; Knust, E. The Crumbs complex: From epithelial-cell polarity to retinal degeneration. *J. Cell Sci.* **2009**, *122*, 2587–2596. [CrossRef]
237. Fan, S.; Fogg, V.; Wang, Q.; Chen, X.-W.; Liu, C.-J.; Margolis, B. A novel Crumbs3 isoform regulates cell division and ciliogenesis via importin beta interactions. *J. Cell Biol.* **2007**, *178*, 387–398. [CrossRef]
238. Bazellières, E.; Aksenova, V.; Barthélémy-Requin, M.; Massey-Harroche, D.; Le Bivic, A. Role of the Crumbs proteins in ciliogenesis, cell migration and actin organization. *Semin. Cell Dev. Biol.* **2018**, *81*, 13–20. [CrossRef]
239. Lee, J.D.; Silva-Gagliardi, N.F.; Tepass, U.; McGlade, C.J.; Anderson, K.V. The FERM protein Epb4.1l5 is required for organization of the neural plate and for the epithelial-mesenchymal transition at the primitive streak of the mouse embryo. *Development* **2007**, *134*, 2007–2016. [CrossRef]
240. Hirano, M.; Hashimoto, S.; Yonemura, S.; Sabe, H.; Aizawa, S. EPB41L5 functions to post-transcriptionally regulate cadherin and integrin during epithelial-mesenchymal transition. *J. Cell Biol.* **2008**, *182*, 1217–1230. [CrossRef]

241. Christensen, A.K.; Jensen, A.M. Tissue-specific requirements for specific domains in the FERM protein Moe/Epb4.1l5 during early zebrafish development. *BMC Dev. Biol.* **2008**, *8*, 3. [CrossRef]
242. Gosens, I.; Sessa, A.; den Hollander, A.I.; Letteboer, S.J.F.; Belloni, V.; Arends, M.L.; Le Bivic, A.; Cremers, F.P.M.; Broccoli, V.; Roepman, R. FERM protein EPB41L5 is a novel member of the mammalian CRB-MPP5 polarity complex. *Exp. Cell Res.* **2007**, *313*, 3959–3970. [CrossRef] [PubMed]
243. Laprise, P.; Beronja, S.; Silva-Gagliardi, N.F.; Pellikka, M.; Jensen, A.M.; McGlade, C.J.; Tepass, U. The FERM protein Yurt is a negative regulatory component of the Crumbs complex that controls epithelial polarity and apical membrane size. *Dev. Cell* **2006**, *11*, 363–374. [CrossRef] [PubMed]
244. Gamblin, C.L.; Parent-Prévost, F.; Jacquet, K.; Biehler, C.; Jetté, A.; Laprise, P. Oligomerization of the FERM-FA protein Yurt controls epithelial cell polarity. *J. Cell Biol.* **2018**, *217*, 3853. [CrossRef] [PubMed]
245. Schell, C.; Rogg, M.; Suhm, M.; Helmstädter, M.; Sellung, D.; Yasuda-Yamahara, M.; Kretz, O.; Küttner, V.; Suleiman, H.; Kollipara, L.; et al. The FERM protein EPB41L5 regulates actomyosin contractility and focal adhesion formation to maintain the kidney filtration barrier. *Proc. Natl. Acad. Sci. USA* **2017**, *114*, E4621–E4630. [CrossRef] [PubMed]
246. Gamblin, C.L.; Hardy, É.J.-L.; Chartier, F.J.-M.; Bisson, N.; Laprise, P. A bidirectional antagonism between aPKC and Yurt regulates epithelial cell polarity. *J. Cell Biol.* **2014**, *204*, 487–495. [CrossRef] [PubMed]
247. Bachmann, A.; Schneider, M.; Theilenberg, E.; Grawe, F.; Knust, E. Drosophila Stardust is a partner of Crumbs in the control of epithelial cell polarity. *Nature* **2001**, *414*, 638–643. [CrossRef]
248. Lemmers, C.; Michel, D.; Lane-Guermonprez, L.; Delgrossi, M.-H.; Médina, E.; Arsanto, J.-P.; Le Bivic, A. CRB3 binds directly to Par6 and regulates the morphogenesis of the tight junctions in mammalian epithelial cells. *Mol. Biol. Cell* **2004**, *15*, 1324–1333. [CrossRef]
249. Roh, M.H.; Fan, S.; Liu, C.-J.; Margolis, B. The Crumbs3-Pals1 complex participates in the establishment of polarity in mammalian epithelial cells. *J. Cell Sci.* **2003**, *116*, 2895–2906. [CrossRef]
250. Roh, M.H.; Makarova, O.; Liu, C.-J.; Shin, K.; Lee, S.; Laurinec, S.; Goyal, M.; Wiggins, R.; Margolis, B. The Maguk protein, Pals1, functions as an adapter, linking mammalian homologues of Crumbs and Discs Lost. *J. Cell Biol.* **2002**, *157*, 161–172. [CrossRef]
251. Kantardzhieva, A.; Alexeeva, S.; Versteeg, I.; Wijnholds, J. MPP3 is recruited to the MPP5 protein scaffold at the retinal outer limiting membrane. *FEBS J.* **2006**, *273*, 1152–1165. [CrossRef]
252. Kantardzhieva, A.; Gosens, I.; Alexeeva, S.; Punte, I.M.; Versteeg, I.; Krieger, E.; Neefjes-Mol, C.A.; den Hollander, A.I.; Letteboer, S.J.F.; Klooster, J.; et al. MPP5 recruits MPP4 to the CRB1 complex in photoreceptors. *Investig. Ophthalmol. Vis. Sci.* **2005**, *46*, 2192–2201. [CrossRef] [PubMed]
253. Suzuki, A.; Yamanaka, T.; Hirose, T.; Manabe, N.; Mizuno, K.; Shimizu, M.; Akimoto, K.; Izumi, Y.; Ohnishi, T.; Ohno, S. Atypical protein kinase C is involved in the evolutionarily conserved PAR protein complex and plays a critical role in establishing epithelia-specific junctional structures. *J. Cell Biol.* **2001**, *152*, 1183–1196. [CrossRef]
254. Suzuki, A.; Akimoto, K.; Ohno, S. Protein kinase C λ/ι (PKCλ/ι: A PKC isotype essential for the development of multicellular organisms. *J. Biochem.* **2003**, *133*, 9–16. [CrossRef] [PubMed]
255. Joberty, G.; Petersen, C.; Gao, L.; Macara, I.G. The cell-polarity protein Par6 links Par3 and atypical protein kinase C to Cdc42. *Nat. Cell Biol.* **2000**, *2*, 531–539. [CrossRef] [PubMed]
256. Lin, D.; Edwards, A.S.; Fawcett, J.P.; Mbamalu, G.; Scott, J.D.; Pawson, T. A mammalian PAR-3-PAR-6 complex implicated in Cdc42/Rac1 and aPKC signalling and cell polarity. *Nat. Cell Biol.* **2000**, *2*, 540–547. [CrossRef] [PubMed]
257. Yamanaka, T.; Horikoshi, Y.; Suzuki, A.; Sugiyama, Y.; Kitamura, K.; Maniwa, R.; Nagai, Y.; Yamashita, A.; Hirose, T.; Ishikawa, H.; et al. PAR-6 regulates aPKC activity in a novel way and mediates cell-cell contact-induces formation of the epithelial junctional complex. *Genes Cells* **2001**, *6*, 721–731. [CrossRef]
258. Atwood, S.X.; Chabu, C.; Penkert, R.R.; Doe, C.Q.; Prehoda, K.E. Cdc42 acts downstream of Bazooka to regulate neuroblast polarity through Par-6 aPKC. *J. Cell Sci.* **2007**, *120*, 3200–3206. [CrossRef]
259. Graybill, C.; Wee, B.; Atwood, S.X.; Prehoda, K.E. Partitioning-defective protein 6 (Par-6) activates atypical protein kinase C (aPKC) by pseudosubstrate displacement. *J. Biol. Chem.* **2012**, *287*, 21003–21011. [CrossRef]
260. Ikenouchi, J.; Umeda, M. FRMD4A regulates epithelial polarity by connecting Arf6 activation with the PAR complex. *Proc. Natl. Acad. Sci. USA* **2010**, *107*, 748–753. [CrossRef]

261. Klarlund, J.K.; Holik, J.; Chawla, A.; Park, J.G.; Buxton, J.; Czech, M.P. Signaling complexes of the FERM domain-containing protein GRSP1 bound to ARF exchange factor GRP1. *J. Biol. Chem.* **2001**, *276*, 40065–40070. [CrossRef]
262. Kong, Y.; Zhao, L.; Charette, J.R.; Hicks, W.L.; Stone, L.; Nishina, P.M.; Naggert, J.K. An FRMD4B variant suppresses dysplastic photoreceptor lesions in models of enhanced S-cone syndrome and of Nrl deficiency. *Hum. Mol. Genet.* **2018**, *27*, 3340–3352. [CrossRef] [PubMed]
263. Aguilar-Aragon, M.; Elbediwy, A.; Foglizzo, V.; Fletcher, G.C.; Li, V.S.W.; Thompson, B.J. Pak1 Kinase Maintains Apical Membrane Identity in Epithelia. *Cell Rep.* **2018**, *22*, 1639–1646. [CrossRef]
264. Belmonte, M.A.; Santos, M.F.; Kihara, A.H.; Yan, C.Y.I.; Hamassaki, D.E. Light-Induced photoreceptor degeneration in the mouse involves activation of the small GTPase Rac1. *Investig. Ophthalmol. Vis. Sci.* **2006**, *47*, 1193–1200. [CrossRef] [PubMed]
265. Hurd, T.W.; Gao, L.; Roh, M.H.; Macara, I.G.; Margolis, B. Direct interaction of two polarity complexes implicated in epithelial tight junction assembly. *Nat. Cell Biol.* **2003**, *5*, 137–142. [CrossRef]
266. Koike, C.; Nishida, A.; Akimoto, K.; Nakaya, M.; Noda, T.; Ohno, S.; Furukawa, T. Function of atypical protein kinase C lambda in differentiating photoreceptors is required for proper lamination of mouse retina. *J. Neurosci.* **2005**, *25*, 10290–10298. [CrossRef]
267. Heynen, S.R.; Tanimoto, N.; Joly, S.; Seeliger, M.W.; Samardzija, M.; Grimm, C. Retinal degeneration modulates intracellular localization of CDC42 in photoreceptors. *Mol. Vis.* **2011**, *17*, 2934–2946.
268. Santos-Bredariol, A.S.; Santos, M.F.; Hamassaki-Britto, D.E. Distribution of the small molecular weight GTP-binding proteins Rac1, CdC42, RhoA and RhoB in the developing chick retina. *J. Neurocytol.* **2002**, *31*, 149–159. [CrossRef]
269. den Hollander, A.I.; Ghiani, M.; de Kok, Y.J.M.; Wijnholds, J.; Ballabio, A.; Cremers, F.P.M.; Broccoli, V. Isolation of Crb1, a mouse homologue of Drosophila crumbs, and analysis of its expression pattern in eye and brain. *Mech. Dev.* **2002**, *110*, 203–207. [CrossRef]
270. Pellissier, L.P.; Lundvig, D.M.S.; Tanimoto, N.; Klooster, J.; Vos, R.M.; Richard, F.; Sothilingam, V.; Garcia Garrido, M.; Le Bivic, A.; Seeliger, M.W.; et al. CRB2 acts as a modifying factor of CRB1-related retinal dystrophies in mice. *Hum. Mol. Genet.* **2014**, *23*, 3759–3771. [CrossRef]
271. van Rossum, A.G.S.H.; Aartsen, W.M.; Meuleman, J.; Klooster, J.; Malysheva, A.; Versteeg, I.; Arsanto, J.-P.; Le Bivic, A.; Wijnholds, J. Pals1/Mpp5 is required for correct localization of Crb1 at the subapical region in polarized Muller glia cells. *Hum. Mol. Genet.* **2006**, *15*, 2659–2672. [CrossRef]
272. Pellissier, L.P.; Quinn, P.M.; Alves, C.H.; Vos, R.M.; Klooster, J.; Flannery, J.G.; Heimel, J.A.; Wijnholds, J. Gene therapy into photoreceptors and Müller glial cells restores retinal structure and function in CRB1 retinitis pigmentosa mouse models. *Hum. Mol. Genet.* **2015**, *24*, 3104–3118. [CrossRef]
273. Herranz-Martín, S.; Jimeno, D.; Paniagua, A.E.; Velasco, A.; Lara, J.M.; Aijón, J.; Lillo, C. Immunocytochemical evidence of the localization of the Crumbs homologue 3 protein (CRB3) in the developing and mature mouse retina. *PLoS ONE* **2012**, *7*, e50511. [CrossRef] [PubMed]
274. Hughes, J.M.; Groot, A.J.; Van Der Groep, P.; Sersansie, R.; Vooijs, M.; Van Diest, P.J.; Van Noorden, C.J.F.; Schlingemann, R.O.; Klaassen, I. Active HIF-1 in the normal human retina. *J. Histochem. Cytochem.* **2010**, *58*, 247–254. [CrossRef]
275. Cabral, T.; Toral, M.A.; Velez, G.; DiCarlo, J.E.; Gore, A.M.; Mahajan, M.; Tsang, S.H.; Bassuk, A.G.; Mahajan, V.B. Dissection of Human Retina and RPE-Choroid for Proteomic Analysis. *J. Vis. Exp.* **2017**, 1–5. [CrossRef]
276. Paniagua, A.E.; Herranz-Martín, S.; Jimeno, D.; Jimeno, Á.M.; López-Benito, S.; Carlos Arévalo, J.; Velasco, A.; Aijón, J.; Lillo, C. CRB2 completes a fully expressed Crumbs complex in the Retinal Pigment Epithelium. *Sci. Rep.* **2015**, *5*, 14504. [CrossRef]
277. Vallespin, E.; Cantalapiedra, D.; Riveiro-Alvarez, R.; Wilke, R.; Aguirre-Lamban, J.; Avila-Fernandez, A.; Lopez-Martinez, M.A.; Gimenez, A.; Trujillo-Tiebas, M.J.; Ramos, C.; et al. Mutation screening of 299 Spanish families with retinal dystrophies by Leber congenital amaurosis genotyping microarray. *Investig. Ophthalmol. Vis. Sci.* **2007**, *48*, 5653–5661. [CrossRef]
278. Corton, M.; Tatu, S.D.; Avila-Fernandez, A.; Vallespín, E.; Tapias, I.; Cantalapiedra, D.; Blanco-Kelly, F.; Riveiro-Alvarez, R.; Bernal, S.; García-Sandoval, B.; et al. High frequency of CRB1 mutations as cause of Early-Onset Retinal Dystrophies in the Spanish population. *Orphanet J. Rare Dis.* **2013**, *8*, 20. [CrossRef]

279. Henderson, R.H.; Mackay, D.S.; Li, Z.; Moradi, P.; Sergouniotis, P.; Russell-Eggitt, I.; Thompson, D.A.; Robson, A.G.; Holder, G.E.; Webster, A.R.; et al. Phenotypic variability in patients with retinal dystrophies due to mutations in CRB1. *Br. J. Ophthalmol.* **2011**, *95*, 811–817. [CrossRef]

280. Mathijssen, I.B.; Florijn, R.J.; van den Born, L.I.; Zekveld-Vroon, R.C.; Ten Brink, J.B.; Plomp, A.S.; Baas, F.; Meijers-Heijboer, H.; Bergen, A.A.; van Schooneveld, M.J. Long-term follow-up of patients with retinitis pigmentosa type 12 caused by CRB1 mutations: A severe phenotype with considerable interindividual variability. *Retina* **2017**, *37*, 161–172. [CrossRef]

281. den Hollander, A.I.; Roepman, R.; Koenekoop, R.K.; Cremers, F.P.M. Leber congenital amaurosis: Genes, proteins and disease mechanisms. *Prog. Retin. Eye Res.* **2008**, *27*, 391–419. [CrossRef]

282. Hasan, S.M.; Azmeh, A.; Mostafa, O.; Megarbane, A. Coat's like vasculopathy in leber congenital amaurosis secondary to homozygous mutations in CRB1: A case report and discussion of the management options. *BMC Res. Notes* **2016**, *9*, 91. [CrossRef] [PubMed]

283. Leber, T. Ueber Retinitis pigmentosa und angeborene Amaurose. *Albr. Von Graefes Arch. Klin Exp. Ophthalmol.* **1869**, *15*, 1–25. [CrossRef]

284. Franceschetti, A.; Dieterle, P. Diagnostic and prognostic importance of the electroretinogram in tapetoretinal degeneration with reduction of the visual field and hemeralopia. *Confin. Neurol.* **1954**, *14*, 184–186. (In French) [CrossRef]

285. Jacobson, S.G.; Cideciyan, A.V.; Aleman, T.S.; Pianta, M.J.; Sumaroka, A.; Schwartz, S.B.; Smilko, E.E.; Milam, A.H.; Sheffield, V.C.; Stone, E.M. Crumbs homolog 1 (CRB1) mutations result in a thick human retina with abnormal lamination. *Hum. Mol. Genet.* **2003**, *12*, 1073–1078. [CrossRef]

286. Richard, M.; Roepman, R.; Aartsen, W.M.; van Rossum, A.G.S.H.; den Hollander, A.I.; Knust, E.; Wijnholds, J.; Cremers, F.P.M. Towards understanding CRUMBS function in retinal dystrophies. *Hum. Mol. Genet.* **2006**, *15*, 235–243. [CrossRef]

287. Aleman, T.S.; Cideciyan, A.V.; Aguirre, G.K.; Huang, W.C.; Mullins, C.L.; Roman, A.J.; Sumaroka, A.; Olivares, M.B.; Tsai, F.F.; Schwartz, S.B.; et al. Human CRB1-associated retinal degeneration: Comparison with the rd8 Crb1-mutant mouse model. *Investig. Ophthalmol. Vis. Sci.* **2011**, *52*, 6898–6910. [CrossRef]

288. McKay, G.J.; Clarke, S.; Davis, J.A.; Simpson, D.A.C.; Silvestri, G. Pigmented paravenous chorioretinal atrophy is associated with a mutation within the crumbs homolog 1 (CRB1) gene. *Investig. Ophthalmol. Vis. Sci.* **2005**, *46*, 322–328. [CrossRef]

289. Simonelli, F.; Ziviello, C.; Testa, F.; Rossi, S.; Fazzi, E.; Bianchi, P.E.; Fossarello, M.; Signorini, S.; Bertone, C.; Galantuomo, S.; et al. Clinical and Molecular Genetics of Leber's Congenital Amaurosis: A Multicenter Study of Italian Patients. *Investig. Opthalmology Vis. Sci.* **2007**, *48*, 4284–4290. [CrossRef]

290. den Hollander, A.I.; ten Brink, J.B.; de Kok, Y.J.; van Soest, S.; van den Born, L.I.; van Driel, M.A.; van de Pol, D.J.; Payne, A.M.; Bhattacharya, S.S.; Kellner, U.; et al. Mutations in a human homologue of Drosophila crumbs cause retinitis pigmentosa (RP12). *Nat. Genet.* **1999**, *23*, 217–221. [CrossRef]

291. Heckenlively, J.R. Preserved para-arteriole retinal pigment epithelium (PPRPE) in retinitis pigmentosa. *Br. J. Ophthalmol.* **1982**, *66*, 26–30. [CrossRef]

292. Talib, M.; Schooneveld, V.M.J.; Genderen, V.M.M.; Wijnholds, J.; Florijn, R.J.; ten Brink, J.B.; Al, E. Genotypic and phenotypic characteristics of CRB1-associated retinal dystrophies: A long-term follow-up study. *Ophthalmology* **2017**, *124*, 884–895. [CrossRef]

293. Tsang, S.H.; Burke, T.; Oll, M.; Yzer, S.; Lee, W.; Xie, Y.A.; Allikmets, R. Whole exome sequencing identifies CRB1 defect in an unusual maculopathy phenotype. *Ophthalmology* **2014**, *121*, 1773–1782. [CrossRef]

294. Tosi, J.; Tsui, I.; Lima, L.H.; Wang, N.-K.; Tsang, S.H. Case report: Autofluorescence imaging and phenotypic variance in a sibling pair with early-onset retinal dystrophy due to defective CRB1 function. *Curr. Eye Res.* **2009**, *34*, 395–400. [CrossRef]

295. Tsang, S.H.; Sharma, T. Leber Congenital Amaurosis. *Adv. Exp. Med. Biol.* **2018**, *1085*, 131–137.

296. Vincent, A.; Ng, J.; Gerth-Kahlert, C.; Tavares, E.; Maynes, J.T.; Wright, T.; Tiwari, A.; Tumber, A.; Li, S.; Hanson, J.V.M.; et al. Biallelic Mutations in CRB1 Underlie Autosomal Recessive Familial Foveal Retinoschisis. *Investig. Opthalmol. Vis. Sci.* **2016**, *57*, 2637–2646. [CrossRef]

297. den Hollander, A.I.; Heckenlively, J.R.; van den Born, L.I.; de Kok, Y.J.M.; van der Velde-Visser, S.D.; Kellner, U.; Jurklies, B.; van Schooneveld, M.J.; Blankenagel, A.; Rohrschneider, K.; et al. Leber congenital amaurosis and retinitis pigmentosa with Coats-like exudative vasculopathy are associated with mutations in the crumbs homologue 1 (CRB1) gene. *Am. J. Hum. Genet.* **2001**, *69*, 198–203. [CrossRef]

298. Quinn, P.M.; Alves, C.H.; Klooster, J.; Wijnholds, J. CRB2 in immature photoreceptors determines the superior-inferior symmetry of the developing retina to maintain retinal structure and function. *Hum. Mol. Genet.* **2018**, *27*, 3137–3153. [CrossRef]
299. Pellissier, L.P.; Alves, C.H.; Quinn, P.M.; Vos, R.M.; Tanimoto, N.; Lundvig, D.M.S.; Dudok, J.J.; Hooibrink, B.; Richard, F.; Beck, S.C.; et al. Targeted ablation of CRB1 and CRB2 in retinal progenitor cells mimics Leber congenital amaurosis. *PLoS Genet.* **2013**, *9*, e1003976. [CrossRef]
300. Yzer, S.; Fishman, G.A.; Racine, J.; Al-Zuhaibi, S.; Chakor, H.; Dorfman, A.; Szlyk, J.; Lachapelle, P.; Van Den Born, L.I.; Allikmets, R.; et al. CRB1 heterozygotes with regional retinal dysfunction: Implications for genetic testing of leber congenital amaurosis. *Investig. Ophthalmol. Vis. Sci.* **2006**, *47*, 3736–3744. [CrossRef]
301. Khan, K.N.; Robson, A.; Mahroo, O.A.R.; Arno, G.; Inglehearn, C.F.; Armengol, M.; Waseem, N.; Holder, G.E.; Carss, K.J.; Raymond, L.F.; et al. A clinical and molecular characterisation of CRB1-associated maculopathy. *Eur. J. Hum. Genet.* **2018**, *26*, 687–694. [CrossRef]
302. Chen, X.; Jiang, C.; Yang, D.; Sun, R.; Wang, M.; Sun, H.; Xu, M.; Zhou, L.; Chen, M.; Xie, P.; et al. CRB2 mutation causes autosomal recessive retinitis pigmentosa. *Exp. Eye Res.* **2018**, *180*, 164–173. [CrossRef] [PubMed]
303. Ray, T.A.; Cochran, K.; Kay, J.N. Single molecule sequencing elucidates retinal mRNA isoform diversity—Implications for CRB1 retinopathies. *Investig. Ophthalmol. Vis. Sci.* **2018**, *59*, 2531.
304. Alves, C.H.; Boon, N.; Mulder, A.A.; Koster, A.J.; Jost, C.R.; Wijnholds, J. CRB2 loss in rod photoreceptors is associated with progressive loss of retinal contrast sensitivity. *Int. J. Mol. Sci.* **2019**, *20*, 4069. [CrossRef]
305. Yuge, K.; Nakajima, M.; Uemura, Y.; Miki, H.; Uyama, M.; Tsubura, A. Immunohistochemical features of the human retina and retinoblastoma. *Virchows Arch* **1995**, *426*, 571–575. [CrossRef] [PubMed]
306. Tulvatana, W.; Adamian, M.; Berson, E.L.; Dryja, T.P. Photoreceptor rosettes in autosomal dominant retinitis pigmentosa with reduced penetrance. *Arch. Ophthalmol.* **1999**, *117*, 399–402. [CrossRef]
307. Lahav, M.; Albert, D.M.; Craft, J.L. Light and electron microscopic study of dysplastic rosette-like structures occurring in the disorganized mature retina. *Albr. Von Graefes Arch. Klin. Exp. Ophthalmol.* **1975**, *195*, 57–68. [CrossRef]
308. Rich, K.A.; Figueroa, S.L.; Zhan, Y.; Blanks, J.C. Effects of müller cell disruption on mouse photoreceptor cell development. *Exp. Eye Res.* **1995**, *61*, 235–248. [CrossRef]
309. West, E.L.; Pearson, R.A.; Tschernutter, M.; Sowden, J.C.; MacLaren, R.E.; Ali, R.R. Pharmacological disruption of the outer limiting membrane leads to increased retinal integration of transplanted photoreceptor precursors. *Exp. Eye Res.* **2008**, *86*, 601–611. [CrossRef]
310. Stuck, M.W.; Conley, S.M.; Naash, M.I. Defects in the outer limiting membrane are associated with rosette development in the Nrl$^{-/-}$ retina. *PLoS ONE* **2012**, *7*, e32484. [CrossRef]
311. Damiani, D.; Alexander, J.J.; O'Rourke, J.R.; McManus, M.; Jadhav, A.P.; Cepko, C.L.; Hauswirth, W.W.; Harfe, B.D.; Strettoi, E. Dicer Inactivation Leads to Progressive Functional and Structural Degeneration of the Mouse Retina. *J. Neurosci.* **2008**, *28*, 4878–4887. [CrossRef]
312. Mehalow, A.K.; Kameya, S.; Smith, R.S.; Hawes, N.L.; Denegre, J.M.; Young, J.A.; Bechtold, L.; Haider, N.B.; Tepass, U.; Heckenlively, J.R.; et al. CRB1 is essential for external limiting membrane integrity and photoreceptor morphogenesis in the mammalian retina. *Hum. Mol. Genet.* **2003**, *12*, 2179–2189. [CrossRef] [PubMed]
313. Krol, J.; Krol, I.; Alvarez, C.P.P.; Fiscella, M.; Hierlemann, A.; Roska, B.; Filipowicz, W. A network comprising short and long noncoding RNAs and RNA helicase controls mouse retina architecture. *Nat. Commun.* **2015**, *6*, 7305. [CrossRef]
314. Serjanov, D.; Bachay, G.; Hunter, D.D.; Brunken, W.J. Laminin β2 Chain Regulates Retinal Progenitor Cell Mitotic Spindle Orientation via Dystroglycan. *J. Neurosci.* **2018**, *38*, 5996–6010. [CrossRef] [PubMed]
315. Li, M.; Sakaguchi, D.S. Inhibition of integrin-mediated adhesion and signaling disrupts retinal development. *Dev. Biol.* **2004**, *275*, 202–214. [CrossRef]
316. Lunardi, A.; Cremisi, F.; Dente, L. Dystroglycan is required for proper retinal layering. *Dev. Biol.* **2006**, *290*, 411–420. [CrossRef]
317. Ouchi, Y.; Baba, Y.; Koso, H.; Taketo, M.M.; Iwamoto, T.; Aburatani, H.; Watanabe, S. β-Catenin signaling regulates the timing of cell differentiation in mouse retinal progenitor cells. *Mol. Cell. Neurosci.* **2011**, *46*, 770–780. [CrossRef]

318. Thompson, B.J.; Pichaud, F.; Röper, K. Sticking together the Crumbs - an unexpected function for an old friend. *Nat. Rev. Mol. Cell Biol.* **2013**, *14*, 307–314. [CrossRef]
319. Röper, K. Anisotropy of Crumbs and aPKC drives myosin cable assembly during tube formation. *Dev. Cell* **2012**, *23*, 939–953. [CrossRef]
320. Kerman, B.E.; Cheshire, A.M.; Myat, M.M.; Andrew, D.J. Ribbon modulates apical membrane during tube elongation through Crumbs and Moesin. *Dev. Biol.* **2008**, *320*, 278–288. [CrossRef]
321. FDA Approves Novel Gene Therapy to Treat Patients with a Rare form of Inherited Vision Loss. [Internet]. *FDA.gov*. 19 December 2017. Available online: https://www.fda.gov/NewsEvents/Newsroom/PressAnnouncements/ucm589467.htm (accessed on 18 August 2019).
322. New Gene Therapy for Rare Inherited Disorder Causing Vision loss Recommended for Approval. [Internet]. *EMA.europa.eu*. 21 September 2019. Available online: https://www.ema.europa.eu/en/news/new-gene-therapy-rare-inherited-disorder-causing-vision-loss-recommended-approval (accessed on 18 August 2019).
323. Henrique Alves, C.; Wijnholds, J. *AAV-Mediated Gene Therapy for CRB1-Hereditary Retinopathies*; Intechopen: London, UK, 2018.
324. Wang, D.; Tai, P.W.L.; Gao, G. Adeno-associated virus vector as a platform for gene therapy delivery. *Nat. Rev. Drug Discov.* **2019**, *18*, 358–378. [CrossRef]
325. Pellissier, L.P.; Hoek, R.M.; Vos, R.M.; Aartsen, W.M.; Klimczak, R.R.; Hoyng, S.A.; Flannery, J.G.; Wijnholds, J. Specific tools for targeting and expression in Müller glial cells. *Mol. Ther. Methods Clin. Dev.* **2014**, *1*, 14009. [CrossRef] [PubMed]
326. Yeste, J.; García-Ramírez, M.; Illa, X.; Guimerà, A.; Hernández, C.; Simó, R.; Villa, R. A compartmentalized microfluidic chip with crisscross microgrooves and electrophysiological electrodes for modeling the blood-retinal barrier. *Lab Chip* **2017**, *18*, 95–105. [CrossRef] [PubMed]
327. Hernandez, M.G.; Guibbal, L.; Toualbi, L.; Routet, F.; Chaffiol, A.; Winckler, C.; Harinquet, M.; Robert, C.; Fouquet, S.; Sahel, J.; et al. Optogenetic light sensors in human retinal organoids. *Front. Neurosci.* **2018**, *12*, 1–12.
328. Held, M.; Santeramo, I.; Wilm, B.; Murray, P.; Lévy, R. Ex vivo live cell tracking in kidney organoids using light sheet fluorescence microscopy. *PLoS ONE* **2018**, *13*, e0199918. [CrossRef]
329. Cora, V.; Haderspeck, J.; Antkowiak, L.; Mattheus, U.; Neckel, P.H.; Mack, A.F.; Bolz, S.; Ueffing, M.; Pashkovskaia, N.; Achberger, K.; et al. A Cleared View on Retinal Organoids. *Cells* **2019**, *8*, 391. [CrossRef]
330. Mongera, A.; Rowghanian, P.; Gustafson, H.J.; Shelton, E.; Kealhofer, D.A.; Carn, E.K.; Serwane, F.; Lucio, A.A.; Giammona, J.; Campàs, O. A fluid-to-solid jamming transition underlies vertebrate body axis elongation. *Nature* **2018**, *561*, 401–405. [CrossRef]
331. Serwane, F.; Mongera, A.; Rowghanian, P.; Kealhofer, D.A.; Lucio, A.A.; Hockenbery, Z.M.; Campàs, O. In vivo quantification of spatially varying mechanical properties in developing tissues. *Nat. Methods* **2017**, *14*, 181–186. [CrossRef]

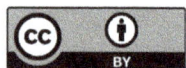

© 2019 by the authors. Licensee MDPI, Basel, Switzerland. This article is an open access article distributed under the terms and conditions of the Creative Commons Attribution (CC BY) license (http://creativecommons.org/licenses/by/4.0/).

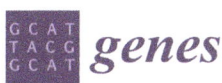

Article

Adeno-Associated Viral Vectors as a Tool for Large Gene Delivery to the Retina

Ivana Trapani [1,2]

[1] Telethon Institute of Genetics and Medicine (TIGEM), 80078 Pozzuoli, Italy; trapani@tigem.it; Tel.: +39-081-1923-0684
[2] Medical Genetics, Department of Translational Medicine, Federico II University, 80131 Naples, Italy

Received: 1 March 2019; Accepted: 5 April 2019; Published: 9 April 2019

Abstract: Gene therapy using adeno-associated viral (AAV) vectors currently represents the most promising approach for the treatment of many inherited retinal diseases (IRDs), given AAV's ability to efficiently deliver therapeutic genes to both photoreceptors and retinal pigment epithelium, and their excellent safety and efficacy profiles in humans. However, one of the main obstacles to widespread AAV application is their limited packaging capacity, which precludes their use from the treatment of IRDs which are caused by mutations in genes whose coding sequence exceeds 5 kb. Therefore, in recent years, considerable effort has been made to identify strategies to increase the transfer capacity of AAV vectors. This review will discuss these new developed strategies, highlighting the advancements as well as the limitations that the field has still to overcome to finally expand the applicability of AAV vectors to IRDs due to mutations in large genes.

Keywords: AAV; retina; gene therapy; dual AAV

1. Introduction

The eye is an ideal target for gene therapy thanks to its small and enclosed structure, relative immune privilege and easy accessibility [1,2]. This has boosted attempts at developing gene therapy approaches for the treatment of a large number of inherited retinal diseases (IRDs) over the recent decades [3,4]. Confirmation of the advancements in the retinal gene therapy field came in the last two years with the approval of the first gene therapy product for an IRD, Luxturna [5]—an adeno-associated viral (AAV) vector-based therapy for a form of Leber Congenital Amaurosis [6]—in the US, first, and then in Europe. The recombinant AAV vector on which Luxturna is based is the most widely used vector for retinal gene delivery. AAV are small (25 nm), nonenveloped, icosahedral viruses belonging to the Parvoviridae family [7]. They package a linear single-stranded DNA genome of ~4.7 kb, flanked by two 145 bp long palindromic inverted terminal repeats (ITRs) [7]. These ITRs form hairpin-loop secondary structures at the strand termini and are the only viral sequences that are retained in cis in the recombinant AAV vector genome [7]. Recombinant vectors based on AAV have fast become popular in the gene therapy field because of their excellent safety profile and low immunogenicity which allows for long-term expression of the therapeutic gene, at least in post-mitotic tissues, so that most experimental therapy studies require only a single vector administration. Additionally, dozens of different AAV variants have been identified thus far, each of them with unique transduction characteristics. This allows the user to select the most appropriate AAV serotype to transduce the retinal cell layer of interest. Indeed, following subretinal delivery, virtually all the AAV serotypes tested efficiently transduced the retinal pigment epithelium (RPE), while the levels of transduction of photoreceptors, which are the main therapeutic target cells in most IRDs, varied significantly among different serotypes [4,8]. AAV5, AAV7, AAV8 and AAV9 serotypes have all been demonstrated to efficiently transduce photoreceptors [4,8]. Additional serotypes with increased retinal transduction abilities have also been identified through either rational design or directed evolution [4,8]. This is one of the most attractive features of AAV vectors for retinal gene therapy, since alternative, both non-viral and viral, vectors tested thus far have shown more limited transduction abilities of adult photoreceptors [2,9]. For all the above described reasons, AAV have been used in many successful preclinical and clinical studies [3,4]. Clinical trial data collected over a decade have confirmed the overwhelming safety of AAV vectors delivered intraocularly and shown many instances of efficacy in treating previously incurable IRDs.

However, one of the main limitations to a broader application of AAV vectors for retinal gene therapy is their packaging capacity, which is restricted to approximately 5 kb of DNA [10]. This vector capacity is a critical issue, given the fact that approximately 6% of all human proteins have a coding sequence (CDS) that exceeds 4 kb [11] and that, in addition to the CDS of the therapeutic gene and the ITRs, a gene therapy vector needs to include, as a minimum, a promoter and a polyadenylation signal (polyA). Thus, the treatment of disorders caused by mutations in genes over 4 kb in size, including those causative of common IRDs, is currently not achievable using standard AAV vector-mediated approaches. The development of strategies to overcome AAV packaging limitation has therefore become a key area of research within the gene therapy field.

2. Strategies for Large Gene Delivery

Two types of strategies have been developed for large gene delivery via AAV: one is based on the "forced" packaging of oversized genomes (i.e., larger than 5 kb) in a single AAV vector (oversized AAV vectors); the other relies on the delivery of portions of large transgenes in two AAV vectors, which recombine through various mechanisms in the target cell, leading to the reconstitution of the full-length gene (dual AAV vectors) (Table 1).

Table 1. Adeno-associated viral (AAV) vector-based strategies for large gene delivery.

Strategy	Advantages	Limitations
Oversized AAV	No need to identify optimal splitting points/region of overlap	Genome highly heterogeneous in size
Trans-Splicing Dual AAV	Genomes with discrete nature	Non-directional concatemerization (with only one concatemer being productive) Need to identify optimal splitting points Efficiency dependent on splicing across the inverted terminal repeat (ITR) junction Potential production of shorter protein products
Overlapping Dual AAV	Genomes with discrete nature No additional foreign or artificial DNA elements required	Need to identify the optimal region of overlap for efficient homologous recombination Potential production of shorter protein products
Hybrid Dual AAV	Genomes with discrete nature Relies on two mechanisms for transgene reconstitution Transgene-independent efficacy of recombination	Need to identify optimal splitting points Efficiency dependent on splicing across the ITR junction Potential production of shorter protein products

2.1. Oversized AAV Vectors

Several research groups have tried to encapsidate large genes in a single AAV vector [12–14]. These "oversized" AAV vectors have been found to successfully express full-length proteins in vitro and in the retina of IRD models to levels which led to significant and stable improvement of the phenotype [12,15]. However, the genome contained in oversized AAV vectors was found to be not a pure population of intact large-sized genomes but rather a mixture of genomes highly heterogeneous in size [14,16–19]. Thus, it was proposed that full-length protein expression from oversized AAV vectors was achieved, following infection, through the re-assembly of truncated genomes in the target cell nucleus [14,16–19]. The efficiency of the transduction of oversized AAV vectors in the retina in comparison to alternative platforms for large gene delivery (i.e., dual AAV vectors, discussed below) has been assessed in various studies and found to be variable. Whereas some studies found considerably high levels of transgene expression from oversized AAV vectors [14,15], others showed efficient large protein reconstitution only upon dual AAV vector delivery [20,21]. Both the design and purification process of oversized AAV vectors were hypothesized to be critical for the success of the strategy, as the use of transgenes slightly above 5 kb can give rise to genomes with longer overlaps compared to the use of transgenes largely exceeding AAV cargo capacity, and this can drive more efficient re-assembly of oversized AAV vectors. Along this line, it was shown that the fractionation of oversized AAV vector preparations can be explored to promote selection of the genomes with the highest transduction properties in the final viral preparation [14]. However, despite the optimization and ability of this strategy to reconstitute large genes expression in vivo, consistently shown in various studies, the heterogenous nature of oversized AAV genomes poses major safety concerns, limiting their further application in clinical settings.

2.2. Dual AAV Vectors

An alternative strategy for AAV-mediated large gene delivery is the generation of dual AAV vectors. In this strategy, large transgenes are split into two separate AAV vectors that, upon co-infection of the same cell, reconstitute the expression of a full-length gene via intermolecular recombination between the two AAV vector genomes. This ideally doubles AAV cargo capacity, allowing delivery of transgenes up to about 9 kb. Various dual AAV vector strategies have been developed (referred to as trans-splicing [22], overlapping [23] and hybrid [24] dual AAV vector strategies), which differ in the mechanism they use to reconstitute the transgene.

2.2.1. Trans-Splicing Dual AAV Vectors

The trans-splicing approach relies on the natural ability of AAV ITRs to concatemerize in order to reconstitute full-length genomes [22,25]. In this approach, the two vectors carry two separate halves of the transgene, without regions of sequence overlap; the 5'-half vector has a splice donor (SD) signal at the 3' end of the AAV genome, while the 3'-half vector carries a splice acceptor (SA) signal at the 5' end of the AAV genome (Figure 1).

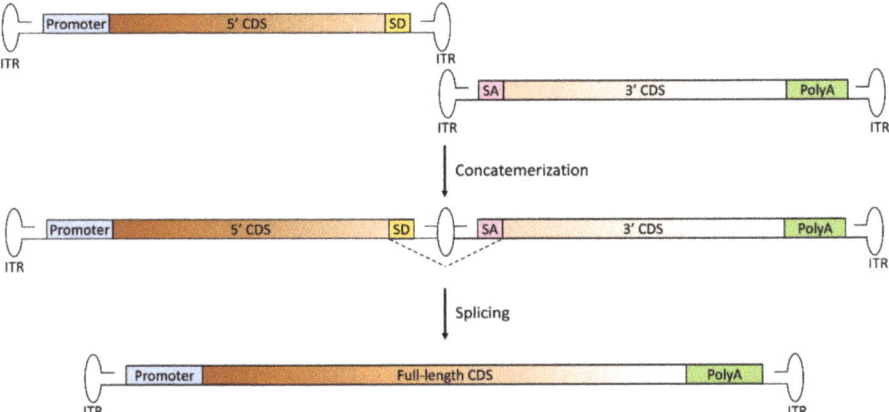

Figure 1. Schematic representation of the trans-splicing dual AAV approach for large gene reconstitution. The first vector includes the promoter, the 5'-half of the coding sequence (CDS) and the splicing donor (SD) signal; the second vector includes the splicing acceptor (SA) signal, the 3'-half of the CDS and the polyadenylation signal (PolyA). Concatemerization of the two vectors, involving the right-hand inverted terminal repeat (ITR) of the first vector and the left-hand ITR of the second vector, reconstitutes the full-length gene. After transcription, splicing leads to the removal of the ITR structure at the junction point, with restoration of the full-length, mature RNA of the transgene.

This allows splicing of the concatemerized ITR structure that forms in the middle of the therapeutic CDS following tail-to-head concatemerization of the two AAV genomes to obtain a single large mRNA molecule. This approach was first tested about 20 years ago, and historically represents the first developed approach for AAV-mediated large gene delivery. Since then, many studies have shown the efficacy of this strategy to reconstitute large genes. The major limitation of this platform, however, is that concatemerization can occur between any of the ITR of the two vectors. This may lead to the formation of both forms of circular monomers of each AAV, as well as two-vector linear concatemers in a number of orientations of which only one (i.e., tail-to-head concatemer) is productive to restore full-length gene expression [26]. Attempts at favoring the formation of concatemers in the correct orientation have been made (as discussed in the "Limitations of dual AAV vectors" paragraph). An additional limiting step of trans-splicing vectors is splicing across the ITR junction, the efficiency of which is dependent on both selection of the optimal exon–exon junction for splitting the large therapeutic gene [27] as well as the efficiency of splicing across the ITR structure [28]. To overcome the first issue, synthetic SD and SA signals have been developed, which mediate high rates of splicing independently of the gene that needs to be delivered [29]. Yet, since the sequence surrounding the splicing signals has an impact on splicing efficiency, careful selection of the splitting point is required.

2.2.2. Overlapping Dual AAV Vectors

In the overlapping approach, the transgene is split into two halves sharing homologous overlapping sequences, such that the reconstitution of the large gene expression cassette relies on homologous recombination [23] (Figure 2).

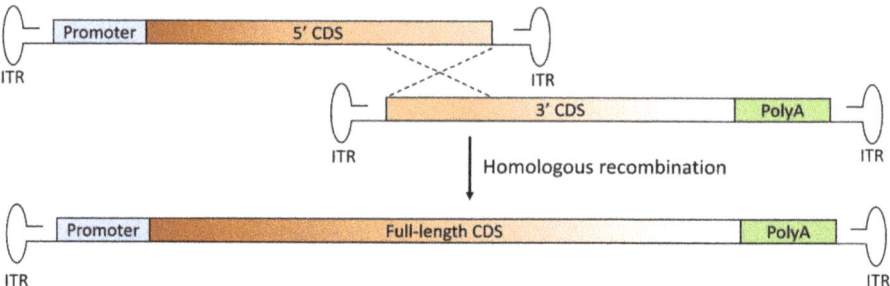

Figure 2. Schematic representation of the overlapping dual AAV approach for large gene reconstitution. The first vector includes the promoter and the 5'-half of the coding sequence (CDS) and the second vector includes the 3'-half of the CDS and the polyadenylation signal (PolyA). A portion of the sequence of the large transgene is repeated in both vectors (at the 3' end of the CDS of the first vector and at the 5' end of the CDS of the second vector). Thus, the full-length transgene expression cassette is reconstituted through homologous recombination of the overlapping regions in the two vectors. ITR: inverted terminal repeat.

As it has been designed, the overlapping approach is the simplest in design and requires less foreign or artificial DNA elements when compared to the other approaches. However, as the success of this strategy is critically dependent upon the ability of the overlapping region to mediate efficient homologous recombination, much work is needed to determine the optimal CDS overlapping region to be used for each transgene. Furthermore, data obtained so far have also highlighted that the success of this strategy is dependent on the retinal cell type being targeted, since the efficiency of the repair mechanism on which overlapping dual AAV vectors rely for large gene reconstitution is tissue dependent, as discussed below.

2.2.3. Hybrid Dual AAV Vectors

To overcome the main limitations of the previously described platforms (i.e., the lack of preference for directional tail-to-head concatemerization of the trans-splicing approach and the need for optimization of the CDS overlap for each transgene in the overlapping approach), a third transgene-independent dual AAV approach was developed: the hybrid dual AAV vectors. This approach is a combination of the trans-splicing and overlapping approaches, as it is based on the addition of a highly recombinogenic exogenous sequence to the trans-splicing vectors in order to increase recombination efficiency [24]. This recombinogenic sequence is placed downstream of the SD signal in the 5′-half vector and upstream of the SA signal in the 3′-half vector, so to be spliced out from the mRNA after recombination and transcription (Figure 3).

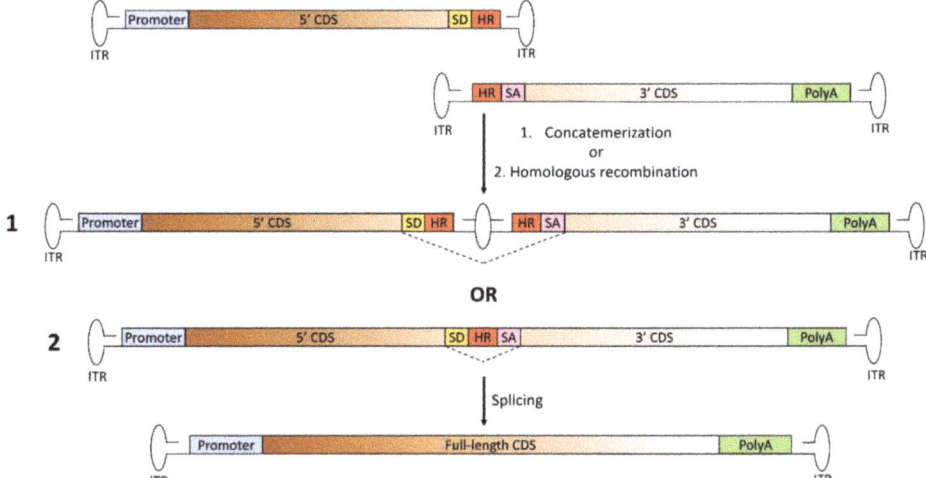

Figure 3. Schematic representation of the hybrid dual AAV approach for large gene reconstitution. The first vector includes the promoter, the 5′-half of the coding sequence (CDS), the splicing donor (SD) signal and the highly recombinogenic exogenous sequence (HR); the second vector includes the highly recombinogenic exogenous sequence, the splicing acceptor (SA) signal, the 3′-half of the CDS and the polyadenylation signal (PolyA). Joining of the two AAV vector genomes to reconstitute the full-length gene can occur through either: 1. concatemerization of the two vectors through the inverted terminal repeats (ITR), as for trans-splicing dual AAV vectors; or 2. homologous recombination mediated by the region of homology included in both vectors. In both cases, after transcription, splicing leads to the removal of the junction point, with restoration of the full-length, mature RNA of the transgene.

The hybrid dual AAV approach is potentially more effective than the other dual AAV vector approaches, since full-length gene reconstitution can occur through both homologous recombination mediated by the highly recombinogenic exogenous sequence as well as concatemerization through the ITRs [24]. The recombinogenic sequences used thus far to induce the recombination between hybrid dual AAV vectors have been derived from regions of either the alkaline phosphatase gene (AP) [24,30] or the F1 phage genome (AK) [21]. The inclusion of the exogenous sequence allows the promotion of high levels of homologous recombination between the two vector genomes, independently of the transgene to be delivered. However, similarly to the trans-splicing approach, the sequences surrounding the splicing signals still have an impact on splicing efficiency. Thus, careful selection of the splitting point is recommended to achieve maximal efficacy of large gene reconstitution.

3. The Choice of the Best Platform for Large Gene Delivery to the Retina

The efficacy of both oversized and dual AAV vectors in the retina has been evaluated in a number of studies using different reporter and therapeutic genes, such as *ABCA4* and *MYO7A* mutated in Stargardt disease (STGD1) [31] and Usher syndrome type 1B (USH1B) [32], respectively. However, literature describing these platforms is often conflicting. Initial studies in the retina reported a better performance of oversized AAV vectors compared to dual AAV strategies [14,15]. These results, however, might be due to both design and purification processes, which favor the generation of oversized vectors with high transduction properties [14], as well as to the less than optimal design of the dual AAV platform that was used as a comparison. One study, as an example, relied on the use of overlapping dual AAV vectors with a large region of overlap (1365 bases) that had not been optimized and, therefore, might potentially have a low efficiency of recombination [15]. Reconstitution from overlapping dual AAV vectors has also been found to occur at variable levels in different studies [15,20,21,26,33]. The most critical aspect of an overlapping dual AAV vector strategy is the event of recombination between the two halves of the transgene. This is influenced by both the sequence of the transgene and the cell type that is targeted, since different cell types could possibly deploy different DNA repair mechanisms. Some studies have found that long regions of overlap may lead to higher levels of transgene reconstitution [26]. However, it has recently been shown that optimization of the overlapping region is a prerequisite to achieve sustained levels of transgene expression in photoreceptors, since the efficiency of reconstitution is not directly proportional to the length of the regions of overlap [33]. It has been suggested that if the regions are too short, they might not be able to efficiently mediate interactions with the opposing viral genome, whereas longer regions of overlap may be less available for such interactions due to secondary structure formation. In line with this hypothesis, a screening of overlapping regions ranging from 23 to 1173 bp identified an overlap of 207–505 bp as the best performing for overlapping dual AAV-mediated reconstitution of *ABCA4* at therapeutic levels [33]. Thus, optimization of the overlapping region is essential to achieve sustained levels of transgene expression in photoreceptors. The targeted tissue also plays an important role in the success of the overlapping dual AAV approach since homologous recombination is typically associated with dividing cells, while low levels of homologous recombination are found in post-mitotic cells as neurons [34]. Along this line, studies have reported inefficient transduction of photoreceptors mediated by overlapping dual AAV vectors [15,21,26], whilst more efficient reconstitution was found in the RPE [21]. Other groups, however, have found efficient transduction of photoreceptors using overlapping dual AAV vectors [20,33], highlighting that the identification of highly recombinogenic regions of overlap in the transgene overcomes the limitations related to the inability of specific cell types to mediate efficient homologous recombination [33].

More consensus on the efficacy of trans-splicing and hybrid dual AAV vectors can be found in literature. A number of studies have indeed shown the ability of these strategies to reconstitute large transgenes in the retina [20,21,26,35,36] at levels which were higher compared to the other dual AAV strategies tested side by side [20,21,26], and which resulted in improvement of the retinal phenotype of animal models of IRDs [21,37]. This is possibly due to a more limited requirement of the optimization of these platforms compared to the others, since joining of the two halves of the transgene, with a discrete nature, occurs through the ITRs and/or a region of overlap known to be highly recombinogenic. Notably, the success obtained in the delivery of the large *MYO7A* gene to the retina [21] has led to the planning of a Phase I/II clinical trial, which will test the safety and efficacy of the hybrid dual AAV platform developed in the retina of USH1B patients (https://cordis.europa.eu/project/rcn/212674_it.html). Importantly, the results of this trial will definitively shed light on the efficiency of dual AAV vectors-mediated large gene delivery in the human retina.

Prompted by the success shown by dual AAV strategies, researchers have attempted at further expanding AAV cargo capacity in the retina up to 14 kb by adding a third vector to the dual system, generating triple AAV vectors [38]. This was found to be achievable, but at the expense of efficiency. Indeed, the levels of transduction achieved in the retina of a mouse model of Alstrom syndrome with triple AAV vectors have led to only a modest and transient improvement of the phenotype [38]. On the other hand, the levels of transduction mediated by triple AAV vectors in the large pig retina were found to be significantly higher than in the mouse retina, as also observed with dual AAV vectors [38]. These results bode well for further optimization of this platform.

4. Limitations of Dual AAV Vectors

Currently, all the dual AAV vector approaches have shown similar issues: variable success and expression of unwanted truncated products from single half-vectors. For all dual AAV platforms to be successful, a cell must necessarily be co-infected by at least one AAV vector including the 5'- and one including the 3'-half of the expression cassette. We and others have shown that co-transduction by two AAV vectors is quite efficient in the small subretinal space [11,21,36], which thus represents a favorable environment for developing dual AAV vector-based gene therapy approaches.

So far, however, all the studies performed have shown that none of the dual AAV approach matches the levels of expression achieved with a single AAV vector [21,26,36]. Various strategies have been explored to increase the efficiency of dual AAV vector-mediated large gene reconstitution.

One option is to increase vector dose and/or use AAV serotypes with higher tropism for the target cells in order to maximize rates of co-infection by both half vectors. A recent study has, however, suggested that an increase in vector dose does not proportionally correlate with increased levels of protein expression in the retina [26]. This suggests that, once efficient co-transduction is achieved, a further increase in vector genome amounts does not provide significant advantages [26]. Attempts at achieving higher levels of transduction by using alternative AAV serotypes have not been found consistently to result in higher transduction levels. Some studies have shown that use of capsid-engineered AAV variants with higher retinal transduction abilities, as tyrosine mutants capsids [39], led to higher levels of transgene expression from overlapping dual AAV vectors compared to naturally occurring AAV serotypes [20,33]. However, delivery of hybrid dual AAV vectors using an in-silico designed, synthetic vector (Anc80L65), which has also been shown to transduce retinal cells with a higher efficiency than AAV8 [40], led to almost identical levels of protein reconstitution compared to dual AAV8 vectors [26].

Another approach explored to increase transduction levels from dual AAV vectors has been maximizing the chances of both trans-splicing and hybrid AAV vectors to generate concatemers in the productive orientation, by forcing concatemerization of the ITRs, through the use of vectors carrying heterologous ITRs (i.e., ITR from different AAV serotypes at the opposite ends of the viral genome) [41]. Indeed, by generating trans-splicing vectors with heterologous ITR from serotypes 2 and 5 it has been shown that it is possible to reduce both the ability of each vector to form circular monomers and to increase directional tail-to-head concatemerization. This resulted in increased levels of transgene reconstitution compared to the use of vectors with homologous ITRs [41,42]. However, we have later shown that inclusion of heterologous ITRs in hybrid dual AAV vectors does not provide a significant advantage in full-length transgene reconstitution over the use of vectors with homologous ITRs [37]. This is consistent with the idea that hybrid dual AAV concatemerization is already partially driven in the correct orientation by the presence of highly recombinogenic regions. An additional strategy which has been used to direct AAV vectors concatemerization in the proper orientation is the use of a single-strand DNA oligonucleotide displaying homology to both of the distinct AAV genomes [43]. Alternatively, strategies that can improve dual AAV vector transduction efficiency by positively modulating AAV transduction steps, as the delivery of kinase inhibitors along with AAV vectors, have also been tested [44].

Another major drawback of dual AAV vectors, observed in some studies, is the production of truncated protein products from each of the single AAV vectors [20,21,33,37]. We and others have shown that, both in vitro and in the retina, truncated proteins from the 5' half vector that contains the promoter sequence and/or from the 3' half vector, due to the low promoter activity of the ITR, are produced. This issue can however be efficiently overcome by the use of the CL1 degron, a C-terminal destabilizing peptide that shares structural similarities with misfolded proteins and is thus recognized by the ubiquitination system [45,46]. Inclusion of this short (16 amino acids in length) degron mediates selective degradation of the truncated product from the 5′ half vector [37], without either affecting full-length protein reconstitution or significantly reducing the packaging capacity of the platform. More recently, McClements et al. have shown how the design of dual AAV vectors can also influence production of truncated proteins by the generation of unintended cryptic translation start sites and/or polyA signals [33]. Thus, the design of these platforms requires multiple considerations and adaptation, which may include codon optimizations to remove cryptic genetic signals. Furthermore, given the expression of such unwanted protein products, confirmation of the safety of dual AAV vectors is an important open question. While our preliminary data have shown no evident alterations of retinal morphology and functionality in mouse and pig eyes injected with dual AAV vectors [21,37], formal toxicity studies are required to elucidate this aspect.

5. Alternative Strategies to Allow AAV-Mediated Large Gene Delivery

Additional strategies to deliver large transgenes via AAV vectors are being actively investigated. Attempts at identifying AAV vectors with expanded cargo capacity, based on either protein libraries and directed evolution [47] or site directed mutagenesis to add positively-charged residues at lumenally exposed sites within the capsid [48], have been described. Alternatively, it has been shown that oversized AAV2 vector genomes can be effectively packaged in the capsid of human Bocavirus 1 (HBoV1) [49,50], an autonomous parvovirus relative of AAV, with a 5.5 kb genome. Testing of these vectors in the retina might lead to the identification of novel suitable vectors for large gene delivery.

The development of different short regulatory elements has also been attempted to reduce the size of the expression cassette and allow delivery of transgenes that exceed the AAV packaging capacity [51–55]. However, this often led to reduced levels of transgene expression. The combination of short synthetic enhancers and promoters was found to be useful for providing increased levels of expression of large transgenes [56]. Other studies have however shown that, despite optimization, some transgenes were more difficult than others to reconstitute from oversized AAV vectors when using short promoters [57].

The use of cDNA encoding for truncated versions of large proteins, which retain their functionality (i.e., a minigene), has also been achieved with some success [58]. However, all these approaches still cannot be easily applied to a large number of genes that exceed the AAV cargo capacity, since extensive optimization and testing would be required for each one of them.

6. Conclusions and Outlook

The growing number of clinical trials that show good safety and efficacy of the subretinal delivery of AAV vectors are contributing to the establishment of AAV as vectors of choice for retinal gene transfer. Expanding AAV cargo capacity over 5 kb is however a prerequisite to allow this platform to be used as a tool for the efficient delivery of a larger number of therapeutic genes. Recent proof-of-concept studies that used dual and triple AAV vectors to deliver large genes to the retina have shown that it is feasible to transfer genes with a CDS larger than 5 kb. Yet, these studies have highlighted that there is no one-fits-all dual AAV vector system, since dual AAV approaches have shown different relative efficiency in different studies. Clearly, the tissue being targeted, as well as the transgene that needs to be delivered, drastically influences transduction efficiency. Thus, careful design of the platform for each therapeutic application is required to achieve maximal efficacy. The planned clinical trial for USH1B will help defining whether the levels of expression achieved with dual AAV vectors are therapeutically relevant in humans. While the need of manufacturing two or more vectors to treat each disorder might represent a challenge of dual/triple AAV platforms, yet the retina is a favorable tissue for development of these approaches due to the fact that it requires delivery of only a small amount of vector. This reduces the total amount of vectors that needs to be produced.

Retinal transduction with multiple AAV vectors has been shown to reach lower levels compared to a single AAV vector. These levels were not sufficient to result in therapeutic efficacy for some diseases [38]. Consequently, alternative strategies should be explored.

Systems that rely on mechanisms different than those exploited by dual AAV vectors for large gene reconstitution might be investigated, including trans-splicing of pre-mRNAs [59] or intein-mediated protein trans-splicing [60]. Genome editing is also a rapidly expanding field of research, and could represent an interesting option for correction of mutations in genes whose delivery through AAV vectors is precluded by the large CDS size. A number of aspects for this approach however still need to be further explored. First, in the retina, where homologous recombination occurs at low rates, genome editing tools for the precise correction of a mutation will most probably need to exploit alternative repair mechanisms such as non-homologous end joining used for homology-independent targeted integration [61]. The efficiency of such approaches in the retina is still unknown. Secondly, the delivery of genome editing tools in post-mitotic tissues, such as the retina, might not be as safe as delivery in more proliferative tissues, considering the fact that their expression will persist long term after a single subretinal injection.

In conclusion, important steps forward have been made towards the treatment of IRDs due to mutations in large genes, which now seems an achievable goal. The optimization of these and the newly emerging platforms will allow expansion of the number of IRDs that are treatable using AAV-mediated gene therapy.

Funding: This work was supported by "Università degli Studi di Napoli Federico II" under the STAR Program.

Acknowledgments: We thank Raffaele Castello (Scientific Office, TIGEM, Pozzuoli, Italy) for critical reading of the manuscript.

Conflicts of Interest: The author is the co-inventor on patent applications on the dual AAV vector platform.

References

1. Auricchio, A.; Smith, A.J.; Ali, R.R. The Future Looks Brighter After 25 Years of Retinal Gene Therapy. *Hum. Gene Ther.* **2017**, *28*, 982–987. [CrossRef] [PubMed]
2. Trapani, I.; Auricchio, A. Seeing the Light after 25 Years of Retinal Gene Therapy. *Trends Mol. Med.* **2018**, *24*, 669–681. [CrossRef] [PubMed]
3. Moore, N.A.; Morral, N.; Ciulla, T.A.; Bracha, P. Gene therapy for inherited retinal and optic nerve degenerations. *Expert. Opin. Biol. Ther.* **2018**, *18*, 37–49. [CrossRef] [PubMed]
4. Trapani, I.; Puppo, A.; Auricchio, A. Vector platforms for gene therapy of inherited retinopathies. *Prog. Retin. Eye Res.* **2014**, *43*, 108–128. [CrossRef] [PubMed]
5. FDA approves hereditary blindness gene therapy. *Nat. Biotechnol* **2018**, *36*, 6. [CrossRef] [PubMed]
6. Pierce, E.A.; Bennett, J. The Status of RPE65 Gene Therapy Trials: Safety and Efficacy. *Cold Spring Harb. Perspect Med.* **2015**, *5*, a017285. [CrossRef]
7. Wang, D.; Tai, P.W.L.; Gao, G. Adeno-associated virus vector as a platform for gene therapy delivery. *Nat. Rev. Drug Discov.* **2019**. [CrossRef] [PubMed]
8. Day, T.P.; Byrne, L.C.; Schaffer, D.V.; Flannery, J.G. Advances in AAV vector development for gene therapy in the retina. *Adv. Exp. Med. Biol.* **2014**, *801*, 687–693.
9. Planul, A.; Dalkara, D. Vectors and Gene Delivery to the Retina. *Annu. Rev. Vis. Sci.* **2017**, *3*, 121–140. [CrossRef]
10. Salganik, M.; Hirsch, M.L.; Samulski, R.J. Adeno-associated Virus as a Mammalian DNA Vector. *Microbiol. Spectr.* **2015**, *3*. [CrossRef]
11. Palfi, A.; Chadderton, N.; McKee, A.G.; Blanco Fernandez, A.; Humphries, P.; Kenna, P.F.; Farrar, G.J. Efficacy of codelivery of dual AAV2/5 vectors in the murine retina and hippocampus. *Hum. Gene. Ther.* **2012**, *23*, 847–858. [CrossRef] [PubMed]
12. Allocca, M.; Doria, M.; Petrillo, M.; Colella, P.; Garcia-Hoyos, M.; Gibbs, D.; Kim, S.R.; Maguire, A.; Rex, T.S.; Di Vicino, U.; et al. Serotype-dependent packaging of large genes in adeno-associated viral vectors results in effective gene delivery in mice. *J. Clin. Invest.* **2008**, *118*, 1955–1964. [CrossRef] [PubMed]

13. Grieger, J.C.; Samulski, R.J. Packaging capacity of adeno-associated virus serotypes: Impact of larger genomes on infectivity and postentry steps. *J. Virol.* **2005**, *79*, 9933–9944. [CrossRef]
14. Hirsch, M.L.; Li, C.; Bellon, I.; Yin, C.; Chavala, S.; Pryadkina, M.; Richard, I.; Samulski, R.J. Oversized AAV transductifon is mediated via a DNA-PKcs-independent, Rad51C-dependent repair pathway. *Mol. Ther.* **2013**, *21*, 2205–2216. [CrossRef]
15. Lopes, V.S.; Boye, S.E.; Louie, C.M.; Boye, S.; Dyka, F.; Chiodo, V.; Fofo, H.; Hauswirth, W.W.; Williams, D.S. Retinal gene therapy with a large MYO7A cDNA using adeno-associated virus. *Gene. Ther.* **2013**, *20*, 824–833. [CrossRef] [PubMed]
16. Dong, B.; Nakai, H.; Xiao, W. Characterization of genome integrity for oversized recombinant AAV vector. *Mol. Ther.* **2010**, *18*, 87–92. [CrossRef] [PubMed]
17. Hirsch, M.L.; Agbandje-McKenna, M.; Samulski, R.J. Little vector, big gene transduction: Fragmented genome reassembly of adeno-associated virus. *Mol. Ther.* **2010**, *18*, 6–8. [CrossRef]
18. Lai, Y.; Yue, Y.; Duan, D. Evidence for the failure of adeno-associated virus serotype 5 to package a viral genome > or = 8.2 kb. *Mol. Ther.* **2010**, *18*, 75–79. [CrossRef]
19. Wu, Z.; Yang, H.; Colosi, P. Effect of genome size on AAV vector packaging. *Mol. Ther.* **2010**, *18*, 80–86. [CrossRef]
20. Dyka, F.M.; Boye, S.L.; Chiodo, V.A.; Hauswirth, W.W.; Boye, S.E. Dual adeno-associated virus vectors result in efficient in vitro and in vivo expression of an oversized gene, MYO7A. *Hum. Gene. Ther. Methods* **2014**, *25*, 166–177. [CrossRef]
21. Trapani, I.; Colella, P.; Sommella, A.; Iodice, C.; Cesi, G.; de Simone, S.; Marrocco, E.; Rossi, S.; Giunti, M.; Palfi, A.; et al. Effective delivery of large genes to the retina by dual AAV vectors. *EMBO Mol. Med.* **2014**, *6*, 194–211. [CrossRef]
22. Yan, Z.; Zhang, Y.; Duan, D.; Engelhardt, J.F. Trans-splicing vectors expand the utility of adeno-associated virus for gene therapy. *Proc. Natl. Acad. Sci. USA* **2000**, *97*, 6716–6721. [CrossRef]
23. Duan, D.; Yue, Y.; Engelhardt, J.F. Expanding AAV packaging capacity with trans-splicing or overlapping vectors: A quantitative comparison. *Mol. Ther.* **2001**, *4*, 383–391. [CrossRef]
24. Ghosh, A.; Yue, Y.; Lai, Y.; Duan, D. A hybrid vector system expands adeno-associated viral vector packaging capacity in a transgene-independent manner. *Mol. Ther.* **2008**, *16*, 124–130. [CrossRef]
25. Yang, J.; Zhou, W.; Zhang, Y.; Zidon, T.; Ritchie, T.; Engelhardt, J.F. Concatamerization of adeno-associated virus circular genomes occurs through intermolecular recombination. *J. Virol.* **1999**, *73*, 9468–9477.
26. Carvalho, L.S.; Turunen, H.T.; Wassmer, S.J.; Luna-Velez, M.V.; Xiao, R.; Bennett, J.; Vandenberghe, L.H. Evaluating Efficiencies of Dual AAV Approaches for Retinal Targeting. *Front Neurosci.* **2017**, *11*, 503. [CrossRef]
27. Lai, Y.; Yue, Y.; Liu, M.; Ghosh, A.; Engelhardt, J.F.; Chamberlain, J.S.; Duan, D. Efficient in vivo gene expression by trans-splicing adeno-associated viral vectors. *Nat. Biotechnol.* **2005**, *23*, 1435–1439. [CrossRef] [PubMed]
28. Xu, Z.; Yue, Y.; Lai, Y.; Ye, C.; Qiu, J.; Pintel, D.J.; Duan, D. Trans-splicing adeno-associated viral vector-mediated gene therapy is limited by the accumulation of spliced mRNA but not by dual vector coinfection efficiency. *Hum. Gene. Ther.* **2004**, *15*, 896–905. [CrossRef] [PubMed]
29. Lai, Y.; Yue, Y.; Liu, M.; Duan, D. Synthetic intron improves transduction efficiency of trans-splicing adeno-associated viral vectors. *Hum. Gene. Ther.* **2006**, *17*, 1036–1042. [CrossRef]
30. Ghosh, A.; Yue, Y.; Duan, D. Efficient transgene reconstitution with hybrid dual AAV vectors carrying the minimized bridging sequences. *Hum. Gene. Ther.* **2011**, *22*, 77–83. [CrossRef]
31. Tanna, P.; Strauss, R.W.; Fujinami, K.; Michaelides, M. Stargardt disease: clinical features, molecular genetics, animal models and therapeutic options. *Br. J. Ophthalmol.* **2017**, *101*, 25–30. [CrossRef]
32. Williams, D.S. Usher syndrome: Animal models, retinal function of Usher proteins, and prospects for gene therapy. *Vision Res.* **2008**, *48*, 433–441. [CrossRef]
33. McClements, M.E.; Barnard, A.R.; Singh, M.S.; Charbel Issa, P.; Jiang, Z.; Radu, R.A.; MacLaren, R.E. An AAV Dual Vector Strategy Ameliorates the Stargardt Phenotype in Adult Abca4(-/-) Mice. *Hum. Gene. Ther.* **2018**. [CrossRef]
34. Fishel, M.L.; Vasko, M.R.; Kelley, M.R. DNA repair in neurons: so if they don't divide what's to repair? *Mutat. Res.* **2007**, *614*, 24–36. [CrossRef] [PubMed]

35. Reich, S.J.; Auricchio, A.; Hildinger, M.; Glover, E.; Maguire, A.M.; Wilson, J.M.; Bennett, J. Efficient trans-splicing in the retina expands the utility of adeno-associated virus as a vector for gene therapy. *Hum. Gene. Ther.* **2003**, *14*, 37–44. [CrossRef]
36. Colella, P.; Trapani, I.; Cesi, G.; Sommella, A.; Manfredi, A.; Puppo, A.; Iodice, C.; Rossi, S.; Simonelli, F.; Giunti, M.; et al. Efficient gene delivery to the cone-enriched pig retina by dual AAV vectors. *Gene. Ther.* **2014**, *21*, 450–456. [CrossRef] [PubMed]
37. Trapani, I.; Toriello, E.; de Simone, S.; Colella, P.; Iodice, C.; Polishchuk, E.V.; Sommella, A.; Colecchi, L.; Rossi, S.; Simonelli, F.; et al. Improved dual AAV vectors with reduced expression of truncated proteins are safe and effective in the retina of a mouse model of Stargardt disease. *Hum. Mol. Genet.* **2015**, *24*, 6811–6825. [CrossRef]
38. Maddalena, A.; Tornabene, P.; Tiberi, P.; Minopoli, R.; Manfredi, A.; Mutarelli, M.; Rossi, S.; Simonelli, F.; Naggert, J.K.; Cacchiarelli, D.; et al. Triple Vectors Expand AAV Transfer Capacity in the Retina. *Mol. Ther.* **2018**, *26*, 524–541. [CrossRef]
39. Petrs-Silva, H.; Dinculescu, A.; Li, Q.; Min, S.H.; Chiodo, V.; Pang, J.J.; Zhong, L.; Zolotukhin, S.; Srivastava, A.; Lewin, A.S.; et al. High-efficiency transduction of the mouse retina by tyrosine-mutant AAV serotype vectors. *Mol. Ther.* **2009**, *17*, 463–471. [CrossRef]
40. Zinn, E.; Pacouret, S.; Khaychuk, V.; Turunen, H.T.; Carvalho, L.S.; Andres-Mateos, E.; Shah, S.; Shelke, R.; Maurer, A.C.; Plovie, E.; et al. In Silico Reconstruction of the Viral Evolutionary Lineage Yields a Potent Gene Therapy Vector. *Cell Rep.* **2015**, *12*, 1056–1068. [CrossRef]
41. Yan, Z.; Zak, R.; Zhang, Y.; Engelhardt, J.F. Inverted terminal repeat sequences are important for intermolecular recombination and circularization of adeno-associated virus genomes. *J. Virol.* **2005**, *79*, 364–379. [CrossRef] [PubMed]
42. Yan, Z.; Lei-Butters, D.C.; Zhang, Y.; Zak, R.; Engelhardt, J.F. Hybrid adeno-associated virus bearing nonhomologous inverted terminal repeats enhances dual-vector reconstruction of minigenes in vivo. *Hum. Gene. Ther.* **2007**, *18*, 81–87. [CrossRef]
43. Hirsch, M.L.; Storici, F.; Li, C.; Choi, V.W.; Samulski, R.J. AAV recombineering with single strand oligonucleotides. *PLoS ONE* **2009**, *4*, e7705. [CrossRef]
44. Maddalena, A.; Dell'Aquila, F.; Giovannelli, P.; Tiberi, P.; Wanderlingh, L.G.; Montefusco, S.; Tornabene, P.; Iodice, C.; Visconte, F.; Carissimo, A.; et al. High-Throughput Screening Identifies Kinase Inhibitors That Increase Dual Adeno-Associated Viral Vector Transduction In Vitro and in Mouse Retina. *Hum. Gene. Ther.* **2018**, *29*, 886–901. [CrossRef]
45. Bence, N.F.; Sampat, R.M.; Kopito, R.R. Impairment of the ubiquitin-proteasome system by protein aggregation. *Science* **2001**, *292*, 1552–1555. [CrossRef]
46. Gilon, T.; Chomsky, O.; Kulka, R.G. Degradation signals for ubiquitin system proteolysis in Saccharomyces cerevisiae. *EMBO J.* **1998**, *17*, 2759–2766. [CrossRef] [PubMed]
47. Turunen, H.T.; Vandenberghe, L.H. Generating Novel AAV Capsid Mutants for Large Genome Packaging Through Protein Libraries and Directed Evolution. In Proceedings of the American Society of Gene & Cell Therapy 17th Annual Meeting, Washigton, DC, USA, 21–24 May 2014; p. S118.
48. Tiffany, M.; Kay, M.A. Expanded Packaging Capacity of AAV by Lumenal Charge Alteration. In Proceedings of the American Society of Gene & Cell Therapy 19th Annual Meeting, Washigton, DC, USA, 22 April 2016; pp. S99–S100.
49. Yan, Z.; Keiser, N.W.; Song, Y.; Deng, X.; Cheng, F.; Qiu, J.; Engelhardt, J.F. A novel chimeric adenoassociated virus 2/human bocavirus 1 parvovirus vector efficiently transduces human airway epithelia. *Mol. Ther.* **2013**, *21*, 2181–2194. [CrossRef]
50. Fakhiri, J.; Schneider, M.A.; Puschhof, J.; Stanifer, M.; Schildgen, V.; Holderbach, S.; Voss, Y.; El Andari, J.; Schildgen, O.; Boulant, S.; et al. Novel Chimeric Gene Therapy Vectors Based on Adeno-Associated Virus and Four Different Mammalian Bocaviruses. *Mol. Ther. Methods Clin. Dev.* **2019**, *12*, 202–222. [CrossRef] [PubMed]
51. Ostedgaard, L.S.; Rokhlina, T.; Karp, P.H.; Lashmit, P.; Afione, S.; Schmidt, M.; Zabner, J.; Stinski, M.F.; Chiorini, J.A.; Welsh, M.J. A shortened adeno-associated virus expression cassette for CFTR gene transfer to cystic fibrosis airway epithelia. *Proc. Natl. Acad. Sci. USA* **2005**, *102*, 2952–2957. [CrossRef] [PubMed]

52. McFarland, T.J.; Zhang, Y.; Atchaneeyaskul, L.O.; Francis, P.; Stout, J.T.; Appukuttan, B. Evaluation of a novel short polyadenylation signal as an alternative to the SV40 polyadenylation signal. *Plasmid* **2006**, *56*, 62–67. [CrossRef]
53. Pellissier, L.P.; Hoek, R.M.; Vos, R.M.; Aartsen, W.M.; Klimczak, R.R.; Hoyng, S.A.; Flannery, J.G.; Wijnholds, J. Specific tools for targeting and expression in Muller glial cells. *Mol. Ther. Methods Clin. Dev.* **2014**, *1*, 14009. [CrossRef]
54. Choi, J.H.; Yu, N.K.; Baek, G.C.; Bakes, J.; Seo, D.; Nam, H.J.; Baek, S.H.; Lim, C.S.; Lee, Y.S.; Kaang, B.K. Optimization of AAV expression cassettes to improve packaging capacity and transgene expression in neurons. *Mol. Brain* **2014**, *7*, 17. [CrossRef]
55. Wang, D.; Fischer, H.; Zhang, L.; Fan, P.; Ding, R.X.; Dong, J. Efficient CFTR expression from AAV vectors packaged with promoters—The second generation. *Gene. Ther.* **1999**, *6*, 667–675. [CrossRef] [PubMed]
56. Yan, Z.; Sun, X.; Feng, Z.; Li, G.; Fisher, J.T.; Stewart, Z.A.; Engelhardt, J.F. Optimization of Recombinant Adeno-Associated Virus-Mediated Expression for Large Transgenes, Using a Synthetic Promoter and Tandem Array Enhancers. *Hum. Gene. Ther.* **2015**, *26*, 334–346. [CrossRef] [PubMed]
57. Holehonnur, R.; Lella, S.K.; Ho, A.; Luong, J.A.; Ploski, J.E. The production of viral vectors designed to express large and difficult to express transgenes within neurons. *Mol. Brain* **2015**, *8*, 12. [CrossRef]
58. Lai, Y.; Thomas, G.D.; Yue, Y.; Yang, H.T.; Li, D.; Long, C.; Judge, L.; Bostick, B.; Chamberlain, J.S.; Terjung, R.L.; et al. Dystrophins carrying spectrin-like repeats 16 and 17 anchor nNOS to the sarcolemma and enhance exercise performance in a mouse model of muscular dystrophy. *J. Clin. Invest.* **2009**, *119*, 624–635. [CrossRef]
59. Yang, Y.; Walsh, C.E. Spliceosome-mediated RNA trans-splicing. *Mol. Ther.* **2005**, *12*, 1006–1012. [CrossRef]
60. Li, Y. Split-inteins and their bioapplications. *Biotechnol. Lett.* **2015**, *37*, 2121–2137. [CrossRef] [PubMed]
61. Suzuki, K.; Tsunekawa, Y.; Hernandez-Benitez, R.; Wu, J.; Zhu, J.; Kim, E.J.; Hatanaka, F.; Yamamoto, M.; Araoka, T.; Li, Z.; et al. In vivo genome editing via CRISPR/Cas9 mediated homology-independent targeted integration. *Nature* **2016**, *540*, 144–149. [CrossRef]

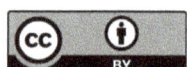

© 2019 by the author. Licensee MDPI, Basel, Switzerland. This article is an open access article distributed under the terms and conditions of the Creative Commons Attribution (CC BY) license (http://creativecommons.org/licenses/by/4.0/).

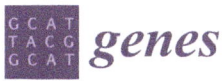

Review

Molecular Therapies for Choroideremia

Jasmina Cehajic Kapetanovic [1,2,*], Alun R. Barnard [1,2] and Robert E. MacLaren [1,2]

[1] Nuffield Laboratory of Ophthalmology, University of Oxford, Oxford OX3 9DU, UK; alun.barnard@eye.ox.ac.uk (A.R.B.); robert.maclaren@eye.ox.ac.uk (R.E.M.)
[2] Oxford Eye Hospital, Oxford University Hospitals NHS Foundation Trust, Oxford OX3 9DU, UK
* Correspondence: enquiries@eye.ox.ac.uk

Received: 31 July 2019; Accepted: 20 September 2019; Published: 23 September 2019

Abstract: Advances in molecular research have culminated in the development of novel gene-based therapies for inherited retinal diseases. We have recently witnessed several groundbreaking clinical studies that ultimately led to approval of Luxturna, the first gene therapy for an inherited retinal disease. In parallel, international research community has been engaged in conducting gene therapy trials for another more common inherited retinal disease known as choroideremia and with phase III clinical trials now underway, approval of this therapy is poised to follow suit. This chapter discusses new insights into clinical phenotyping and molecular genetic testing in choroideremia with review of molecular mechanisms implicated in its pathogenesis. We provide an update on current gene therapy trials and discuss potential inclusion of female carries in future clinical studies. Alternative molecular therapies are discussed including suitability of *CRISPR* gene editing, small molecule nonsense suppression therapy and vision restoration strategies in late stage choroideremia.

Keywords: choroideremia; gene therapy; REP1; inherited retinal disease; treatment

1. Introduction

Choroideremia is a rare X-linked recessive inherited retinal disease caused by sequence variations or deletions in the *CHM* gene which are usually functionally null mutations, leading to deficiency in Rab escort protein 1 (REP1) [1–3]. The estimated prevalence is 1 in 50,000 males. Although REP1 is expressed ubiquitously, in humans choroideremia appears only to affect the retinal pigment epithelium (RPE) layer of the eye, leading to a characteristic clinical phenotype of progressive centripetal retinal degeneration. In Ancient Greek, the name choroid derives from χόριον (khórion, "skin") and εἶδος (eîdos, "resembling"). The suffix 'eremia' (ἐρημία) was added to describe the barren appearance (from the root word meaning wasteland or desert). Hence the literal translation of choroideremia is, in relation to the eye, 'the skin-resembling part is deserted'. Interestingly, the incorrect spelling '*choroideraemia*' has been used previously, but this may be based on misinterpretation of the suffix being derived from αἷμα (haima, blood), into which the 'ae' diphthong is still substituted in many non-US English usages. Importantly however, despite reference to the choroid in the name, the disease is now known to be driven primarily by the loss of the RPE, followed by the secondary degeneration of photoreceptors and choroidal atrophy [4]. Recent evidence has shed light on the molecular mechanisms of REP1 contribution to retinal degeneration in choroideremia, describing its essential role in post-translational modification of proteins and in intracellular trafficking of molecules [5]. The process affects primarily the RPE and pigment clumping is the first sign, long before photoreceptor loss. However, since the RPE has an essential role in retinal isomerization in the visual cycle which is more important for rod compared to cone function and hence rod function is impaired quite early in the disease process. As a result, the disease presents with early childhood nyctalopia, but the majority of patients retain excellent visual acuity until the very end stages of disease, presumably because Müller cells can still contribute to the cone visual cycle in the absence of RPE [6–8].

In this chapter we review advances in molecular therapies that have resulted in the development of adeno-associated vector (AAV) gene replacement therapy for choroideremia. The therapy is currently being explored in multiple clinical trials worldwide, having recently reached phase III in the development (Table 1). We discuss new insights into the clinical phenotyping and genotyping of choroideremia male patients and female carriers, including progress from the natural history studies, that will aid disease characterisation, monitoring of disease progression and interpretation of clinical trial endpoints. The review discusses current knowledge and progress in molecular mechanisms of choroideremia and the development of emerging potential therapies.

Table 1. Summary of interventional gene therapy clinical trials in choroideremia.

Clinical trial	Intervention	Clinical centre	References
Phase I/II NCT01461213 Start date: 2011 Completed 2018	Gene therapy involving subretinal delivery of AAV2-REP1	University of Oxford, UK	Lancet, 2014 [9] NEJM, 2016 [10] Nat Med, 2018 [11]
Phase I/II NCT02341807 Start date: 2015 Ongoing	Gene therapy involving subretinal delivery of AAV2-REP1	Philadelphia, USA Spark Therapeutics	No reports to date
Phase I/II NCT02077361 Start date: 2015 Completed 2018	Gene therapy involving subretinal delivery of AAV2-REP1	University of Alberta, Canada	Am J Ophthalmol, 2018 [12]
Phase II NCT02553135 Start date: 2015 Completed 2019	Gene therapy involving subretinal delivery of AAV2-REP1	University of Miami, USA	Am J Ophthalmol, 2019 [13]
Phase II NCT02671539 THOR TRIAL Start date: 2016 Completed 2018	Gene therapy involving subretinal delivery of AAV2-REP1	University of Tubingen, Germany	Retina, 2018 [14]
Phase II NCT02407678 REGENERATE TRIAL Start date: 2016 Ongoing	Gene therapy involving subretinal delivery of AAV2-REP1	University of Oxford and Moorfields Eye Hospital, UK	No reports to date
Phase II NCT03507686 GEMINI TRIAL Start date: 2017 Ongoing	Gene therapy involving bilateral subretinal delivery of AAV2-REP1	Nightstar Therapeutics (now Biogen) International, Multi-centre	No reports to date
Phase III NCT03496012 STAR TRIAL Start date: 2017 Ongoing	Gene therapy involving subretinal delivery of AAV2-REP1	Nightstar Therapeutics (now Biogen), International, Multi-centre	No reports to date
Observational NCT03584165 SOLSTICE TRIAL Start date: 2018 Ongoing	Long-term follow up study evaluating the safety and efficacy of AAV2-REP1 used in antecedent interventional choroideremia studies, 100 participants	Nightstar Therapeutics (now Biogen), International, Multi-centre	No reports to date

2. Choroideremia Phenotype

Choroideremia manifests with a pathognomonic fundus appearance characterised by progressive degeneration of retina and choroid (Figure 1). The degeneration starts in a ring around the mid-periphery of the retina and expands both centripetally towards the fovea and anteriorly to the pars plana [7,15,16]. The anatomical changes are accompanied by loss of functional scotopic vision and the reduction of the mid-peripheral visual field that begins during the first and second decade of life. The visual acuity is generally well preserved until late in the disease process, usually until the fifth decade of life, when the degeneration starts to encroach onto the fovea [6–8,15,16].

It remains somewhat unclear whether the RPE, the retina and the choroid are all primarily affected, or whether one or more of these tissues is secondarily affected during the pathogenesis of choroideremia [4].

There is however mounting indirect evidence that the RPE is the primary site of the disease in choroideremia, with the inner (photoreceptor) and outer (choroidal) layers degenerating through secondary mechanisms [5]. The unique pattern of preserved retina and RPE, as seen on autofluorescence imaging (Figure 1), with sharply demarcated edges is very different from many other retinal diseases where preserved regions are more circular or oval. This appearance is, however, almost identical in dominantly inherited *RPE65* retinal diseases. Since *RPE65* is only expressed in the RPE, we know that this phenotype is a feature specific to the RPE (presumably, RPE cell death), giving indirect evidence that choroideremia is a disease driven by RPE loss. The confounding variable in choroideremia is that the REP1 protein is expressed throughout the body [17] and the name 'choroideremia' gives the impression that this is primarily a choroidal degeneration. This is not the case, however, because any disease or treatments such as cryotherapy that destroys the RPE layer alone, will eventually lead to secondary atrophy of the underlying choroid, in a similar manner. In other words, choroideremia is the phenotype of complete RPE cell loss. The other relevant factor is that male patients with choroideremia can develop choroidal new vessels (Figure 2) and this clearly shows that the choroidal vasculature has the capacity to regenerate in certain cases. Finally, we know from female carriers (Figure 3) that the pattern of RPE loss is very similar to that in carriers of ocular albinism. There is no evidence of X inactivation leading to patchy loss of the choroid independently in female carriers.

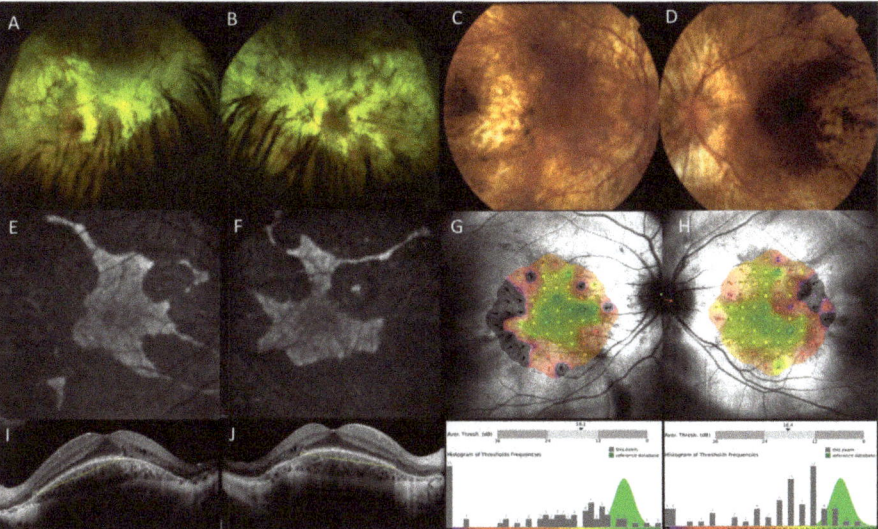

Figure 1. Retinal imaging in choroideremia. Widefield optomaps, Optos, Dumfernline, UK (**A**,**B**) and Heidelberg Spectralis imaging, Heidelberg, Germany (**C**–**F**) showing choroideremia phenotype in an affected male. Colour fundus photographs (**C**,**D**) show extensive retinal degeneration with choroidal atrophy and visualisation of underlying pale sclera. Fundus autofluorescence (**E**,**F**) shows typical patterns of sharply demarcated areas of remaining tissue (hyperfluorescent) against atrophic retina (hypofluorescent background). Mesopic microperimetry, MAIA CenterVue SpA, Padova, Italy (**G**,**H**) measures central retinal sensitivity that closely maps areas of residual retina as seen on autofluorescence. Sensitivity maps are shown with corresponding histograms of threshold frequencies. Spectral domain optical coherence tomography, Heidelberg, Germany (**I**,**J**) shows retinal structure in cross-section with distribution of ellipsoid zone (yellow line) and preserved inner retinal layers.

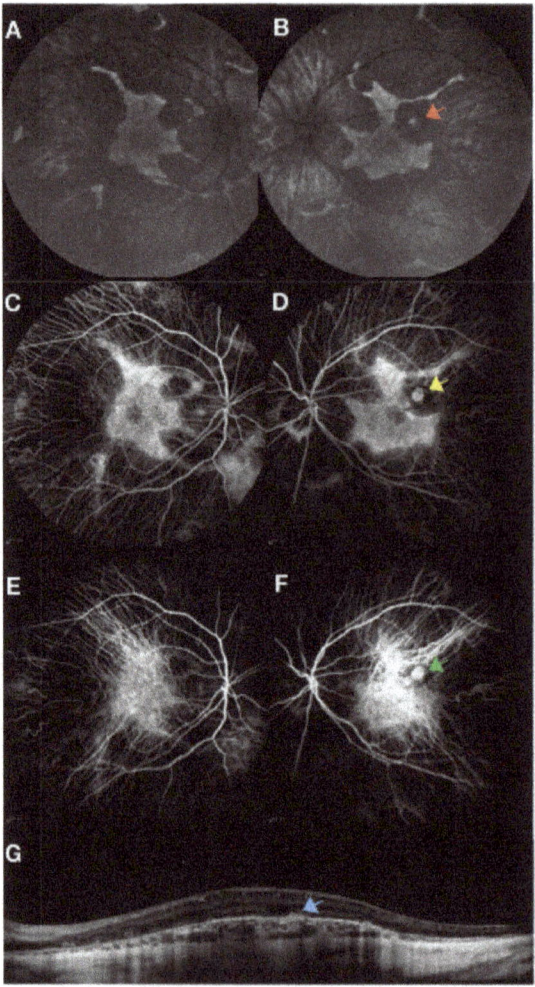

Figure 2. Retinal imaging in a choroideremia patient showing an area of scaring from an old choroidal neovascular membrane in the left eye. Fundus autofluorescence (**A**,**B**), fluorescein angiography (**C**,**D**), indocyanine green angiography (**E**,**F**) and spectral domain optical coherence tomography (**G**) with arrows marking the old scar. Imaging was performed with Heidelberg Spectralis, Heidelberg, Germany.

It is also possible that REP1 expression may be important for rod photoreceptor function [18]. Processing of post-mortem tissue from patients can make histological analyses difficult, and studies using advanced imaging techniques have provided somewhat equivocal results in terms of evidence of independent rod degeneration in humans in areas of the retina where the underlying RPE cells are unaffected by the disease [6,8,18–20]. Since patients with choroideremia maintain excellent visual acuity until the very late stages of the disease [6–8], it is likely that the REP1 deficiency is not a significant factor for the cone photoreceptors.

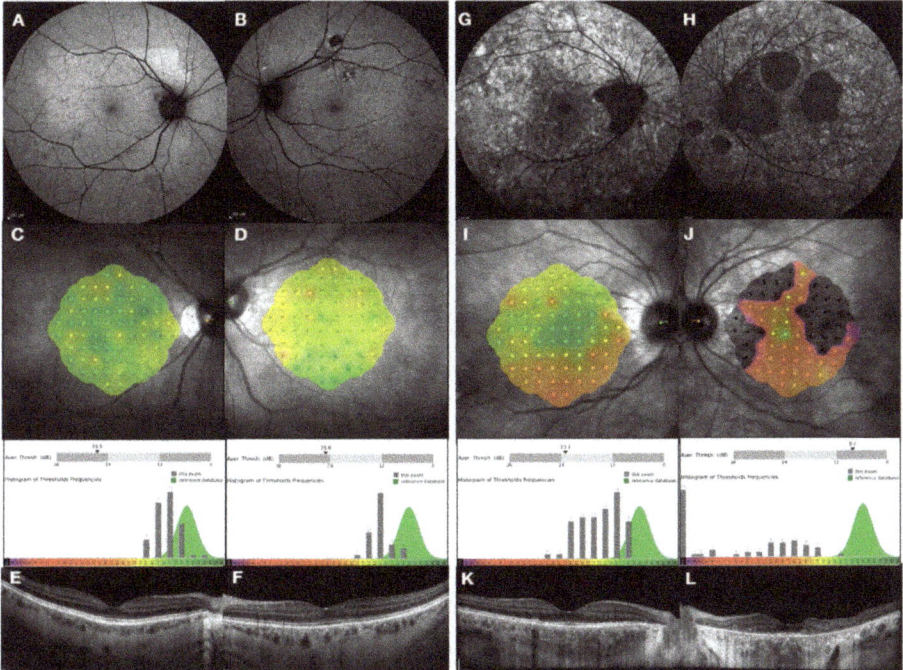

Figure 3. Retinal imaging in two female choroideremia carriers. Phenotype of an asymptomatic mild carrier with Snellen visual acuity of 6/5 in both eyes is shown from (**A–F**) and a carrier with a 'geographic-pattern' phenotype and reduced visual acuity of 6/7.5 in the right eye and 6/12 in the left eye is shown from (**G–L**). Fundus autofluorescence showing very early signs of fine 'salt and pepper' mottling (**A,B**) compared with coarse mottling and atrophic patches resembling geographic patterns (**G,H**). Mesopic microperimetry, MAIA CenterVue SpA, Padova, Italy showing sensitivity maps with corresponding histograms of threshold frequencies. Near-normal central retinal sensitivity is found in mild, asymptomatic carriers (**C,D**) compared to reduced retinal sensitivity in affected carriers especially in the left eye of the above case (**I,J**). OCT imaging is clinically insignificant in mild, asymptomatic carriers (**E,F**) whereas some disruption of retinal pigment epithelium (RPE) and ellipsoid zone is observed in the affected carrier, particularly in the left eye (**K,L**).

Elucidating the pattern of degeneration in choroideremia may help us understand the basis of the disease and how it progresses [16]. It is not known why the degeneration in choroideremia starts in the equatorial region before spreading anteriorly and posteriorly to reach the macula. The retinal pigment epithelial cell density is roughly similar at 5000 cells per mm^2 throughout the posterior eyecup. Gyrate atrophy of the choroid however may develop in a similar distribution, although this is in contrast to age-related macular degeneration, which is very much focused in the region around the fovea. In a recent study it was shown that the rate of degeneration in choroideremia followed an exponential decay function and was very similar across patients of different ages [21], but the key factor that determined the severity of the disease was the age of onset of degeneration. It may therefore be possible to predict the severity of the disease simply by measuring the residual area in a patient at a given age, because the progression is likely to be constant in the absence of treatment.

The centripetal degeneration in choroideremia has two phases by fundus autofluorescence-mottled RPE up to the edge and a more central zone of smooth RPE, both of which shrink progressively. In more advanced stages of the disease there is a total loss of smooth zone. The anatomical basis for these two zones is not immediately clear, but it may be that the slightly increased RPE cell density and much thicker choroid at the posterior pole provides some degree of protection against the metabolic stress caused by REP1 deficiency. Recent evidence suggests that there is less preserved autoflourescence area in nasal macula that may be more vulnerable to degeneration [16]. Further studies are necessary to determine whether the RPE zones can predict the health status of the overlying photoreceptors and how these might be affected following treatment.

3. Choroideremia Genotype

The choroideremia gene, *CHM* (OMIM #300390), encodes the REP1 protein, a 653 amino acid polypeptide essential for intracellular trafficking and post-translational prenylation of proteins within the human eye. Currently, there are 346 mutations registered on Leiden Open Variation Database, LOVD[3] (www.lovd.nl/CHM). Almost all of the identified sequence variations regardless of mechanism, are predicted to be null [3,22–25]. The mechanisms include insertions and deletions (minor, a few nucleotides, and major involving up to the entire gene length), splice site mutations, missense changes and point mutations that result in stop codons (premature termination codons). Novel mutations have recently been identified involving a deep-intronic region [26] and a promoter region [27] of the *CHM* gene.

Compared with other genetic diseases including inherited retinal disease, choroideremia has a surprisingly low number of disease-causing missense mutations. This would suggest that the REP1 protein, with 3 principal domains, has no catalytic domains with corresponding mutational hotspots within the gene. This is in contrast to genes that encode enzymes (such as *retinitis pigmentosa GTPase regulator* gene) that typically have such hotspot regions (e.g., ORF15 region). This supports the role of REP1 as a chaperone protein, enhancing activity of another protein, which is important in cell structure and stability.

Recent evidence shows that the majority of missense mutations are disproportionately found to be single point C to T transitions at C-phosphate-G (CpG) dinucleotides, spread across 5 of only 24 CpG dinucleotides in the entire *CHM* gene [25]. This is consistent with the evolutionary loss of CpG dinucleotides through destabilising methylation and subsequent deamination. Notably, the 5 locations were the only sites at which C to T transitions resulted in a stop codon. Future de novo mutations are likely to arise within these destabilised hotspot loci.

Molecular genetic testing offers means of confirming the clinical diagnosis in choroideremia and is mandatory for the inclusion in gene therapy clinical trials. It also offers a means of identifying carriers and establishing presymptomatic diagnoses in families that carry a pathogenic change. The rate of mutation detection via next generation sequencing has been reported as high as 94% [25]. In cases of unidentified mutations, it is important to request sequencing of the above mentioned deep-intronic and promoter regions, that are not routinely sequenced, to check for pathogenic variations. In addition, functional in-vitro assay that measure levels of REP1 in peripheral blood cells and its prenylation activity [17], can support clinical diagnosis and confirm variants of uncertain pathogenicity. In this regard, choroideremia is different to retinitis pigmentosa, because the unique choroideremia phenotype can justify the additional resources needed to sequence the entire CHM genomic region.

3.1. Genotype–Phenotype Correlation in Choroideremia

Although the clinical phenotype can vary in terms of the age of onset of retinal degeneration and rate of progression, no evidence has been found for genotype–phenotype correlation with regard to onset of symptoms, decline in visual acuity and visual fields [23–25], or in the residual retinal area of fundus autofluorescence [25]. The reasons for this are not fully understood, but the lack of correlation may be due to the near universal absence of REP1 irrespective of the causative mutation that range from single point missense changes to whole gene deletions. The phenotypic variation in choroideremia may in part be explained by the degree to which the absence of REP1 can be compensated by other prenylation proteins such as REP2, which shares 95% of its amino acid sequence with REP1 [26,27].

In addition, genetic modifiers and environmental factors may play roles in the onset and progression of degeneration in choroideremia.

3.2. Molecular Mechanisms of Choroideremia

The molecular mechanisms involved in the pathology of choroideremia have recently been reviewed in great detail [5]. However, some basic concepts are worth re-stating and outlining to aid understanding of the disease. The gene that is disrupted in choroideremia produces REP1 protein. Unlike in many other inherited retinal diseases, this protein is not directly involved in the process of phototransduction or in cellular signalling within the retina. Instead, REP1 is a key player in the addition of prenyl groups (prenylation) to the Rab family of GTPases (Rabs). Such hydrophobic prenyl groups are thought to be necessary to anchor Rabs to the membranes of intracellular organelles and vesicles [28].

In the absence of REP1, there is an observable deficit in the prenylation of several different types of Rabs, and their association with membranes appears to be impaired [29]. Because Rabs themselves act as important regulators of intracellular membrane trafficking, many fundamental cellular processes can potentially be impacted by this deficit. Information from a variety of sources points to a deficit in melanosome trafficking, a delay in phagosome degradation and an accelerated accumulation of intracellular deposits in RPE cells caused by loss of REP1 [4,18,30–33]. The cellular deficits of photoreceptors themselves have been less studied, but it has been suggested that there is mislocalisation of opsin and shortening of photoreceptor outer segments in mice that is independent of RPE degeneration [4].

Fortunately, the absence of REP1 does not appear to be catastrophic for all human cells, which is likely due to the fact that there is a built-in redundancy in this system, provided by the presence of the *CHML* gene [34,35]. The *CHML* gene is thought to be an autosomal retrogene of *CHM*, created by the reverse transcription of the mRNA of the original gene and reinsertion in a new genomic location that occurred sometime during vertebrate evolution. The protein product of *CHML*, known as REP2, appears to be able to largely compensate for the loss of REP1. Although a prenylation deficit of certain Rabs can be detected in several cell types of the body [29,36,37], a single report of a systemic, blood-related, clinical phenotype have not been substantiated [38,39] and loss of REP1 appears to cause cellular dysfunction and death that is limited to specific ocular tissues and manifest as a specific disease of the retina. Differential spatial expression does not provide an obvious answer, as both REP1 and REP2 are expressed ubiquitously.

In truth, the reason why absence of REP1 drives a specific degeneration of the RPE and photoreceptor cells remains a mystery. Perhaps more than other cell types, RPE and photoreceptor cells require acute and sensitive regulation of intracellular membrane trafficking to fulfil their cellular functions. Combined with the fact that there is not any appreciable post-natal replacement of these cells, it may simply be that these cell types are sensitive to the generalised, ongoing prenylation deficit, become 'worn-out' early than usual, and undergo a type of accelerated aging and cell death. Alternatively, it has been proposed that REP1 has a selective affinity to particular Rabs that are of special significance to the cell types affected in the disease. For example, it has been suggested there is a particular requirement for correctly prenylated Rab27a to mediate melanosome trafficking in RPE cells [29,40] and Rab6, 8 and 11 might be important in targeting rhodopsin-bearing vesicles to the photoreceptor outer segment [41,42]. Biochemical assays have suggested that REP1and REP2 have largely overlapping substrate specificities but differences in the association with other catalytic units within the prenylation process might contribute instead [43–45].

3.3. Gene Therapy for Choroideremia

Gene based therapies show great promise for the treatment of inherited retinal disease, including choroideremia [46]. Recent advances have paved a successful progression of gene therapy clinical trials on choroideremia (Table 1). The first phase I/II trial started in Oxford, UK in 2011, using a subretinal delivery of AAV2-REP1 in 14 male patients with choroideremia [9,10]. The two-year trial results were recently reported [11] with median gains in visual acuity (measured by Early Treatment Diabetic Retinopathy Study, ETDRS chart) of 4.5 letters in treated eyes versus 1.5 letter loss in untreated eyes across the cohort at 24 months post treatment. Six treated eyes gained more than 5 ETDRS letters. In two patients with the greatest gains in visual acuity, improvements were noted by 6 months post treatment, and sustained at up to 5 years of follow-up. Two patients in the cohort had complications, one related to surgery (retinal overstretch and incomplete vector dosing) and the other had postoperative inflammation. Both of these events resulted in protocol changes which included developing an automated subretinal injection system and a more prolonged post-operative immunosuppressive regimen.

These encouraging safety and efficacy signals prompted additional trials using the same vector (sponsored by Nightstar Therapeutics, UK) at other international sites including Canada (NCT02077361), USA (NCT02553135) and Germany (NCT02671539) all reporting similar results [12–14], following which a phase III trial started in 2017 at multiple international sites. Independent to the Nightstar led trials, another phase I/II trial (NCT02341807) using a similar AAV vector construct (without the woodchuck hepatitis virus posttranscriptional regulatory element) begun in 2015 in Philadelphia, USA. The results of this trial are expected in the coming years.

The above-mentioned early phase I/II gene therapy clinical trials recruited patients with advanced disease with early efficacy signals suggesting that vision can be restored following treatment. Reassuring safety data, following improvements in the surgical technique, prompted initiation of a phase II trial (NCT02407678) sponsored by University of Oxford that included patients with early central degeneration and normal visual acuity. The REGENERATE trial recently completed recruitment of 30 male patients with choroideremia with prediction that earlier intervention might slow down or halt the degeneration prior to irreversible structural disorganisation.

The solstice study is an observational, long-term follow up study of 100 participants that will evaluate the safety and efficacy of the AAV2-REP1 used in the above-mentioned interventional choroideremia trials.

The outcomes of clinical trials are measured in terms of clearly defined clinical endpoints, which predict the success and ultimately the approval of new treatments. These outcomes must be selected carefully to capture the most sensitive and reliable measures of the disease progression during the course of a clinical trial and will critically depend on the stage of retinal degeneration. In the reported choroideremia trials, the primary endpoint was the change from baseline in best-corrected visual acuity (BCVA) in the treated eye compared to the untreated eye with evidence of gains in vision after gene therapy in treated eyes. This suggests that BCVA can be used as a viable primary outcome in cases of advanced choroideremia, where disease process has already affected the visual acuity. Indeed, the phase III STAR trial is using BCVA as a primary outcome measure. However, in patients with early disease stage with near-normal vision, BCVA may not be the most sensitive outcome measure, especially since the visual loss in choroideremia typically progresses very slowly. Thus, for the REGENERATE trial, secondary endpoints including the measure of central visual field by microperimetry and anatomical measures such as fundus autofluorescence and optical coherence tomography may prove to be additional valuable outcomes. However, measurements of these secondary outcomes may not always be straightforward, and need to be interpreted with caution. For example, the remaining autofluorescence area may not be easily demarcated, even with the use of automated algorithms, which may influence area measurements especially following sub-retinal gene therapy which may differentially affect central (para-foveal) and peripheral areas of the treated island.

4. Should We Treat Female Carriers in the Future?

Heterozygous female choroideremia carriers often show generalized RPE mottling due to random X-inactivation (Figure 3A–F) and are usually asymptomatic or show early deficits in dark adaptation. In some carriers a coarser pattern of degeneration is seen, with patches of atrophy interspersed with normal tissue (Figure 3G–L). Usually, a mild reduction in retinal function is observed with this carrier phenotype. Occasionally, however, female carriers manifest with more severe male-like pattern of retinal degeneration with associated deficit in visual function [47]. This is most likely the result of skewed X-inactivation, or the proportion of cells expressing the mutant X chromosome, which occurs during early retinal development.

Choroideremia gene therapy trials are currently including affected male subjects only. For the majority of female carriers who are mildly affected and asymptomatic or have minor deficits in night vision or visual fields, treatment may not be necessary. Such functional deficits are usually slowly progressing with the majority of cases being able to maintain driving standard vision. However, the more severe female carrier phenotypes, with associated visual field loss and reduction in visual acuity, are likely to benefit from gene therapy and could be included in future clinical trials. Careful characterisation and geneotype-phenotypes correlations will help with the inclusion criteria and give insight into the optimal timing for successful gene therapy.

5. Alternative Therapies

The potential therapy that has been discussed in this review is gene replacement/augmentation therapy. This is the therapy that has advanced the furthest clinically but there are other potential therapies worth considering.

Instead of adding a working copy of the *CHM* gene, it may instead be possible to alter the patient's own copy with gene editing. Techniques to achieve this, such as zinc finger nucleases or Tal-effector nucleases (TALENs), have existed for some time, but the clinical relevance of these techniques has been somewhat limited by the low editing efficiencies generally achieved. The development of CRISPR/Cas (clustered regularly interspaced short palindromic repeats/CRISPR-associated nuclease 9) technology has given gene editing a renaissance for two reasons. Firstly, gene-editing efficiency appears to be generally better, with the potential to be more clinically meaningful. Secondly, in the CRISPR/Cas9 system, most of the investigational medicinal product can remain the same and only a specific RNA guide sequence needs to be developed to target a site within the disease specific gene—this is more attractive in terms of a clinical development pathway. Gene editing therapy is most useful when there is a need to correct or silence a mutated gene, such as when a missense mutation leads to production of dominant negative or toxic gain-of-function protein, which normally manifests as autosomal dominant and semi-dominant disease [48]. Because the vast majority of mutations in choroideremia are effectively null and therefore result in no detectable protein [24] there is no compelling need to develop a gene editing approach, and simply adding a correct copy as an episomal transgene would be sufficient to result in a therapeutic effect. Correcting the genomic copy of the gene might provide higher confidence of a correct and sustained level of expression, given that the gene would be subject to regulation by its normal transcriptional regulation and epigenetic environment. However, there is evidence that expression from a transgene can be sustained for years when using the appropriate delivery vector and expression cassette [49]. For choroideremia, there is no cell type in which ectopic expression may be predicted to cause a problem, as the protein in normally ubiquitously expressed. In terms of the level of expression, we know that the level of restored REP1 expression is inversely proportional to the prenylation deficit, and so far there is no evidence of overexpression causing toxicity [50]. Although it may be theoretically possible to develop a gene editing approach for some mutations that cause choroideremia, using CRISPR/Cas9, the effectiveness of such strategies has not yet been well established in the retina. Therefore, as gene editing might offer only marginal benefits over gene replacement, it is not currently an attractive strategy of treating choroideremia.

Another therapy that has been suggested and developed is the use of drug-stimulated translational read-through (RT) of premature termination codons (PTC). Nonsense mutations arise when a point mutation converts an amino-acid codon into a PTC that can cause premature translational termination of the mRNA, and subsequently inhibit normal full-length protein expression. Occasionally, instead of translational termination, read-through occurs. Here, a partial mispairing of codon–anticodon is successful, an amino acid is incorporated and protein synthesis continues. Small molecule translational read-through inducing drugs (TRIDs) exist that form the basis of the proposed therapy [51]. Nonsense mutations are the cause of choroideremia in over 30% of patients [52], so, although this will not be appropriate for all patients, there is a significant proportion in which it might be used.

Translational read-through inducing drugs have been used in clinical trials for life-limiting congenital diseases, such as Duchenne muscular dystrophy (DMD) and cystic fibrosis. Early trials appeared to successfully suppress premature stop mutations in patients, but there were concerns over toxicity and the need for repeated intramuscular or intravenous dosing. A newer read-through drug, Ataluren (PTC124), showed a good safety profile when administered orally and the clinical benefit shown in DMD has led to its approval in the EU for this disease [53]. Although no adverse effects have been observed so far, even the approximately 48 weeks of administration given in the clinical studies do not approach the decades of treatment that would be necessary for choroideremia. Preclinical work in the lower-vertebrate, zebrafish model has been important in developing the proof-of-concept, as this is currently the only existing model of choroideremia with a nonsense mutation [54,55]. However, absence of the CHML (REP2) gene in zebrafish means that the CHM mutation is lethal—translational read-through inducing drugs increase the lifespan of the zebrafish model but this is outcome is not directly clinically relevant. The ability of TRIDs to rescue the Rab prenylation defect in fibroblast of a patient with a particular choroideremia nonsense mutation is encouraging, despite the fact that levels of full-length REP1 protein remained below the level of detection [55]. Given the relatively slow disease progression and the potential risks and cost to the patient from long-term administration of TRIDs, it would be judicious to establish that the correction of the prenylation deficit by TRIDs is present in fibroblast from patients with the equivalent nonsense mutations in which treatment will be attempted in any clinical study [56].

It might be argued that systemic or ocular administration of TRIDs has the potential to treat a larger area of retina when compared to gene therapy, as the former might spread by local diffusion while the latter is limited by the extent of the subretinal bleb. However, to our knowledge, the local concentration achieved in the posterior segment of the eye has never been measured when TRIDs are taken orally or administered locally. The effect of TRIDs appears to often follow an inverted u-shaped dose-response curve, so the pharmacokinetics of therapy may be critical important [57]. Until such questions are addressed, it would appear that translational read-through inducing drugs do not represent a superior strategy compared to gene replacement therapy.

Recent work has identified that antisense oligonucleotides (AONs) may also provide another potential therapy for choroideremia [58]. In some cases of choroideremia, deep-intronic mutations can create a cryptic splice acceptor site that results in the insertion of a pseudoexon in the *CHM* transcript. This disrupts gene function, and specific AONs can be designed to bind to the pre-mRNA and redirect the splicing process, potentially returning it to a normal, working transcript [59,60]. For choroideremia, AONs therapy has shown some promising in vitro results but is further along the clinical development pathway for several inherited disorders, including other forms of inherited retinal dystrophy [59,60]. As AON therapy relies on particular types of mutations, it will not be relevant for all cases of choroideremia and such a strategy is most attractive when conventional gene replacement therapy is not possible because of the large size of the coding sequence of the genes involved, such as in *CEP290*-associated Leber congenital amaurosis [59,60].

The therapies above aim to slow down or stop the degeneration of the retina and RPE and are obviously the preferred choice. However, it is also worth considering strategies that might restore vision in the late stages of the disease, when the majority of photoreceptors have already been lost. Cell transplantation is an interesting strategy for the treatment of inherited retinal disease, but this might present a significant challenge in late-stage choroideremia, where RPE and choroid have been lost along with the degenerating photoreceptors. A more feasible approach may be to use some form of retinal prosthesis. Although most systems rely on surviving inner retinal layers, with intact ganglion cell nerve conduction, there is no dependence on survival of the RPE, photoreceptors or choroid. The Argus II retinal prosthesis, an epiretinal device approved for commercial use in advanced retinal degeneration in the EU and USA, has been implanted in at least one patient with choroideremia [61]. This device has a very good safety profile and various improvements in visual function have been reported, although these vary widely between individuals [62]. Other devices exist or are in development (44-channel suprachoriodal Bionic Eye Device (NCT03406416) Melbourne, Australia and Intelligent Retinal Implant System, IRIS V1 (NCT01864486) and V2 (NCT02670980) Pixium Vision SA) that could theoretically restore much greater levels of visual function than the Argus II, however, stopping cell loss, even at a late-stage will likely still result in a better functional outcome. Another potential therapy to restore vision in choroideremia is to render the remaining cells of the retina sensitive to light by ectopically expressing light-sensitive ion channels or opsins. This strategy, known as optogenetics, has its own considerations and challenges, which will not be discussed extensively here. Suffice to say, a number of systems are in various stages of pre-clinical development and are beginning to be investigated in clinical trials [63–65]. Again, the level of vision that can be restored by this method is likely to be relatively crude, however, this is likely to be comparable to any retinal prosthesis and may offer specific benefits such as less invasive surgery and potential restoration of a wider visual field.

6. Summary

Molecular mechanisms in choroideremia are well established. Ultimately, the absence or reduced prenylation of REP1 activity disrupts intracellular trafficking pathways leading to accumulation of toxic products and premature degeneration of the retina and vision less. Logically then, replacement of REP1 to the retinal tissue, via gene-based therapy, could restore cellular function and slow down the degeneration. Multiple clinical trials are underway testing this hypothesis. The trials are using subretinal delivery of AAV2-REP1 to target surviving central islands of the retina with promising safety and early efficacy results.

Despite ubiquitous expression of REP1, a robust systemic association with choroideremia has not been identified, although the prenylation defect is visible in assays of the peripheral blood cells. This assay can be used to support the diagnosis of choroideremia. It is not known why the retina is the only part of the body that becomes clinically affected by the lack of REP1 activity. Moreover, the complex interactions between different retinal cell types during the pathogenesis of choroideremia mean that it is difficult to deconvolve the exact order in which RPE, photoreceptors and the choroid degenerate. It appears likely that the RPE is directly affected by the loss of REP1, and is a key driver of pathogenesis, but the importance of primary or secondary degeneration of photoreceptors is less clear. Elucidating these mechanisms may help us to understand what triggers the onset of clinically significant degeneration and how the rate of degeneration in each cell type might be affected following treatment.

Evidence to date has shown no apparent genotype–phenotype correlation within the spectrum of reported *CHM* mutations, with regard to the onset of symptoms and the rate of functional visual decline. Since variations in male phenotypes cannot be explained by mutations in *CHM* only, genetic modifiers or environmental factors must play a role in the onset and progression of degeneration in choroideremia. Ongoing natural history studies are adding insight into the progression of the disease and the characteristics of the clinical phenotype that will help to establish the optimal therapeutic window for choroideremia. Female carriers should be enrolled into natural history studies with aim to offer gene therapy (under the realm of clinical trials) to those affected by skewed X inactivation.

Author Contributions: Writing: J.C.K. and A.R.B. Revision: J.C.K. and A.R.B. Supervision: R.E.M.

Funding: This research was funded by Oxford NIHR Biomedical Research Centre, Oxford, UK and Medical Research Council UK; JCK is also funded by Global Ophthalmology Awards Fellowship, Bayer, Switzerland.

Conflicts of Interest: REM is a founder and receives grant funding from Nightstar Therapeutics (now Biogen Inc.). REM and ARB are consultants to Nightstar Therapeutics and REM is a consultant to Spark Therapeutics. These companies did not have any input into the work presented.

References

1. Cremers, F.P.; van de Pol, D.J.; van Kerkhoff, L.P.; Wieringa, B.; Ropers, H.H. Cloning of a gene that is rearranged in patients with choroideraemia. *Nature* **1990**, *347*, 674–677. [CrossRef] [PubMed]
2. Seabra, M.C.; Brown, M.S.; Goldstein, J.L. Retinal degeneration in choroideremia: Deficiency of rab geranylgeranyl transferase. *Science* **1993**, *259*, 377–381. [CrossRef] [PubMed]
3. Van den Hurk, J.A.; Schwartz, M.; van Bokhoven, H.; Van de Pol, T.J.R.; Bogerd, L.; Pinckers, A.J.L.G.; Bleeker-Wagemakers, E.M.; Pawlowitzki, I.H.; Rüther, K.; Ropers, H.H.; et al. Molecular basis of choroideremia (CHM): Mutations involving the Rab escort protein-1 (*REP-1*) gene. *Hum. Mutat.* **1997**, *9*, 110–117. [CrossRef]
4. Tolmachova, T.; Anders, R.; Abrink, M.; Bugeon, L.; Dallman, M.J.; Futter, C.E.; Ramalho, J.S.; Tonagel, F.; Tanimoto, N.; Seeliger, M.W.; et al. Independent degeneration of photoreceptors and retinal pigment epithelium in conditional knockout mouse models of choroideremia. *J. Clin. Investig.* **2006**, *116*, 386–394. [CrossRef] [PubMed]
5. Patrício, M.I.; Barnard, A.R.; Xue, K.; MacLaren, R.E. Choroideremia: Molecular mechanisms and development of AAV gene therapy. *Expert Opin. Biol. Ther.* **2018**, *18*, 807–820. [CrossRef] [PubMed]
6. Aleman, T.S.; Han, G.; Serrano, L.W.; Fuerst, N.M.; Charlson, E.S.; Pearson, D.J.; Chung, D.C.; Traband, A.; Pan, W.; Ying, G.S.; et al. Natural history of the central structural abnormalities in choroideremia: A Prospective Cross-Sectional Study. *Ophthalmology* **2017**, *124*, 359–373. [CrossRef] [PubMed]
7. Hariri, A.H.; Velaga, S.B.; Girach, A.; Ip, M.S.; Le, P.V.; Lam, B.L.; Fischer, M.D.; Sankila, E.M.; Pennesi, M.E.; Holz, F.G.; et al. Measurement and reproducibility of preserved ellipsoid zone area and preserved retinal pigment epithelium area in eyes with choroideremia. *Am. J. Ophthalmol.* **2017**, *179*, 110–117. [CrossRef] [PubMed]
8. Sun, L.W.; Johnson, R.D.; Williams, V.; Summerfelt, P.; Dubra, A.; Weinberg, D.V.; Stepien, K.E.; Fishman, G.A.; Carroll, J. Multimodal imaging of photoreceptor structure in choroideremia. *PLoS ONE* **2016**, *11*, e0167526. [CrossRef] [PubMed]
9. MacLaren, R.E.; Groppe, M.; Barnard, A.R.; Cottriall, C.L.; Tolmachova, T.; Seymour, L.; Clark, K.R.; During, M.J.; Cremers, F.P.; Black, G.C.; et al. Retinal gene therapy in patients with choroideremia: Initial findings from a phase 1/2 clinical trial. *Lancet* **2014**, *383*, 1129–1137. [CrossRef]
10. Edwards, T.L.; Jolly, J.K.; Groppe, M.; Barnard, A.R.; Cottriall, C.L.; Tolmachova, T.; Black, G.C.; Webster, A.R.; Lotery, A.J.; Holder, G.E.; et al. Visual Acuity after Retinal Gene Therapy for Choroideremia. *N. Engl. J. Med.* **2016**, *374*, 1996–1998. [CrossRef]
11. Xue, K.; Jolly, J.K.; Barnard, A.R.; Rudenko, A.; Salvetti, A.P.; Patrício, M.I.; Edwards, T.L.; Groppe, M.; Orlans, H.O.; Tolmachova, T.; et al. Beneficial effects on vision in patients undergoing retinal gene therapy for choroideremia. *Nat. Med.* **2018**, *24*, 1507–1512. [CrossRef] [PubMed]
12. Dimopoulos, I.S.; Hoang, S.C.; Radziwon, A.; Binczyk, N.M.; Seabra, M.C.; MacLaren, R.E.; Somani, R.; Tennant, M.T.; MacDonald, I.M. Two-year results after aav2-mediated gene therapy for choroideremia: The Alberta experience. *Am. J. Ophthalmol.* **2018**, *193*, 130–142. [CrossRef] [PubMed]
13. Lam, B.L.; Davis, J.L.; Gregori, N.Z.; MacLaren, R.E.; Girach, A.; Verriotto, J.D.; Rodriguez, B.; Rosa, P.R.; Zhang, X.; Feuer, W.J. Choroideremia Gene Therapy Phase 2 Clinical Trial: 24-Month Results. *Am. J. Ophthalmol.* **2019**, *197*, 65–73. [CrossRef] [PubMed]
14. Fischer, M.D.; Ochakovski, G.A.; Beier, B.; Seitz, I.P.; Vaheb, Y.; Kortuem, C.; Reichel, F.F.; Kuehlewein, L.; Kahle, N.A.; Peters, T.; et al. Changes in retinal sensitivity after gene therapy in choroideremia. *Retina* **2018**. [CrossRef] [PubMed]
15. Jolly, J.K.; Xue, K.; Edwards, T.L.; Groppe, M.; MacLaren, R.E. Characterizing the natural history of visual function in choroideremia using microperimetry and multimodal retinal imaging. *Investig. Ophthalmol. Vis. Sci.* **2017**, *58*, 5575–5583. [CrossRef] [PubMed]
16. Hariri, A.H.; Ip, M.S.; Girach, A.; Lam, B.L.; Fischer, M.D.; Sankila, E.M.; Pennesi, M.E.; Holz, F.G.; Maclaren, R.E.; Birch, D.G.; et al. Macular spatial distribution of preserved autofluorescence in patients with choroideremia. For Natural History of the Progression of Choroideremia (NIGHT) Study Group. *Br. J. Ophthalmol.* **2019**, *103*, 933–937. [CrossRef] [PubMed]

17. Patrício, M.I.; Barnard, A.R.; Cox, C.I.; Blue, C.; MacLaren, R.E. The Biological Activity of AAV Vectors for Choroideremia Gene Therapy Can Be Measured by In Vitro Prenylation of RAB6A. *Mol. Ther. Methods Clin. Dev.* **2018**, *9*, 288–295. [CrossRef]
18. Syed, N.; Smith, J.E.; John, S.K.; Seabra, M.C.; Aguirre, G.D.; Milam, A.H. Evaluation of retinal photoreceptors and pigment epithelium in a female carrier of choroideremia. *Ophthalmology* **2001**, *108*, 711–720. [CrossRef]
19. Morgan, J.I.; Han, G.; Klinman, E.; Maguire, W.M.; Chung, D.C.; Maguire, A.M.; Bennett, J. High-resolution adaptive optics retinal imaging of cellular structure in choroideremia. *Investig. Ophthalmol. Vis. Sci.* **2014**, *55*, 6381–6397. [CrossRef]
20. Xue, K.; Oldani, M.; Jolly, J.K.; Edwards, T.L.; Groppe, M.; Downes, S.M.; MacLaren, R.E. Correlation of Optical Coherence Tomography and Autofluorescence in the Outer Retina and Choroid of Patients with Choroideremia. *Investig. Ophthalmol. Vis. Sci.* **2016**, *57*, 3674–3684. [CrossRef]
21. Aylward, J.W.; Xue, K.; Patrício, M.I.; Jolly, J.K.; Wood, J.C.; Brett, J.; Jasani, K.M.; MacLaren, R.E. Retinal Degeneration in Choroideremia follows an Exponential Decay Function. *Ophthalmology* **2018**, *125*, 1122–1124. [CrossRef] [PubMed]
22. Ramsden, S.C.; O'Grady, A.; Fletcher, T.; O'Sullivan, J.; Hart-Holden, N.; Barton, S.J.; Hall, G.; Moore, A.T.; Webster, A.R.; Black, G.C. A clinical molecular genetic service for United Kingdom families with choroideraemia. *Eur. J. Med. Genet.* **2013**, *56*, 432–438. [CrossRef] [PubMed]
23. Freund, P.; Furgoch, M.; MacDonald, I. Genotype—Phenotype analysis of male subjects affected by choroideremia. *Investig. Ophthalmol. Vis. Sci.* **2013**, *54*, 1567.
24. Freund, P.R.; Sergeev, Y.V.; MacDonald, I.M. Analysis of a large choroideremia dataset does not suggest a preference for inclusion of certain genotypes in future trials of gene therapy. *Mol. Genet. Genomic Med.* **2016**, *4*, 344–358. [CrossRef] [PubMed]
25. Simunovic, M.P.; Jolly, J.K.; Xue, K.; Edwards, T.L.; Groppe, M.; Downes, S.M.; MacLaren, R.E. The Spectrum of CHM Gene Mutations in Choroideremia and Their Relationship to Clinical Phenotype. *Investig. Ophthalmol. Vis. Sci.* **2016**, *57*, 6033–6039. [CrossRef] [PubMed]
26. Carss, K.; Arno, G.; Erwood, M.; Stephens, J.; Sanchis-Juan, A.; Hull, S.; Megy, K.; Grozeva, D.; Dewhurst, E.; Malka, S.; et al. Comprehensive rare variant analysis via whole-genome sequencing to determine the molecular pathology of inherited retinal disease. *Am. J. Hum. Genet.* **2017**, *100*, 75–90. [CrossRef]
27. Radziwon, A.; Arno, G.K.; Wheaton, D.; McDonagh, E.M.; Baple, E.L.; Webb-Jones, K.G.; Birch, D.; Webster, A.R.; MacDonald, I.M. Single-base substitutions in the CHM promoter as a cause of choroideremia. *Hum. Mutat.* **2017**, *38*, 704–715. [CrossRef] [PubMed]
28. Zhang, F.L.; Casey, P.J. Protein prenylation: Molecular mechanisms and functional consequences. *Ann. Rev. Biochem.* **1996**, *65*, 241–269. [CrossRef]
29. Seabra, M.C.; Ho, Y.K.; Anant, J.S. Deficient geranylgeranylation of Ram/Rab27 in choroideremia. *J. Biol. Chem.* **1995**, *270*, 24420–24427. [CrossRef]
30. Gordiyenko, N.V.; Fariss, R.N.; Zhi, C.; MacDonald, I.M. Silencing of the CHM gene alters phagocytic and secretory pathways in the retinal pigment epithelium. *Investig. Ophthalmol. Vis. Sci.* **2010**, *51*, 1143–1150. [CrossRef]
31. Tolmachova, T.; Wavre-Shapton, S.T.; Barnard, A.R.; MacLaren, R.E.; Futter, C.E.; Seabra, M.C. Retinal pigment epithelium defects accelerate photoreceptor degeneration in cell type-specific knock-out mouse models of Choroideremia. *Investig. Ophthalmol. Vis. Sci.* **2010**, *51*, 4913–4920. [CrossRef] [PubMed]
32. Wavre-Shapton, S.T.; Tolmachova, T.; da Silva, M.L.; Futter, C.E.; Seabra, M.C. Conditional ablation of the choroideremia gene causes age-related changes in mouse retinal pigment epithelium. *PLoS ONE* **2013**, *8*, e57769. [CrossRef]
33. Flannery, J.G.; Bird, A.C.; Farber, D.B.; Weleber, R.G.; Bok, D. A histopathologic study of a choroideremia carrier. *Investig. Ophthalmol. Vis. Sci.* **1990**, *31*, 229–236.
34. Cremers, F.P.; Molloy, C.M.; van de Pol, D.J.; van den Hurk, J.A.; Bach, I.; Geurts van Kessel, A.H.; Ropers, H.H. An autosomal homologue of the choroideremia gene colocalizes with the Usher syndrome type II locus on the distal part of chromosome 1q. *Hum. Mol. Genet.* **1992**, *1*, 71–75. [CrossRef] [PubMed]
35. Cremers, F.P.M.; Armstrong, S.A.; Seabra, M.C.; Brown, M.S.; Goldstein, J.L. REP-2, a Rab escort protein encoded by the choroideremia-like gene. *J. Biol. Chem.* **1994**, *269*, 2111–2117. [PubMed]
36. Anand, V.; Barral, D.C.; Zeng, Y.; Brunsmann, F.; Maguire, A.M.; Seabra, M.C.; Bennett, J. Gene therapy for choroideremia: In vitro rescue mediated by recombinant adenovirus. *Vis. Res.* **2003**, *43*, 919–926. [CrossRef]

37. Tolmachova, T.; Tolmachov, O.E.; Wavre-Shapton, S.T.; Tracey-White, D.; Futter, C.E.; Seabra, M.C. CHM/REP1 cDNA delivery by lentiviral vectors provides functional expression of the transgene in the retinal pigment epithelium of choroideremia mice. *J. Gene Med.* **2012**, *14*, 158–168. [CrossRef]
38. Zhang, A.Y.; Mysore, N.; Vali, H.; Koenekoop, J.; Cao, S.N.; Li, S.; Ren, H.; Keser, V.; Lopez-Solache, I.; Siddiqui, S.N.; et al. Choroideremia Is a Systemic Disease with Lymphocyte Crystals and Plasma Lipid and RBC Membrane Abnormalities. *Investig. Ophthalmol. Vis. Sci.* **2015**, *56*, 8158–8165. [CrossRef]
39. Radziwon, A.; Cho, W.J.; Szkotak, A.; Suh, M.; MacDonald, I.M. Crystals and Fatty Acid Abnormalities Are Not Present in Circulating Cells from Choroideremia Patients. *Investig. Ophthalmol. Vis. Sci.* **2018**, *59*, 4464–4470. [CrossRef]
40. Futter, C.E.; Ramalho, J.S.; Jaissle, G.B.; Seeliger, M.W.; Seabra, M.C. The role of Rab27a in the regulation of melanosome distribution within retinal pigment epithelial cells. *Mol. Biol. Cell* **2004**, *15*, 2264–2275. [CrossRef]
41. Kwok, M.C.M.; Holopainen, J.M.; Molday, L.L.; Foster, L.J.; Molday, R.S. Proteomics of photoreceptor outer segments identifies a subset of SNARE and Rab proteins implicated in membrane vesicle trafficking and fusion. *Mol. Cell Proteom.* **2008**, *7*, 1053–1066. [CrossRef] [PubMed]
42. Wang, J.; Deretic, D. Molecular complexes that direct rhodopsin transport to primary cilia. *Prog. Retin. Eye Res.* **2014**, *38*, 1–19. [CrossRef] [PubMed]
43. Larijani, B.; Hume, A.N.; Tarafder, A.K.; Seabra, M.C. Multiple factors contribute to inefficient prenylation of Rab27a in Rab Prenylation diseases. *J. Biol. Chem.* **2003**, *278*, 46798–46804. [CrossRef] [PubMed]
44. Rak, A.; Pylypenko, O.; Niculae, A.; Pyatkov, K.; Goody, R.S.; Alexandrov, K. Structure of the Rab7: REP-1 Complex. *Cell* **2004**, *117*, 749–760. [CrossRef] [PubMed]
45. Köhnke, M.; Delon, C.; Hastie, M.L.; Nguyen, U.T.; Wu, Y.W.; Waldmann, H.; Goody, R.S.; Gorman, J.J.; Alexandrov, K. Rab GTPase prenylation hierarchy and its potential role in choroideremia disease. *PLoS ONE* **2013**, *8*, e81758. [CrossRef] [PubMed]
46. Barnard, A.R.; Groppe, M.; MacLaren, R.E. Gene therapy for choroideremia using an adeno-associated viral (AAV) vector. *Cold Spring Harb. Perspect. Med.* **2014**, *5*, a017293. [CrossRef] [PubMed]
47. Edwards, T.L.; Groppe, M.; Jolly, J.K.; Downes, S.M.; MacLaren, R.E. Correlation of retinal structure and function in choroideremia carriers. *Ophthalmology* **2015**, *122*, 1274–1276. [CrossRef]
48. Diakatou, M.; Manes, G.; Bocquet, B.; Meunier, I.; Kalatzis, V. Genome Editing as a Treatment for the Most Prevalent Causative Genes of Autosomal Dominant Retinitis Pigmentosa. *Int. J. Mol. Sci.* **2019**, *20*, 2542. [CrossRef]
49. Cideciyan, A.V.; Jacobson, S.G.; Beltran, W.A.; Sumaroka, A.; Swider, M.; Iwabe, S.; Roman, A.J.; Olivares, M.B.; Schwartz, S.B.; Komaromy, A.M.; et al. Human retinal gene therapy for Leber congenital amaurosis shows advancing retinal degeneration despite enduring visual improvement. *Proc. Natl. Acad. Sci. USA* **2013**, *110*, E517–E525. [CrossRef]
50. Tolmachova, T.; Tolmachov, O.E.; Barnard, A.R.; de Silva, S.R.; Lipinski, D.M.; Walker, N.J.; Maclaren, R.E.; Seabra, M.C. Functional expression of Rab escort protein 1 following AAV2-mediated gene delivery in the retina of choroideremia mice and human cells ex vivo. *J. Mol. Med.* **2013**, *91*, 825–837. [CrossRef]
51. Nagel-Wolfrum, K.; Möller, F.; Penner, I.; Baasov, T.; Wolfrum, U. Targeting Nonsense Mutations in Diseases with Translational Read-Through-Inducing Drugs (TRIDs). *BioDrugs* **2016**, *30*, 49–74. [CrossRef]
52. Moosajee, M.; Ramsden, S.C.; Black, G.C.; Seabra, M.C.; Webster, A.R. Clinical utility gene card for: Choroideremia. *Eur. J. Hum. Genet.* **2014**, *22*, 572. [CrossRef]
53. McDonald, C.M.; Campbell, C.; Torricelli, R.E.; Finkel, R.S.; Flanigan, K.M.; Goemans, N.; Heydemann, P.; Kaminska, A.; Kirschner, J.; Muntoni, F.; et al. Clinical Evaluator Training Group; ACT DMD Study Group. Ataluren in patients with nonsense mutation Duchenne muscular dystrophy (ACT DMD): A multicentre, randomised, double-blind, placebo-controlled, phase 3 trial. *Lancet* **2017**, *390*, 1489–1498. [CrossRef]
54. Moosajee, M.; Gregory-Evans, K.; Ellis, C.D.; Seabra, M.C.; Gregory-Evans, C.Y. Translational bypass of nonsense mutations in zebrafish rep1, pax2.1 and lamb1 highlights a viable therapeutic option for untreatable genetic eye disease. *Hum. Mol. Genet.* **2008**, *17*, 3987–4000. [CrossRef]
55. Moosajee, M.; Tracey-White, D.; Smart, M.; Weetall, M.; Torriano, S.; Kalatzis, V.; da Cruz, L.; Coffey, P.; Webster, A.R.; Welch, E. Functional rescue of REP1 following treatment with PTC124 and novel derivative PTC-414 in human choroideremia fibroblasts and the nonsense-mediated zebrafish model. *Hum. Mol. Genet.* **2016**, *25*, 3416–3431. [CrossRef]

56. Torriano, S.; Erkilic, N.; Baux, D.; Cereso, N.; De Luca, V.; Meunier, I.; Moosajee, M.; Roux, A.F.; Hamel, C.P.; Kalatzis, V. The effect of PTC124 on choroideremia fibroblasts and iPSC-derived RPE raises considerations for therapy. *Sci. Rep.* **2018**, *8*, 8234. [CrossRef]
57. Dabrowski, M.; Bukowy-Bieryllo, Z.; Zietkiewicz, E. Advances in therapeutic use of a drug-stimulated translational readthrough of premature termination codons. *Mol. Med.* **2018**, *24*, 25. [CrossRef]
58. Garanto, A.; van der Velde-Visser, S.D.; Cremers, F.P.M.; Collin, R.W.J. Antisense Oligonucleotide-Based Splice Correction of a Deep-Intronic Mutation in CHM Underlying Choroideremia. *Adv. Exp. Med. Biol.* **2018**, *1074*, 83–89.
59. Collin, R.W.; den Hollander, A.I.; van der Velde-Visser, S.D.; Bennicelli, J.; Bennett, J.; Cremers, F.P. Antisense Oligonucleotide (AON)-based Therapy for Leber Congenital Amaurosis Caused by a Frequent Mutation in CEP290. *Mol. Ther. Nucleic Acids.* **2012**, *1*, e14. [CrossRef]
60. Gerard, X.; Perrault, I.; Hanein, S.; Silva, E.; Bigot, K.; Defoort-Delhemmes, S.; Rio, M.; Munnich, A.; Scherman, D.; Kaplan, J.; et al. AON-mediated Exon Skipping Restores Ciliation in Fibroblasts Harboring the Common Leber Congenital Amaurosis CEP290 Mutation. *Mol. Ther. Nucleic Acids.* **2012**, *1*, e29. [CrossRef]
61. Parmeggiani, F.; De Nadai, K.; Piovan, A.; Binotto, A.; Zamengo, S.; Chizzolini, M. Optical coherence tomography imaging in the management of the Argus II retinal prosthesis system. *Eur. J. Ophthalmol.* **2017**, *27*, e16–e21. [CrossRef]
62. Luo, Y.H.; da Cruz, L. The Argus® II Retinal Prosthesis System. *Prog. Retin. Eye Res.* **2016**, *50*, 89–107. [CrossRef]
63. Simunovic, M.P.; Shen, W.; Lin, J.Y.; Protti, D.A.; Lisowski, L.; Gillies, M.C. Optogenetic approaches to vision restoration. *Exp. Eye Res.* **2019**, *178*, 15–26. [CrossRef]
64. Cehajic-Kapetanovic, J.; Eleftheriou, C.; Allen, A.E.; Milosavljevic, N.; Pienaar, A.; Bedford, R.; Davis, K.E.; Bishop, P.N.; Lucas, R.J. Restoration of Vision with Ectopic Expression of Human Rod Opsin. *Curr. Biol.* **2015**, *25*, 2111–2122. [CrossRef]
65. Eleftheriou, C.G.; Cehajic-Kapetanovic, J.; Martial, F.P.; Milosavljevic, N.; Bedford, R.A.; Lucas, R.J. Meclofenamic acid improves the signal to noise ratio for visual responses produced by ectopic expression of human rod opsin. *Mol. Vis.* **2017**, *23*, 334–345.

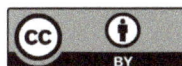

© 2019 by the authors. Licensee MDPI, Basel, Switzerland. This article is an open access article distributed under the terms and conditions of the Creative Commons Attribution (CC BY) license (http://creativecommons.org/licenses/by/4.0/).

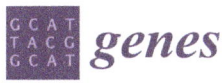

Review

Molecular Strategies for *RPGR* Gene Therapy

Jasmina Cehajic Kapetanovic [1,2,*], Michelle E McClements [1], Cristina Martinez-Fernandez de la Camara [1,2] and Robert E MacLaren [1,2]

1. Nuffield Laboratory of Ophthalmology, University of Oxford, Oxford OX3 9DU, UK
2. Oxford Eye Hospital, Oxford University Hospitals NHS Foundation Trust, Oxford OX3 9DU, UK
* Correspondence: FRCOphthenquiries@eye.ox.ac.uk

Received: 31 July 2019; Accepted: 1 September 2019; Published: 4 September 2019

Abstract: Mutations affecting the *Retinitis Pigmentosa GTPase Regulator* (*RPGR*) gene are the commonest cause of X-linked and recessive retinitis pigmentosa (RP), accounting for 10%–20% of all cases of RP. The phenotype is one of the most severe amongst all causes of RP, characteristic for its early onset and rapid progression to blindness in young people. At present there is no cure for *RPGR*-related retinal disease. Recently, however, there have been important advances in *RPGR* research from bench to bedside that increased our understanding of *RPGR* function and led to the development of potential therapies, including the progress of adeno-associated viral (AAV)-mediated gene replacement therapy into clinical trials. This manuscript discusses the advances in molecular research, which have connected the RPGR protein with an important post-translational modification, known as glutamylation, that is essential for its optimal function as a key regulator of photoreceptor ciliary transport. In addition, we review key pre-clinical research that addressed challenges encountered during development of therapeutic vectors caused by high infidelity of the *RPGR* genomic sequence. Finally, we discuss the structure of three current phase I/II clinical trials based on three AAV vectors and *RPGR* sequences and link the rationale behind the use of the different vectors back to the bench research that led to their development.

Keywords: *Retinitis Pigmentosa GTPase Regulator*; gene therapy; adeno-associated viral; Retinitis Pigmentosa (RP)

1. Introduction

Inherited retinal diseases, most of which are retinitis pigmentosa (RP), affect 1 in 4000 people worldwide. The hallmark of this heterogeneous group of disorders is premature degeneration of rod and cone photoreceptors that leads to early vision loss. RP can be inherited as an autosomal recessive, dominant, X-linked, oligogenic, or mitochondrial trait. X-linked RP is one of the most severe forms of retinal degeneration and it accounts for 10%–20% of all RP cases [1–3]. To date, only 3 genes have been identified to be associated with X-linked pattern of inheritance. Mutations in the *Retinitis pigmentosa GTPase regulator* (*RPGR*) gene accounts for over 70% of X-linked RP cases whereas less common forms of the disease are caused by retinitis pigmentosa 2 (*RP2*) and 23 (*RP23* or *OFD1*) genes [4,5].

RPGR-related X-linked RP is characterised by severe disease in males with early onset and rapidly progressing sight loss that leads to legal blindness commonly by the fourth decade of life [2]. The classic rod-cone phenotype with peripheral pigmentary retinopathy, waxy optic disc pallor and vascular attenuation makes it often indistinguishable from other forms of RP. Less commonly, a cone-rod phenotype manifests with early central cone degeneration and accompanying loss of visual acuity. Female carriers of the *RPGR* disease are typically asymptomatic with a characteristic phenotype that manifests as a radial streak pattern originating from the fovea [6,7]. Rarely, however, skewed X-inactivation leads to more severe male-like phenotype with associated visual impairment [8].

At present, there is no approved treatment for retinitis pigmentosa caused by mutations in *RPGR*. Several treatment options have been under investigation and with the emergence of novel gene-based therapies for inherited retinal disease, this seems the most logical strategy to develop for the *RPGR* disease. Due to its severe phenotype, relatively high incidence and the fact that more commonly mutated genes such as *ABCA4* or *USH2A* are too large to be packaged into AAV vectors, the *RPGR* disease has drawn significant interest amongst scientific and clinical research communities over the last years. However, due to the inherent instability in the retina-specific RPGR^{ORF15} isoform sequence [9–12] the production of the therapeutic AAV-mediated *RPGR* vector has been very challenging. In attempts to improve the sequence stability and fidelity several approaches have been explored including codon optimisation [13–15], which has allowed generation of vectors for use in human trials. In this review we discuss recent advances in the understanding of *RPGR* gene structure and its evolutionary conservation that has led to an improved understanding of protein's molecular function and mechanisms implicated in the pathogenesis of RPRG-related retinal dystrophy. The pre-clinical development of gene therapy vectors that has resulted in their progression into three phase I/II clinical trials is covered in detail, including discussion on three different *RPGR* cDNA sequences used in the trials.

2. Structure and Function of *Retinitis Pigmentosa GTPase Regulator (RPGR)*

The human *RPGR* gene is located on the short arm of the X-chromosome (Xp21.1). The gene exhibits a complex expression pattern with 10 alternatively spliced isoforms, five of which are protein coding [16]. The first transcript to be identified in association with X-linked retinitis pigmentosa, was the constitutive RPGR^{Ex1-19} isoform. In humans, the RPGR^{Ex1-19} isoform contains 19 exons and expresses a full-length messenger RNA transcript of 2448 bp, which generates an 815 amino acid sequence that forms ~90 kDa protein in a variety of tissues [17]. Since this initial characterisation, multiple alternative transcripts have been identified, including the retina-specific RPGR^{ORF15} variant [10,16,18]. This variant contains exons 1–14 of constitutive RPGR with the exon ORF15 derived from alternatively spliced exon 15 and intron 15 (Figure 1A). The RPGR^{ORF15} isoform is 3459 bp, encoding a 1152 amino acid sequence which forms a ~200 kDa protein. As with the widely expressed variant, amino acids 54–367 (exons 3–10) form a regulator of chromosome condensation 1 (RCC1)-like domain. The alternative ORF15 exon consists of a highly repetitive purine-rich sequence coding for multiple acidic glutamate-glycine repeats. This is followed by a C-terminal tail region rich in basic amino acid residues, called the basic domain.

The reason for this complex expression pattern of the RPGR protein remains largely unknown, but may be related to the functional role of its splice isoforms in various cell types. The RPGR protein is widely expressed in vertebrate tissue including eye, brain, lung, testis and kidney. In the eye, the two major isoforms, RPGR^{Ex1-19} and RPGR^{ORF15} are predominantly localised to the photoreceptor connecting cilia [19] and less consistently, to the nuclei and photoreceptor outer segments of some species [20]. The connecting cilium is a critical junction between the inner and outer photoreceptor segments, controlling the bidirectional transport of opsin and other proteins involved in the phototransduction cascade and the overall health and viability of the photoreceptors. Attempts are ongoing to elucidate further the expression patterns of RPGR through evolutionary characterisation of RPGR domains across species and via molecular interactions of RPGR with other proteins in order to shed light on the exact role of the RPGR protein.

The RCC1-like domain, present in both major splice forms, adopts a seven-bladed β-propeller structure and it is strongly conserved across evolution, in vertebrates and invertebrates [9]. This domain has been implicated in a regulatory role of small GTPases. It is thought to enable RPGR to act as a Ran guanine nucleotide exchange factor and RPGR has been shown to upregulate the guanine nucleotide exchange factor RAB8A, associating with the GDP-bound form of RAB8A to stimulate GDP/GTP nucleotide exchange [21]. The RCC1-like region also interacts with: RPGR interaction protein 1 (RPGRIP1), which links it to the connecting cilium of photoreceptor cells [19]; the lipid trafficking protein phosphodiesterase 6D (PDE6D) [22]; two chromosome-associated proteins important for the structural maintenance of chromosomes, SMC1 and SMC3 [23] and two ciliary disease-associated proteins nephrocystin-5 (NPHP5) [24] and centrosomal protein 290 (CEP290) [25].

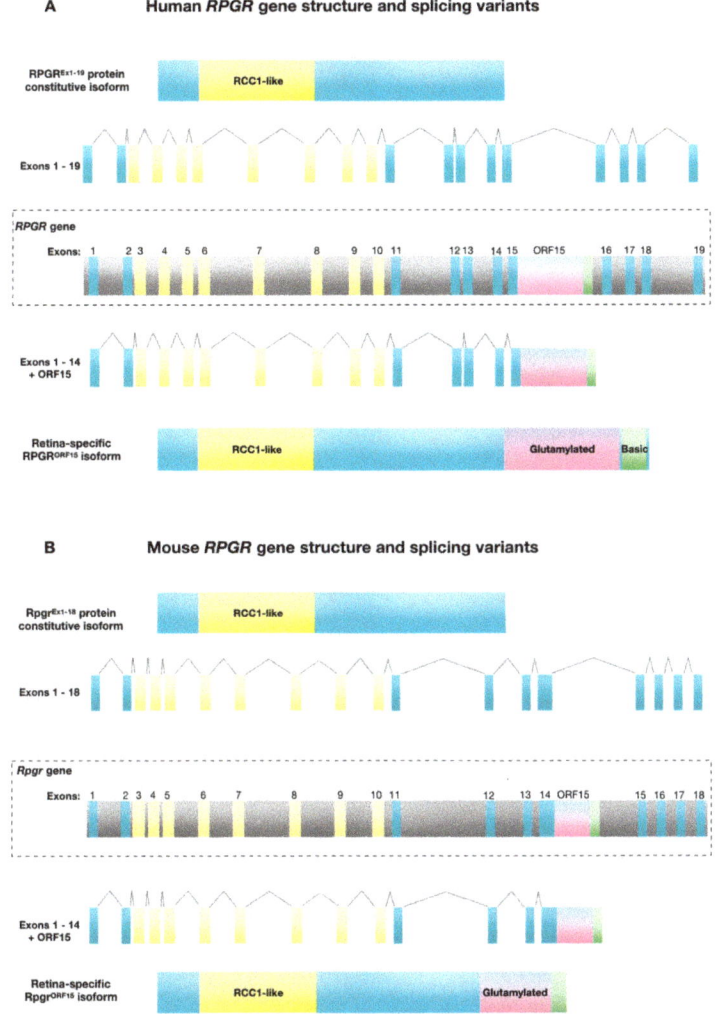

Figure 1. *Retinitis Pigmentosa GTPase Regulator (RPGR)* gene structure and splicing variants. (**A**) Human *RPGR* gene exon-intron structure showing the combination of exons 1 to 19 to create the constitutive protein isoform, and alternative splicing of exon 15/intron 15 that creates the RPGR^{ORF15} variant. (**B**) Mouse RPGR gene exon-intron structure showing the combination of exons 1 to 18 to create the constitutive protein isoform and alternative splicing of intron 14 creates the RPGR^{OFR15} variant.

The retina-specific ORF15 domain is also highly evolutionarily conserved across varied species, indicating a functional importance (Table 1). However, in contrast to the RCC1-like domain, the ORF15 domain is unique to vertebrates, suggesting a role that is unique to the ciliary-derived photoreceptors of "simple" vertebrate eyes, compared to the rhabdomeric photoreceptors of "compound" invertebrate eyes. Hence, the ciliary-based transport of cargoes such as rhodopsin, which is at least 10 times more abundant in vertebrates than invertebrates, fits with this hypothesis. ORF15 homology and a region of high AG content of >80% is identifiable in a range of species although the length varies—the mouse

ORF15 is shorter than the human ORF15, Figure 1A). This purine-rich region of ORF15 (97.5% purines within 1kb in humans) encodes the glutamine-glycine rich domain that ends in a basic C-terminal domain, which is also highly conserved, suggesting that it constitutes another functional region. This basic domain, which is unique to RPGR^{ORF15}, interacts with at least two proteins, a chaperone protein nucleophosmin and a scaffold protein whirlin [26]. Neither protein is unique to vertebrate photoreceptors, but nucleophosmin is present in metaphase centrosomes during cell division, while whirlin helps to maintain ciliary structures within the eye and ear.

Table 1. Evolutionary conservation of DNA and amino acid sequences of RPGR^{ORF15} variants across selected species. All data were extracted from NCBI database files with comparisons performed in Geneious Prime 2017.10.2. For *Homo sapiens*, details were extracted from gene files NG_009553.1 and 6103 combined with mRNA file NM_001034853.2. * The conserved basic domain of the human *RPGR^{ORF15}* coding sequence was used for predictions of ORF15 locations in all other species sequences by homology alignment. For *Mus musculus* data, gene files NC_000086.7 and 19893 were aligned with the basic domain of human *RPGR^{ORF15}* and the partial sequence file AF286473.1 to identify the predicted ORF15 variant. For *Canis lupus familiaris* data, gene files 403726 and AF148801.1 were aligned with the basic domain of human *RPGR^{ORF15}* and the partial sequence file AF385629.1. For *Pan troglodytes* data, files 4465569 and XM_024352988 were used. For *Gorilla gorilla gorilla*, files 101149059, the basic domain of human *RPGR^{ORF15}* and the partial sequence AY855163.1 were combined. For *Macaca mulatta*, files 714316, the basic domain of human *RPGR^{ORF15}* and the partial sequence file AY855162.1 were combined. Finally, *Xenopus tropicalis* sequence predictions were achieved from files 733454 and XM_018091818.1.

	DNA Sequence				Amino Acid Sequence	
Species	Coding Sequence Prior to ORF15	Percentage of Purine Bases	Region with Homology to Human ORF15 *	Percentage of Purine Bases	ORF15 Amino Acid Length (Percentage Glu-Gly) *	Glutamylation Region (Percentage Glu-Gly) *
Homo sapiens	1 to 14 1.7 kb	54%	ORF15 1.7 kb	89%	567 (67%)	351 (88%)
Mus musculus	1 to 14 2.5 kb	57%	Intron 14 1.5 kb	86%	488 (60%)	273 (84%)
Canis lupus familiaris	1 to 13 2.5 kb	58%	Exon 14/ Intron 14 1.5 kb	88%	522 (66%)	331 (72%)
Pan troglodytes	1 to 14 1.7 kb	54%	Exon 15/ Intron 15 1.7 kb	89%	560 (66%)	330 (88%)
Gorilla gorilla gorilla	1 to 14 1.7 kb	54%	Exon 15/ Intron 15 1.7 kb	89%	549 (66%)	321 (88%)
Macaca mulatta	1 to 14 1.7 kb	53%	Exon 15/ Intron 15 1.7 kb	89%	549 (65%)	323 (86%)
Xenopus tropicalis	1 to 13 1.6 kb	57%	Exon 14/ Intron 14/ Exon 15 2.0 kb	77%	679 (45%)	232 (82%)

The function of the repetitive glutamine-glycine-rich domain itself has been difficult to establish due to its variable length and relatively poor conservation at the individual amino acid level, although the overall charge and repeat structure length remain conserved in vertebrates. However, recent evidence shows that this intrinsically disordered region is heavily glutamylated [27], a post-translational protein modification that adds glutamates to target proteins to affect their stabilisation and folding. This process is known to be essential for the function of tubulins in intracellular trafficking [28]. Furthermore, this glutamylation has been shown to be achieved by tubulin tyrosine ligase like-5

(TTLL5) enzyme, which interacts directly with the basic domain of the OFR15 to bring it into the proximity of glutamylation sites along the glutamine-glycine-rich repetitive region [29]. The role of the ORF15 region is of course critically important to photoreceptor function, because otherwise ORF15 mutations would not be pathogenic since the RPGR^{Ex1-19} variant is still expressed in these cells. Hence in-frame deletions in the ORF15 region lead to progressive loss of function as the deletion length increases [13].

3. Molecular Mechanisms and Pathogenesis of RPGR-Related X-Linked Retinitis Pigmentosa (RP)

Molecular mechanisms and pathogenesis of RPGR-related X-linked RP have been under investigation for several decades. The drive to better understand the disease process comes from the high incidence with mutations in the gene encoding RPGR accounting at least 70% of X-linked RP and up to 20% of all RP cases [2–4]. Moreover, the disease is associated with one of the most severe phenotypes among inherited retinal diseases with central visual loss occurring early in adult life [2]. This coupled with the developments in genetic therapies has given impetus to a large number of studies aimed to uncover the pathogenic mechanisms.

Despite ubiquitous expression of the constitutive RPGR variant in ciliated cells throughout the body, the RPGR^{Ex1-19} has yet to show a firm association with any human disease. The RPGR-related phenotype seems to be confined to the retina and several studies have established an essential role for RPGR^{ORF15} in photoreceptor function and survival [10,11]. Genetic studies have shown that mutations in the RPGR^{ORF15} result in abnormal protein transport across the connecting cilium, which can lead to photoreceptor cell death [12,30,31]. However, there are reports in the literature that describe RPGR-related X-linked retinitis pigmentosa syndrome comprising of retinitis pigmentosa, recurrent respiratory tract infections and hearing loss [32,33]. These findings point to the abnormalities in respiratory and auditory cilia in addition to the photoreceptors. In addition, as photoreceptors develop from ciliated progenitors, it has been postulated that the axoneme may play a role in their early development. Sperm axonemes were thus studies in patients with X-linked retinitis pigmentosa and a significant increase in abnormal sperm tails was observed [34]. Similar findings have been reported in another syndromic ciliopathy, the Usher syndrome [35].

Mutations in *RPGR* account for ~70% of cases of X-linked RP and have been identified across exons 1–15, yet up to 60% of mutations occur in the ORF15 region [10,30]. The repetitive nature of the glutamate-glycine region in ORF15 is prone to adopt unusual double helix DNA conformations or triplexes that are thought to promote polymerase arrest and block replication and transcription. These imperfections are likely to contribute to genome instability and account for the high frequency of mutations in this region, known as the mutation 'hot spot' of the *RPGR*. Surprisingly, no disease-causing mutations have been reported in exons 16–19 [36].

The most common mutations are small deletions that lead to frameshifts followed by nonsense mutations [30]. Within ORF15, the most common mutations are microdeletions 1–2, or 4–5 bp [10], that cause frameshifts leading to truncated forms of the protein and in particular, loss of the C-terminus. Small in-frame deletions or insertions (and missense changes) that can alter the length of ORF15 region by a few base-pairs (e.g., up to 36, equivalent to 9 amino acids in this population based study [37], are seemingly well tolerated [38]. Thus, despite being a coding region, this domain has a surprisingly high rate of tolerable indels within primate lineages, suggesting a rapidly evolving region [9]. However, recent evidence shows that larger deletions in the ORF15 region significantly affect the degree of RPGR glutamylation, which may subsequently influence its function and ability to associate with the cilium and other interacting factors [29]. Thus, frame shift mutations that lead to loss of the C-terminal basic domain are invariably disease causing [12]. In addition, mutations that lead to the loss of TTLL5 enzyme, the basic domain-binding partner that mediates RPGR glutamylation, abort glutamylation process and cause RPGR-like phenotype in humans [39]. This further supports the critical role of glutamylation in normal RPGR^{ORF15} function. It remains intriguing that despite its ubiquitous expression, the RPGR^{Ex1-19} is unable to compensate for the loss of function of RPGR^{ORF15} in the retina to rescue the phenotype. It is possible that the alternative splicing in the retina could favour the RPGR^{ORF15} variant, so the majority of transcripts will be the RPGR^{ORF15} isoform, with few constitutive variants available to compensate. One study failed to identify the constitutive transcript in the retina [18], which supports the finding that the constitutive isoform is expressed early in development in a mouse before its levels decline and the RPGR^{ORF15} becomes the predominant isoform [26]. Notably, the constitutive variant lacks the glutamate-glycine repetitive region and given the importance of this domain for the normal function of RPGR^{ORF15} in the photoreceptors, perhaps it is not so surprising that the constitutive variant cannot offer the same functional benefit as the RPGR^{ORF15} variant.

4. Clinical and Genetic Diagnosis of RPGR-Related X-Linked RP

The diagnosis of RPGR-related retinal dystrophy is made on the basis of presenting symptoms and retinal signs seen on clinical examination and various imaging modalities. In addition, study of family history showing X-linked inheritance (no male to male transmission) and genetic testing identifying the pathogenic mutation are important in confirming the diagnosis. In cases of uncertain diagnosis and unequivocal genetic test results we have adopted several important steps, which are discussed below, in order to minimise the risk of establishing an incorrect diagnosis, and administering the patient with an incorrect gene if recruited into a gene therapy clinical trial.

RPGR-related retinal dystrophy is associated with a very heterogeneous phenotype that ranges from pan-retinal rod-cone to predominant cone dystrophy (Figure 2). The phenotype is generally more severe with faster progression compared to other forms of RP and median age of legal blindness of approximately 45 years old, which is much younger than in other RP genotypes [40]. Most patients lose their peripheral vision first, followed by the loss of central vision. Recent evidence suggests that the rod-cone phenotype is found in 70% of patients, the cone-rod in 23% and the cone phenotype in 7% of patients with X-linked RPGR related retinal dystrophy [2]. The study shows that the onset of symptoms was in early childhood in rod-cone dystrophy (median age 5 years) and in third decade in cone-rod and cone dystrophy, although the age range was very wide (between 0 and 60 years). However, cone-rod and cone dystrophies were associated with a more severe phenotype and the probability of being blind at the age of 40, with visual acuity of less than 0.05 LogMAR (3/60 or 20/400) observed in 55% of patients with cone-rod and cone dystrophy compared to only 20% in rod-cone dystrophy.

The RPGR phenotype (Figure 2) has been associated with anatomical changes including central retinal thinning of the outer nuclear layer as seen on retinal cross-sections taken by optical coherence tomography [40,41]. The junction between the inner and outer photoreceptor segments, better known as the ellipsoid zone, can be used as an important predictor of central retinal function and for monitoring of disease progression. [42]. Thus, the disruption of the ellipsoid zone can be detected with corresponding early reduction in visual acuity and retinal sensitivity as measured by microperimetry. In addition, autofluorescence can be used to assess the health of the retinal pigment epithelium with early signs of hyper-autofluorescence indicating accumulation of lipofuscin and related metabolites as a by-product of photoreceptor outer segment degradation. Later in the disease process, areas of hypo-autofluorescence become evident indicating outer retinal atrophy with loss of retinal pigment epithelium cells. The RPGR phenotype is often associated with para-foveal hyper-autofluorescent rings, which decline exponentially with disease progression [43]. Constriction areas are correlated highly with baseline area and age, where younger subjects had greatest rate of progression. No correlation with genotype was observed in this study. In the cone-rod phenotype, however, the area of hypo-autofluorescence associated with a surrounding hyper-autofluorescent ring tends to increase in size with disease progression and is inversely related to electroretinogram amplitude [44]. Ongoing natural history studies are promising to shed more light on the natural progression of the RPGR disease phenotypes and provide better understanding and interpretation of clinical trial endpoints used in current interventional gene therapy trials (Table 2).

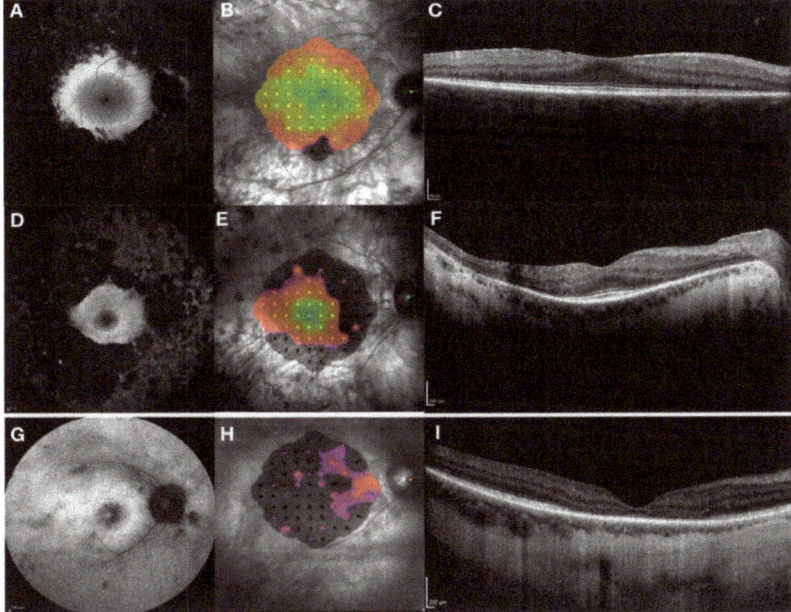

Figure 2. Clinical phenotypes associated with *RPGR* retinal degeneration—rod-cone phenotype (early stage (**A–C**) and a more advanced stage (**D–F**)) and cone-rod phenotype (**G–I**). The phenotypes are captured by Heidelberg fundus autofluorescence, (left column), MAIA microperimetry measuring central retinal sensitivity (central column; sensitivity is represented by a heat map: green/yellow—normal/mildly reduced; red/purple—reduced; black—not measurable) and Heidelberg optical coherence tomography showing retinal structures in cross-section (right column). In rod-cone phenotype there is extensive peripheral retinal atrophy with relative preservation of central retina as seen on autofluorescence associated with para-foveal hyper-autofluorescent ring (**A**). This is confirmed by near normal central retinal sensitivity (**B**) and preservation of ellipsoid zone (**C**). In more advanced stages of the disease there is reduction in size of the para-foveal hyper-autofluorescent ring (**D**) with corresponding reduction in retinal sensitivity (**E**) and length of ellipsoid zone (**F**). In contrast, in cone-rod phenotype there is early loss of para-foveal photoreceptors with associated hypo-fluorescent ring and marked reduction of retinal sensitivity with corresponding loss of the ellipsoid zone.

Female carriers of *RPGR* mutations also show high phenotypic variability [7] (Figure 3). The carrier phenotype includes asymptomatic females with near-normal clinical appearance, macular pattern reflex with different degrees of pigmentary retinopathy and severely affected females with clinical phenotype that results from skewed X chromosome inactivation and is indistinguishable from the male pattern. Female carriers with male pattern dystrophy should be considered for *RPGR* gene therapy as discussed below.

The molecular diagnosis using next-generation sequencing (NGS) is usually a robust approach in determining pathogenic variants in RP. However, the ORF15 region of RPGR is not normally sequenced with NGS methods and is currently only performed upon specific request. Moreover, sequencing of the ORF15 region in *RPGR* is notoriously difficult and error-prone. Overlapping reading frames and polymorphic deletions/insertions add further complexity to the detection of true mutations. Additional precautions must, therefore, be taken with interpreting the sequencing data so that small deletions are not confused with artefacts that would lead to spurious results. In cases of uncertainty, testing should be repeated. In addition, the full RP panel should be performed to exclude other pathogenic variants including the sequencing of *RP2* and *OFD1* X-linked genes. This comprehensive molecular genetic analysis together with the *RPGR* phenotype and a clear family history of X-linked inheritance, including evidence of a carrier phenotype, forms the basis of inclusion criteria into gene therapy clinical trials. In addition, a recent study describes an in vitro assay for determining the pathogenicity of *RPGR* missense variations [45]. The strategy is based on the RPGR protein interaction network, which is disrupted by missense variations in RCC1-like domain in RPGR, and could help to differentiate between causative missense mutations and non-disease-causing polymorphisms.

Table 2. Summary of clinical trials for RPGR-related X-linked retinitis pigmentosa (RP).

Clinical Trial (clinicaltrials.gov)	Intervention/ Observation	Clinical Centre/s	Sponsor
Phase I/II/III NCT03116113 multicenter, open-label Part 1: non-randomised, dose-selection study 18 participants Part 2: dose expansion study (randomised to low dose, high dose, control) 63 participants Start date: March 2017	Subretinal delivery of AAV8-hRK-coRPGR^{ORF15}	Oxford, UK Manchester, UK Southampton, UK Florida, USA Oregon, USA Pennsylvania, USA	Nightstar Therapeutics (now Biogen Inc), UK
Phase I/II NCT03252847 Non-randomised, open-label, dose-escalation trial 36 participants Start date: July 2017	Subretinal delivery of AAV2/5-hRK-RPGR^{ORF15}	London, UK	MeiraGTx, UK
Phase I/II NCT03316560 Non-randomised, open-label, multicenter, dose-escalation trial 30 participants with RPGR ORF15 mutations Start date: April 2018	Subretinal delivery of rAAV2tYF-GRK1-coRPGR^{ORF15}	Colorado, USA Massachusetts, USA New York, USA North Carolina, USA Ohio, USA Oregon, USA Pennsylvania, USA Texas, USA	Applied Genetic Technologies Corporation (AGTC), USA
Prospective natural history study of XLRP with genetically confirmed mutation in RPGR 150 participants Start date: December 2017	Observational study	Multiple centres in UK, Germany, Holland, France, USA	Nightstar Therapeutics (now Biogen Inc), UK
Prospective natural history study of XLRP NCT03349242 Start date: December 2017	Observational study	Massachusetts, USA Michigan, USA	MeiraGTx, UK
Prospective natural history study of XLRP caused by RPGR-ORF15 mutations 45 participants NCT03314207 Start date: December 2017	Observational study	New York, USA North Carolina, USA Ohio, USA Oregon, USA Texas, USA	Applied Genetic Technologies Corporation (AGTC), USA

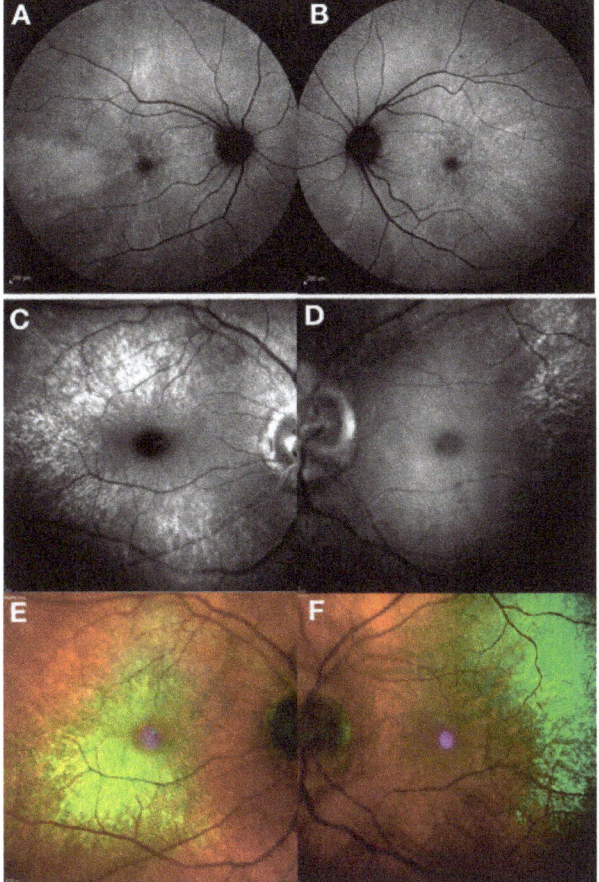

Figure 3. Clinical phenotype of *RPGR* female carriers. Fundus autofluorescence (Heidelberg) showing a typical macular radial pattern or 'tapetal' reflex in a female carrier of an *RPGR* mutation (**A,B**). Random X-chromosome inactivation generates clones of normal or affected photoreceptors giving rise to this mosaic pattern. Blue reflectance (**C,D**) and multicoloured (**E,F**) modes using Heidelberg scanning laser ophthalmoscope can be very helpful in showing the macular reflex.

5. Treatment Options for RPGR-Related X-Linked RP

Several non-gene based treatment approaches have been investigated for the preservation of vision in X-linked RP including a nutritional supplement, docosahexaenoic acid [46] and a ciliary neurotrophic factor [47] both of which were unable to prevent photoreceptor degeneration and visual loss. For patients with advanced disease, electronic retinal devices have demonstrated proof-of-concept in their ability to restore crude vision [48,49]. However, the unpredictability of benefit for individual patients and the high price of these devices make it economically difficult to maintain their availability for the treatment of patients with RP. Another potential strategy, optogenetics, is under investigation and has shown promising results for vision restoration in advanced retinal degeneration [50,51].

Emerging gene-based therapy using the AAV vector is currently the most promising therapeutic strategy for RPGR X-linked RP. The size of the coding sequence of RPGR^{ORF15} (3.5 kb) is within the AAV carrying capacity and the relatively high prevalence and disease severity have justified development of this therapy. However, the repetitive sequence of ORF15 not only makes it a hotspot for mutations but also creates challenges for therapeutic vector production. Attempts to generate AAV vectors for RPGR gene-supplementation strategies have been thwarted by the poor sequence stability of the ORF15 region and transgene production has struggled to control spontaneous mutations and maintain the complete sequence [13,52–55]. AAV gene therapy in two RPGR X-linked RP canine models that carry different ORF15 mutations [55] provided proof of concept for treating RPGR mutations within the ORF15 region. AAV2/5-mediated sub retinal gene delivery of a full-length human RPGR-ORF15 cDNA [10], driven by either the human interphotoreceptor retinoid-binding protein (hIRBP) promoter or the human G-protein-coupled receptor kinase 1 (hGRK1) promoter, prevented photoreceptor degeneration and preserved retinal function in both canine models. However, the AAV2/5.RPGR vector was found to have multiple mutations within the purine-rich exon 15 region that led to toxic effects in mice at higher doses [52] thus posing safety questions for human applications. In an attempt to improve the sequence stability, a step-wise cloning approach was used to generate the correct full-length RPGR^{ORF15} coding sequence (the purine-rich region was generated first and then ligated to the rest of the DNA sequence) [53], which was packaged into the AAV8.GRK1.*RPGR*^{ORF15} vector and evaluated in the *Rpgr*-KO mouse. However, despite improved stability, some vector preparations were still ridden with micro-deletions that led to expression of alternatively spliced truncated forms of the RPGR protein that was mislocalised to photoreceptor inner segments and only a partial rescue of the phenotype in treated mice. The truncated forms of the protein were further investigated for their ability to rescue the RPGR phenotype in the *Rpgr*-KO mouse [13]. The short (314 out of 348 ORF15 codons deleted) and the long (126 out of 348 codons deleted) forms of the *RPGR*^{ORF15} were tested. The long form demonstrated significant improvement in the disease phenotype, whilst the short form failed to localise correctly in the photoreceptors and showed no functional rescue of the phenotype. Importantly, as discussed above, large deletions in the ORF15 region can affect the glutamylation of the protein and lead to impaired function. Indeed, a follow-up study by the same group tested these truncated vectors [29] for their glutamylation capacity. Unsurprisingly, the long form demonstrated significantly impaired glutamylation (only 30% of the full length protein), whereas the short form showed no detectable glutamylation of the RPGR protein.

To circumvent these issues, the research team of Fischer and colleagues (2017) generated a full-length, human, codon-optimised version of RGPR^{ORF15} to stabilise the sequence, remove cryptic splice sites and increase expression levels from the therapeutic transgene [14]. This enabled reliable cloning and vector production. The resulting AAV8.coRPGR^{ORF15} vector was shown to offer therapeutic rescue in two mouse models of X-linked RP (*Rpgr*$^{-/y}$ and *Rd9*). This vector is now being used in a Phase I/II/III gene therapy clinical trial in humans (NCT03116113). In addition, the codon optimised form of the RPGR vector used in the canine studies [15] and the truncated form of the RPGR with near-total OFR15 deletion [13] are also being tested in ongoing clinical trials (NCT03316560 and NCT03252847 respectively) as will be discussed further in the next section. A very recent study used a bioinformatics approach as an alternative method to develop a molecularly stable *RPGR* gene therapy vector [56]. The strategy identified regions of genomic instability within ORF15 and made synonymous substitutions to reduce the repetitive sequence and thus increase the molecular stability of *RPGR*. The codon optimized construct was validated in vitro in pull-down experiments and in a murine model, demonstrating production of functional RPGR protein.

6. Gene Therapy Clinical Trials for RPGR-Related X-Linked RP

The results of the pre-clinical studies described above support the use of AAV-based gene therapy for RPGR-related X-linked RP in humans, in the early to mid-stage of the disease. Ideally, patients with moderately reduced visual acuity and constricted visual fields, but a preserved central ellipsoid zone, should be recruited into gene therapy trials for best expected therapeutic benefits. Interestingly, development of RPGR therapy from bench to bedside has resulted in setting-up of three multi-centre dose-escalation gene-therapy clinical trials (see Table 2 for details). Each trial is using a different combination of AAV vector variant and *RPGR* coding sequence (Figure 4). Specifically, the Nightstar

Therapeutics (now Biogen Inc) sponsored trial (NCT03116113) is using the wild-type AAV8 vector with a human rhodopsin kinase promoter and a human codon optimised full-length RPGR^{ORF15} cDNA sequence (AAV2/8.hRK.*coRPGR^{ORF15}*). The second trial sponsored by Meira GTx (NCT03252847) is using a wild-type AAV2/5 capsid with a truncated, non-codon optimised *RPGR* sequence under control of the human rhodopsin kinase promoter (AAV2/5.hRK.*RPGR^{ORF15}*). The third trial conducted by Applied Genetic Technologies Corporation (NCT03316560) is using mutated AAV2 capsids (capsids with single tyrosine to phenylalanine (YF) mutations) packaged with full-length, codon optimised human *RPGR^{ORF15}* sequence also driven by the rhodopsin kinase promoter (AAV2tYF.GRK1.*coRPGR^{ORF15}*).

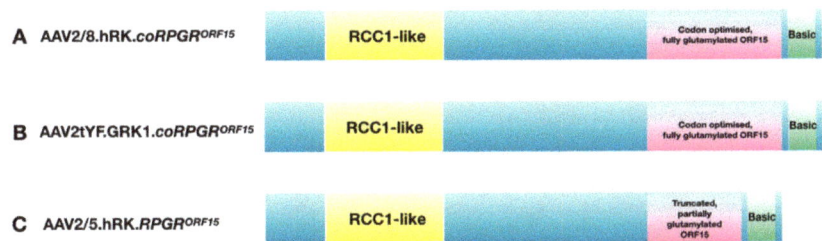

Figure 4. AAV vector constructs used in current gene therapy trials: (**A**) the Nightstar Therapeutics (now Biogen Inc) trial, NCT03116113; (**B**) the Applied Genetic Technologies Corporation trial, NCT03316560; (**C**) the MeiraGTx trial, NCT03252847.

The pre-clinical studies that led to the development of vectors used in human trials were described in detail in the previous section. However, the rationale for using the three different vectors deserves further discussion. The coding sequence used in the Meira GTx trial is an abbreviated form of human *RPGR^{ORF15}* sequence. The rationale provided for using the truncated form, which arose through a spontaneous mutation resulting in deletion of one third of the ORF15 region, was because the deletion led it to become more stable, thereby reducing the rate of further recombination errors and potential mutations. Interestingly, the authors also showed that further shortening of this critical ORF15 region significantly affects the protein function, leading to mislocalisation of the protein in photoreceptors and no functional or morphological rescue in a mouse model, confirming the importance of the ORF15 region for photoreceptor function. Importantly, a further study demonstrated that the post-translational glutamylation is reduced by over 70% in this abbreviated form of the RPGR^{ORF15}, significantly affecting trafficking of molecules critical for photoreceptor function [29]. However, since RPGR is not expressed highly in photoreceptors, it is possible that over-expression of RPGR with gene therapy can compensate for the reduced trafficking ability. The truncated construct was shown to rescue the photoreceptor function in a murine model of X-linked RP [13]. However, the mouse *RPGR^{ORF15}* is naturally shorter than the human *RPGR^{ORF15}* with an abbreviated ORF15 region (see Figure 2 and Table 1) much like the engineered abbreviated human construct used in the human trial. Thus, it may not be so surprising that the abbreviated human construct led to the rescue in a murine model, as the two sequences are very similar and the murine model has a milder phenotype compared to humans. The efficacy of this shortened version of *RPGR^{ORF15}* has not been evaluated in canine models of X-linked RP and the results from human trials are awaited in anticipation.

The constructs used in the AGTC and the Nightstar Therapeutics (now Biogen Inc.) trials are very similar and encode the full-length human wild-type RPGR^{ORF15} protein. Both constructs applied codon optimisation that was shown by Fischer et al. to confer greater sequence stability with higher expression levels than wild-type RPGR sequence, whilst not affecting the glutamylation pattern in the RPGR protein. The codon-optimised RPGR rescued the disease phenotype in two mouse models of X-linked RP [14] and was recently also validated in the RPGR canine model [15] showing transduction of both rods and cones and preserving the outer nuclear layer structure in the treated retina. The results of the phase I/II trials are expected in the near future.

7. Summary

X-linked RPGR-related RP is a heterogenous group of disorders with no clear genotype–phenotype correlation. Both rod-cone and cone-rod retinal dystrophies are seen with relatively early onset and rapid progression to blindness that is related to mutations that cause loss of function of this key photoreceptor protein. The complex expression pattern of the *RPGR* gene through cryptic splice sites that create multiple isoforms poses challenges in elucidating its function. However, mounting evidence suggests that retina-specific RPGR^{ORF15} is unique to vertebrates and plays a crucial role in regulating protein trafficking between inner and outer segments as well as in microtubular organisation. Importantly, RPGR^{ORF15} contains a characteristic repetitive purine-rich region that is highly glutamylated and only the glutamylated RPGR^{ORF15} is fully functional. Thus, any mutations that reduce the glutamylation process adversely affect RPGR protein function. In addition, the ORF15 region created challenges for the researches interested in developing *RPGR* gene-based therapies as the repetitive region made it unstable and prone to mutations. The current approach in developing a codon-optimised version of the RGPR^{ORF15} to stabilise the sequence, remove cryptic splice sites and increase expression levels from the therapeutic transgene is now being used in humans, following proof-of-concept studies in murine and canine models of X-linked RP. This approach has allowed the rapid progression towards the first in-human gene therapy trial (NCT03116113) for X-linked RP, which began in March 2017. In parallel, two additional independent research consortia have been developing gene therapies for the RPGR disease. With recent approval of gene replacement therapy Luxturna, for the treatment of *RPE65*-related retinal disease, the precedence for approval of future gene-based therapies has been set and results of the RPGR early phase clinical trials are awaited with great expectation.

Funding: This research was funded by Oxford NIHR Biomedical Research Centre, Oxford, UK and Medical Research Council UK; JCK is also funded by Global Ophthalmology Awards Fellowship, Bayer, Switzerland.

Conflicts of Interest: REM receives grant funding from Nightstar Therapeutics (now Biogen Inc.). REM is a consultant to Nightstar Therapeutics and Spark Therapeutics. These companies did not have any input into the work presented. No other authors have a conflict of interest.

References

1. Tee, J.J.; Smith, A.J.; Hardcastle, A.J.; Michaelides, M. *RPGR*-associated retinopathy: Clinical features, molecular genetics, animal models and therapeutic options. *Br. J. Ophthalmol.* **2016**, *100*, 1022–1027. [CrossRef]
2. Talib, M.; van Schooneveld, M.J.; Thiadens, A.A.; Fiocco, M.; Wijnholds, J.; Florijn, R.J.; Schalij-Delfos, N.E.; van Genderen, M.M.; Putter, H.; Cremers, F.P.M.; et al. Clinical and genetic characteristics of male patients with *RPGR*-associated retinal dystrophies: A long-term follow-up study. *Retina* **2019**, *39*, 1186–1199. [CrossRef]
3. Pelletier, V.; Jambou, M.; Delphin, N.; Zinovieva, E.; Stum, M.; Gigarel, N.; Dollfus, H.; Hamel, C.; Toutain, A.; Dufier, J.L.; et al. Comprehensive survey of mutations in RP2 and RPGR in patients affected with distinct retinal dystrophies: Genotype-phenotype correlations and impact on genetic counseling. *Hum. Mutat.* **2007**, *28*, 81–91. [CrossRef]
4. Branham, K.; Othman, M.; Brumm, M.; Karoukis, A.J.; Atmaca-Sonmez, P.; Yashar, B.M.; Schwartz, S.B.; Stover, N.B.; Trzupek, K.; Wheaton, D.; et al. Mutations in *RPGR* and *RP2* account for 15% of males with simplex retinal degenerative disease. *Investig. Ophthalmol. Vis. Sci.* **2012**, *53*, 8232–8237. [CrossRef]
5. Webb, T.R.; Parfitt, D.A.; Gardner, J.C.; Martinez, A.; Bevilacqua, D.; Davidson, A.E.; Zito, I.; Thiselton, D.L.; Ressa, J.H.; Apergi, M.; et al. Deep intronic mutation in *OFD1*, identified by targeted genomic next-generation sequencing, causes a severe form of X-linked retinitis pigmentosa (RP23). *Hum. Mol. Genet.* **2012**, *21*, 3647–3654. [CrossRef]
6. Comander, J.; Weigel-DiFranco, C.; Sandberg, M.A.; Berson, E.L. Visual function in carriers of X-linked retinitis pigmentosa. *Ophthalmology* **2015**, *122*, 1899–1906. [CrossRef]
7. Nanda, A.; Salvetti, A.P.; Clouston, P.; Downes, S.M.; MacLaren, R.E. Exploring the Variable Phenotypes of *RPGR* Carrier Females in Assessing their Potential for Retinal Gene Therapy. *Genes* **2018**, *9*, 643. [CrossRef]

8. Wu, H.; Luo, J.; Yu, H.; Rattner, A.; Mo, A.; Wang, Y.; Smallwood, P.M.; Erlanger, B.; Wheelan, S.J.; Nathans, J. Cellular resolution maps of X chromosome inactivation: Implications for neural development, function, and disease. *Neuron* **2014**, *81*, 103–119. [CrossRef]
9. Raghupathy, R.K.; Gautier, P.; Soares, D.C.; Wright, A.F.; Shu, X. Evolutionary characterization of the retinitis pigmentosa GTPase regulator gene. *Investig. Ophthalmol. Vis. Sci.* **2015**, *56*, 6255–6264. [CrossRef]
10. Vervoort, R.; Lennon, A.; Bird, A.C.; Tulloch, B.; Axton, R.; Miano, M.G.; Meindl, A.; Meitinger, T.; Ciccodicola, A.; Wright, A.F. Mutational hot spot within a new *RPGR* exon in X-linked retinitis pigmentosa. *Nat. Genet.* **2000**, *25*, 462–466. [CrossRef]
11. Vervoort, R.; Wright, A.F. Mutations of *RPGR* in X-linked retinitis pigmentosa (RP3). *Hum. Mutat.* **2002**, *19*, 486–500. [CrossRef]
12. Megaw, R.D.; Soares, D.C.; Wright, A.F. RPGR: Its role in photoreceptor physiology, human disease, and future therapies. *Exp. Eye Res.* **2015**, *138*, 32–41. [CrossRef]
13. Pawlyk, B.S.; Bulgakov, O.V.; Sun, X.; Adamian, M.; Shu, X.; Smith, A.J.; Berson, E.L.; Ali, R.R.; Khani, S.; Wright, A.F.; et al. Photoreceptor rescue by an abbreviated human *RPGR* gene in a murine model of X-linked retinitis pigmentosa. *Gene. Ther.* **2015**, *23*, 196–204. [CrossRef]
14. Fischer, M.D.; McClements, M.E.; Martinez-Fernandez De La Camara, C.; Bellingrath, J.S.; Dauletbekov, D.; Ramsden, S.C.; Hickey, D.G.; Barnard, A.R.; MacLaren, R.E. Codon-optimized RPGR improves stability and efficacy of AAV8 gene therapy in two mouse models of X-linked retinitis pigmentosa. *Mol. Ther.* **2017**, *25*, 1854–1865. [CrossRef]
15. Beltran, W.A.; Cideciyan, A.V.; Boye, S.E.; Ye, G.J.; Iwabe, S.; Dufour, V.L.; Marinho, L.F.; Swider, M.; Kosyk, M.S.; Sha, J.; et al. Optimization of retinal gene therapy for X-linked retinitis pigmentosa due to *RPGR* mutations. *Mol. Ther.* **2017**, *25*, 1866–1880. [CrossRef]
16. Hong, D.H.; Li, T. Complex expression pattern of RPGR reveals a role for purine-rich exonic splicing enhancers. *Investig. Ophthalmol. Vis. Sci.* **2002**, *43*, 3373–3382.
17. Meindl, A.; Dry, K.; Herrmann, K.; Manson, E.; Ciccodicola, A.; Edgar, A.; Carvalho, M.R.; Achatz, H.; Hellebrand, H.; Lennon, A.; et al. A gene (RPGR) with homology to the RCC1 guanine nucleotide exchange factor is mutated in X–linked retinitis pigmentosa (RP3). *Nat. Genet.* **1996**, *13*, 35–42. [CrossRef]
18. Kirschner, R.; Erturk, D.; Zeitz, C.; Sahin, S.; Ramser, J.; Cremers, F.P.; Ropers, H.H.; Berger, W. DNA sequence comparison of human and mouse retinitis pigmentosa GTPase regulator (*RPGR*) identifies tissue-specific exons and putative regulatory elements. *Hum. Genet.* **2001**, *109*, 271–278. [CrossRef]
19. Hong, D.H.; Pawlyk, B.; Sokolov, M.; Strissel, K.J.; Yang, J.; Tulloch, B.; Wright, A.F.; Arshavsky, V.Y.; Li, T. RPGR isoforms in photoreceptor connecting cilia and the transitional zone of motile cilia. *Investig. Ophthalmol. Vis. Sci.* **2003**, *44*, 2413–2421. [CrossRef]
20. Mavlyutov, T.A.; Zhao, H.; Ferreira, P.A. Species-specific subcellular localization of RPGR and RPGRIP isoforms: Implications for the phenotypic variability of congenital retinopathies among species. *Hum. Mol. Genet.* **2002**, *11*, 1899–1907. [CrossRef]
21. Murga-Zamalloa, C.A.; Atkins, S.J.; Peranen, J.; Swaroop, A.; Khanna, H. Interaction of retinitis pigmentosa GTPase regulator (RPGR) with RAB8A GTPase: Implications for cilia dysfunction and photoreceptor degeneration. *Hum. Mol. Genet.* **2010**, *19*, 3591–3598. [CrossRef]
22. Zhang, H.; Liu, X.-H.; Zhang, K.; Chen, C.-K.; Frederick, J.M.; Prestwich, G.D.; Baehr, W. Photoreceptor cGMP phosphodiesterase delta subunit (PDEδ) functions as a prenyl-binding protein. *J. Biol. Chem.* **2004**, *279*, 407–413. [CrossRef]
23. Khanna, H.; Hurd, T.W.; Lillo, C.; Shu, X.; Parapuram, S.K.; He, S.; Akimoto, M.; Wright, A.F.; Margolis, B.; Williams, D.S.; et al. RPGR-ORF15, which is mutated in retinitis pigmentosa, associates with SMC1, SMC3, and microtubule transport proteins. *J. Biol. Chem.* **2005**, *280*, 33580–33587. [CrossRef]
24. Otto, E.A.; Loeys, B.; Khanna, H.; Hellemans, J.; Sudbrak, R.; Fan, S.; Muerb, U.; O'Toole, J.F.; Helou, J.; Attanasio, M.; et al. Nephrocystin-5, a ciliary IQ domain protein, is mutated in Senior-Loken syndrome and interacts with RPGR and calmodulin. *Nat. Genet.* **2005**, *37*, 282–288. [CrossRef]
25. Chang, B.; Khanna, H.; Hawes, N.; molecular, D.J.H. In-frame deletion in a novel centrosomal/ciliary protein CEP290/NPHP6 perturbs its interaction with RPGR and results in early-onset retinal degeneration in the rd16 mouse. *Hum. Mol. Genet.* **2006**, *15*, 1847–1857. [CrossRef]
26. Wright, R.N.; Hong, D.-H.; Perkins, B. RpgrORF15 Connects to the usher protein network through direct interactions with multiple whirlin isoforms. *Investig. Opthalmol. Vis. Sci.* **2012**, *53*, 1519. [CrossRef]

27. Rao, K.N.; Anand, M.; Khanna, H. The carboxyl terminal mutational hotspot of the ciliary disease protein RPGRORF15 (retinitis pigmentosa GTPase regulator) is glutamylated in vivo. *Biol. Open* **2016**, *5*, 424–428. [CrossRef]
28. Natarajan, K.; Gadadhar, S.; Souphron, J.; Magiera, M.M.; Janke, C. Molecular interactions between tubulin tails and glutamylases reveal determinants of glutamylation patterns. *EMBO Rep.* **2017**, *18*, 1013–1026. [CrossRef]
29. Sun, X.; Park, J.H.; Gumerson, J.; Wu, Z.; Swaroop, A.; Qian, H.; Roll-Mecak, A.; Li, T. Loss of RPGR glutamylation underlies the pathogenic mechanism of retinal dystrophy caused by TTLL5 mutations. *Proc. Natl. Acad. Sci. USA* **2016**, *113*, E2925–E2934. [CrossRef]
30. Shu, X.; McDowall, E.; Brown, A.F.; Wright, A.F. The human retinitis pigmentosa GTPase regulator gene variant database. *Hum. Mutat.* **2008**, *29*, 605–608. [CrossRef]
31. Hosch, J.; Lorenz, B.; Stieger, K. RPGR: Role in the photoreceptor cilium, human retinal disease, and gene therapy. *Ophthalmic Genet.* **2011**, *32*, 1–11. [CrossRef]
32. Iannaccone, A.; Breuer, D.K.; Wang, X.F.; Kuo, S.F.; Normando, E.M.; Filippova, E.; Baldi, A.; Hiriyanna, S.; MacDonald, C.B.; Baldi, F.; et al. Clinical and immunohistochemical evidence for an X linked retinitis pigmentosa syndrome with recurrent infections and hearing loss in association with an RPGR mutation. *J. Med. Genet.* **2003**, *40*, e118. [CrossRef]
33. Zito, I.; Downes, S.M.; Patel, R.J.; Cheetham, M.E.; Ebenezer, N.D.; Jenkins, S.A.; Bhattacharya, S.S.; Webster, A.R.; Holder, G.E.; Bird, A.C.; et al. RPGR mutation associated with retinitis pigmentosa, impaired hearing, and sinorespiratory infections. *J. Med. Genet.* **2003**, *40*, 609–615. [CrossRef]
34. Hunter, D.G.; Fishman, G.A.; Kretzer, F.L. Abnormal axonemes in X-linked retinitis pigmentosa. *Arch. Ophthal.* **1988**, *106*, 362–368. [CrossRef]
35. Hunter, D.G.; Fishman, G.A.; Mehta, R.S.; Kretzer, F.L. Abnormal sperm and photoreceptor axonemes in Usher's syndrome. *Arch. Ophthalmol.* **1986**, *104*, 385–389. [CrossRef]
36. He, S.; Parapuram, S.K.; Hurd, T.W.; Behnam, B.; Margolis, B.; Swaroop, A.; Khanna, H. Retinitis pigmentosa GTPase regulator (RPGR) protein isoforms in mammalian retina: Insights into X-linked retinitis pigmentosa and associated ciliopathies. *Vision Res.* **2008**, *48*, 366–376. [CrossRef]
37. Jacobi, F.K.; Karra, D.; Broghammer, M.; Blin, N.; Pusch, C.M. Mutational risk in highly repetitive exon ORF15 of the RPGR multidisease gene is not associated with haplotype background. *Int. J. Mol. Med.* **2005**, *16*, 1175–1178. [CrossRef]
38. Karra, D.; Jacobi, F.K.; Broghammer, M.; Blin, N.; Pusch, C.M. Population haplotypes of exon ORF15 of the retinitis pigmentosa GTPase regulator gene in Germany: Implications for screening for inherited retinal disorders. *Mol. Diagn. Ther.* **2006**, *10*, 115–123. [CrossRef]
39. Sergouniotis, P.I.; Chakarova, C.; Murphy, C.; Becker, M.; Lenassi, E.; Arno, G.; Lek, M.; MacArthur, D.G.; Bhattacharya, S.S.; Moore, A.T.; et al. UCL-Exomes Consortium Biallelic variants in TTLL5, encoding a tubulin glutamylase, cause retinal dystrophy. *Am. J. Hum. Genet.* **2014**, *94*, 760–769. [CrossRef]
40. Sandberg, M.A.; Rosner, B.; Weigel-DiFranco, C.; Dryja, T.P.; Berson, E.L. Disease course of patients with X-linked retinitis pigmentosa due to RPGR gene mutations. *Investig. Ophthalmol. Vis. Sci.* **2007**, *48*, 1298–1304. [CrossRef]
41. Huang, W.C.; Wright, A.F.; Roman, A.J.; Cideciyan, A.V.; Manson, F.D.; Gewaily, D.Y.; Schwartz, S.B.; Sadigh, S.; Limberis, M.P.; Bell, P.; et al. RPGR-associated retinal degeneration in human X-linked RP and a murine model. *Investig. Ophthalmol. Vis. Sci.* **2012**, *53*, 5594–5608. [CrossRef]
42. Mitamura, Y.; Mitamura-Aizawa, S.; Nagasawa, T.; Katome, T.; Eguchi, H.; Naito, T. Diagnostic imaging in patients with retinitis pigmentosa. *J. Med. Investig.* **2012**, *59*, 1–11. [CrossRef]
43. Tee, J.J.L.; Kalitzeos, A.; Webster, A.R.; Peto, T.; Michaelides, M. Quantitative analysis of hyperautofluorescent rings to characterize the natural history and progression in RPGR-associated retinopathy. *Retina* **2018**, *38*, 2401–2414. [CrossRef]
44. Robson, A.G.; Michaelides, M.; Luong, V.A.; Holder, G.E.; Bird, A.C.; Webster, A.R.; Moore, A.T.; Fitzke, F.W. Functional correlates of fundus autofluorescence abnormalities in patients with RPGR or RIMS1 mutations causing cone or cone rod dystrophy. *Br. J. Ophthalmol.* **2008**, *92*, 95–102. [CrossRef]
45. Zhang, Q.; Giacalone, J.C.; Searby, C.; Stone, E.M.; Tucker, B.A.; Sheffield, V.C. Disruption of RPGR protein interaction network is the common feature of RPGR missense variations that cause XLRP. *Proc. Natl. Acad. Sci. USA* **2019**, *116*, 1353–1360. [CrossRef]

46. Hoffman, D.R.; Hughbanks-Wheaton, D.K.; Pearson, N.S.; Fish, G.E.; Spencer, R.; Takacs, A.; Klein, M.; Locke, K.G.; Birch, D.G. Four-year placebo-controlled trial of docosahexaenoic acid in X-linked retinitis pigmentosa (DHAX trial): A randomized clinical trial. *JAMA Ophthalmol.* **2014**, *132*, 866–873. [CrossRef]
47. Beltran, W.A.; Wen, R.; Acland, G.M.; Aguirre, G.D. Intravitreal injection of ciliary neurotrophic factor (CNTF) causes peripheral remodeling and does not prevent photoreceptor loss in canine RPGR mutant retina. *Exp. Eye Res.* **2007**, *84*, 753–771. [CrossRef]
48. Ho, A.C.; Humayun, M.S.; Dorn, J.D.; da Cruz, L.; Dagnelie, G.; Handa, J.; Barale, P.O.; Sahel, J.A.; Stanga, P.E.; Hafezi, F.; et al. Long-term results from an epiretinal prosthesis to restore sight to the blind. *Ophthalmology* **2015**, *122*, 1547–1554. [CrossRef]
49. Edwards, T.L.; Cottriall, C.L.; Xue, K.; Simunovic, M.P.; Ramsden, J.D.; Zrenner, E.; MacLaren, R.E. Assessment of the Electronic Retinal Implant α AMS in Restoring Vision to Blind Patients with End-Stage Retinitis Pigmentosa. *Ophthalmology* **2018**, *125*, 432–443. [CrossRef]
50. Cehajic-Kapetanovic, J.; Eleftheriou, C.; Allen, A.E.; Milosavljevic, N.; Pienaar, A.; Bedford, R.; Davis, K.E.; Bishop, P.N.; Lucas, R.J. Restoration of Vision with Ectopic Expression of Human Rod Opsin. *Curr. Biol.* **2015**, *25*, 2111–2122. [CrossRef]
51. Eleftheriou, C.G.; Cehajic-Kapetanovic, J.; Martial, F.P.; Milosavljevic, N.; Bedford, R.A.; Lucas, R.J. Meclofenamic acid improves the signal to noise ratio for visual responses produced by ectopic expression of human rod opsin. *Mol. Vis.* **2017**, *23*, 334–345.
52. Hong, D.H.; Pawlyk, B.S.; Adamian, M.; Sandberg, M.A.; Li, T. A single, abbreviated RPGR-ORF15 variant reconstitutes RPGR function in vivo. *Investig. Ophthalmol. Vis. Sci.* **2005**, *46*, 435–441. [CrossRef]
53. Deng, W.T.; Dyka, F.M.; Dinculescu, A.; Li, J.; Zhu, P.; Chiodo, V.A.; Boye, S.L.; Conlon, T.J.; Erger, K.; Cossette, T.; et al. Stability and Safety of an AAV Vector for Treating RPGR-ORF15 X-Linked Retinitis Pigmentosa. *Hum. Gene. Ther.* **2015**, *26*, 593–602. [CrossRef]
54. Wu, Z.; Hiriyanna, S.; Qian, H.; Mookherjee, S.; Campos, M.M.; Gao, C.; Fariss, R.; Sieving, P.A.; Li, T.; Colosi, P.; et al. A long-term efficacy study of gene replacement therapy for RPGR-associated retinal degeneration. *Hum. Mol. Genet.* **2015**, *24*, 3956–3970. [CrossRef]
55. Beltran, W.A.; Cideciyan, A.V.; Lewin, A.S.; Iwabe, S.; Khanna, H.; Sumaroka, A.; Chiodo, V.A.; Fajardo, D.S.; Román, A.J.; Deng, W.T.; et al. Gene therapy rescues photoreceptor blindness in dogs and paves the way for treating human X-linked retinitis pigmentosa. *Proc. Natl. Acad. Sci. USA* **2012**, *109*, 2132–2137. [CrossRef]
56. Giacalone, J.C.; Andorf, J.L.; Zhang, Q.; Burnight, E.R.; Ochoa, D.; Reutzel, A.J.; Collins, M.M.; Sheffield, V.C.; Mullins, R.F.; Han, I.C.; et al. Development of a Molecularly Stable Gene Therapy Vector for the Treatment of *RPGR*-Associated X-Linked Retinitis Pigmentosa. *Hum. Gene. Ther.* **2019**, *30*, 967–974. [CrossRef]

© 2019 by the authors. Licensee MDPI, Basel, Switzerland. This article is an open access article distributed under the terms and conditions of the Creative Commons Attribution (CC BY) license (http://creativecommons.org/licenses/by/4.0/).

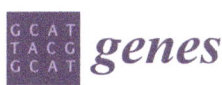

Article

Correction of NR2E3 Associated Enhanced S-cone Syndrome Patient-specific iPSCs using CRISPR-Cas9

Laura R. Bohrer, Luke A. Wiley, Erin R. Burnight, Jessica A. Cooke, Joseph C. Giacalone, Kristin R. Anfinson, Jeaneen L. Andorf, Robert F. Mullins, Edwin M. Stone and Budd A. Tucker *

Institute for Vision Research, Department of Ophthalmology and Visual Sciences, University of Iowa, Iowa City, IA 52241, USA; laura-bohrer@uiowa.edu (L.R.B.); luke-wiley@uiowa.edu (L.A.W.); erin-burnight@uiowa.edu (E.R.B.); jessica-cooke@uiowa.edu (J.A.C.); joseph-giacalone@uiowa.edu (J.C.G.); kristin-anfinson@uiowa.edu (K.R.A.); jeaneen-andorf@uiowa.edu (J.L.A.); robert-mullins@uiowa.edu (R.F.M.); edwin-stone@uiowa.edu (E.M.S.)
* Correspondence: budd-tucker@uiowa.edu

Received: 15 March 2019; Accepted: 3 April 2019; Published: 5 April 2019

Abstract: Enhanced S-cone syndrome (ESCS) is caused by recessive mutations in the photoreceptor cell transcription factor *NR2E3*. Loss of *NR2E3* is characterized by repression of rod photoreceptor cell gene expression, over-expansion of the S-cone photoreceptor cell population, and varying degrees of M- and L-cone photoreceptor cell development. In this study, we developed a CRISPR-based homology-directed repair strategy and corrected two different disease-causing *NR2E3* mutations in patient-derived induced pluripotent stem cells (iPSCs) generated from two affected individuals. In addition, one patient's iPSCs were differentiated into retinal cells and *NR2E3* transcription was evaluated in CRISPR corrected and uncorrected clones. The patient's c.119-2A>C mutation caused the inclusion of a portion of intron 1, the creation of a frame shift, and generation of a premature stop codon. In summary, we used a single set of CRISPR reagents to correct different mutations in iPSCs generated from two individuals with ESCS. In doing so we demonstrate the advantage of using retinal cells derived from affected patients over artificial in vitro model systems when attempting to demonstrate pathophysiologic mechanisms of specific mutations.

Keywords: induced pluripotent stem cell (iPSC); clustered regularly interspaced short palindromic repeats (CRISPR); homology-directed repair (HDR); Enhanced S-Cone Syndrome (ESCS); *NR2E3*

1. Introduction

Enhanced S-cone syndrome (ESCS) is an autosomal recessive retinopathy that results from mutations in the photoreceptor cell transcription factor, *NR2E3* (Nuclear Receptor Subfamily 2, Group E, Member 3). *NR2E3*, which is specifically expressed in the outer nuclear layer of the human retina [1], is a direct transcriptional target of NRL, a key regulator of photoreceptor cell genesis. Work in animal models has shown that *NR2E3* acts to repress cone photoreceptor cell gene expression and promote rod photoreceptor cell fate commitment. Specifically, loss of *NR2E3* function hinders rod photoreceptor cell development and drives over-expansion of the S-opsin-positive cone photoreceptor cell population (i.e., blue cones) [2–6], which is normally the least prevalent of the photoreceptor cell subtypes.

Patients with ESCS present with increased sensitivity to blue light (due to overabundance of short wavelength sensitive S-cones), early onset impairment of night vision (due primarily to lack of functional rod development) and varying degrees of sensitivity to green and red light (due to varying abundance of medium wavelength sensitive M-cones and long wavelength sensitive L-cones). Although the disease is progressive in nature, clinically evident retinal degeneration is often highly-variable, ranging from a relatively mild and nearly static disorder in some individuals to a very severe and progressive disease in others [1,7–10].

To date, more than 33 different disease-causing mutations in *NR2E3* have been described [1,11,12]. In addition to ESCS, mutations in NR2E3 can also cause more severe forms of retinal disease, including Goldmann-Farve syndrome (GFS) or autosomal dominant retinitis pigmentosa (adRP). Of these mutations, the majority are in either DNA- (e.g., c.219G>C; p.(Arg73Ser)) or ligand-binding (e.g., c.932G>A; p.(Arg311Gln)) domains of the NR2E3 protein [11,13]. That said, one of the most common *NR2E3* mutations reported in the United States is c.119-2A>C [13], which falls within the canonical splice acceptor site of intron 1. To demonstrate the functional effect of this mutation, Bernal and colleagues transiently transfected COS7 cells with an expression plasmid containing a copy of the *NR2E3* gene harboring the c.119-2A>C variant [14]. Sequence analysis revealed that in addition to the normal transcript, an aberrant transcript that lacked exon 2 and contained a premature stop codon in exon 3 was also present [14].

Understanding how different disease-causing *NR2E3* genotypes alter retinal development and give rise to the observed spectrum of clinical outcomes is of particular interest and relevance to investigators attempting to develop treatments based on photoreceptor cell replacement. Specifically, by understanding exactly how genes such as *NR2E3* function, we may be able to strategically guide developing photoreceptor cells down a more cone-selective path (i.e., alter *NR2E3* function to increase cone genesis without causing widespread photoreceptor cell degeneration). To evaluate the effects of different *NR2E3* variants on photoreceptor cell fate, we have used CRISPR-based genome editing of human patient-derived induced pluripotent stem cells (iPSC). Human iPSCs have several advantages over animal models for this type of work. Unlike animal models, iPSCs can be generated from patients with known disease-causing variants on genetic backgrounds that are demonstrably permissive of the disease. By correcting the patients' mutations one at a time, one can readily evaluate the role of a specific variant on gene expression and phenotypic outcome. Correlating these in vitro findings with the patients' clinical history may provide a better understanding of how variants in each of the different *NR2E3* domains influence photoreceptor cell fate decisions.

To correct retinal disease-causing variants in patient-derived iPSCs, we and others have used CRISPR-based genome editing [15–22]. Unlike the more cumbersome ZFN- and TALEN-based approaches, which require the development of elaborate genomic targeting complexes, the CRISPR method relies on the use of small single guide RNAs (sgRNAs) that can be easily synthesized to direct human codon-optimized Cas9 nuclease to specific genomic targets. Cas9 induces double-strand DNA breaks that can subsequently be repaired via fairly error-prone non-homologous end joining (NHEJ), or via the more precise homology-directed repair (HDR) mechanism [15]. The advantage of the HDR-based strategy, even for mutations within the deep intronic space where NHEJ could be used, is that a single HDR repair template and set of sgRNAs is often sufficient to correct a variety of different mutations that are contained within a limited genomic space (e.g., an HDR template spanning exons 1 through 3 would cover both the above-mentioned c.119-2A>C splice site mutation and the p.(Arg73Ser) variant contained within the *NR2E3*-DNA binding element). By using the same set of reagents to correct a variety of mutations in different cell lines, one can control for differences related to reagent variability while increasing throughput.

In this study, we developed a CRISPR-Cas9-based HDR strategy to correct two different *NR2E3* mutations in iPSCs generated from two patients with clinically-diagnosed and molecularly-confirmed ESCS: Patient 1 harbors homozygous c.119-2A>C mutations, and Patient 2 harbors compound heterozygous p.(Arg73Ser) and p.(Arg311Gln) mutations. The close proximity of c.119-2A>C and p.(Arg73Ser) allowed the same sgRNA and HDR reagents to be used to correct iPSC lines generated from both individuals. Genomic correction of both mutations was confirmed by PCR and Sanger sequencing. To demonstrate the utility of this system for elucidating disease mechanism, iPSCs obtained from Patient 1, both before and after CRISPR correction, were differentiated down a photoreceptor cell lineage. Analysis of the *NR2E3* transcript revealed that, prior to CRISPR correction, patient-derived retinal cells completely lack wild-type messages and instead express a mutant transcript that contains a portion of intron 1, which causes a frameshift and the creation of a premature stop codon. Following monoallelic CRISPR correction, the expression of the wild-type *NR2E3* transcript was restored.

2. Materials and Methods

2.1. Patient-Derived iPSCs

This study was approved by the Institutional Review Board of the University of Iowa (project approval #200202022) and adhered to the tenets set forth in the Declaration of Helsinki. The dermal fibroblast-derived iPSCs used in this study were generated from two patients with molecularly confirmed ESCS. These previously described cell lines were generated using current good manufacturing practices in a clean room environment and validated using scorecard and karyotypic analysis [23]. Consistent with the patients' clinical diagnoses and unlike control individuals, differentiation of these lines gave rise to S-opsin-positive blue cone photoreceptor cell-dominated retinal organoids, which lack rod photoreceptor cells [24].

2.2. Cloning of CRISPR-Cas9 and HDR Donor Constructs

The sgRNAs used in this study were designed to target the region of *NR2E3* that contains the c.119-2A>C (Patient 1) and c.219G>C; p.(Arg73Ser) (Patient 2) mutations using the Benchling platform (www.benchling.com) or the Optimized CRISPR Design Tool (crispr.mit.edu). Guides were cloned into our previously described bicistronic construct expressing a human codon-optimized *Streptococcus pyogenes Cas9* (*spCas9*) nuclease [17,18]. A homology-directed repair (HDR) construct was synthesized by GenScript. As described previously, the HDR plasmid contains 450–750 bp of homologous sequence flanking a floxed puromycin resistance gene followed by the Herpes Simplex Virus type 1 thymidine kinase (vTK) gene [16].

2.3. Screening of NR2E3-specific sgRNAs

sgRNA and CRISPR-Cas9 constructs were transfected into HEK293T cells (ATCC) using Lipofectamine 2000 (Thermo Fisher Scientific) and cleavage was assessed via a T7 endonuclease 1 (T7E1) assay using *NR2E3*-specific primers (Table S1) as described previously [17,18]. Control iPSCs were transfected with 2 µg of plasmid using the Neon transfection system as described previously [16].

2.4. Delivery of sgRNA-Cas9 and the HDR Contruct to NR2E3-Patient-Specific iPSCs

The CRISPR-Cas9 machinery was delivered to iPSCs and analyzed as described previously [16–18]. Briefly, the sg4-spCas9 and HDR plasmids were transfected at a 1:2 molar ratio into patient iPSCs with Lipofectamine Stem (Thermo Fisher Scientific; Patient 1) or Neon electroporation (Thermo Fisher Scientific; Patient 2). Puromycin (0.5 µg/mL) selection was performed as previously described [16], and surviving colonies were PCR screened for HDR incorporation and sequenced to confirm correction. The puroR-vTK cassette was removed by Lipofectamine Stem transfection of Cre recombinase, and cells were treated with 40–400 nM Ganciclovir to select for those with vTK removal. The top off-target sites (Table S2) were determined using the Benchling platform (https://benchling.com/) and analyzed using the T7E1 assays as described above.

2.5. Retinal Differentiation

Undifferentiated iPSCs cultured on Laminin-521 coated culture dishes in Essential 8 medium (Thermo Fisher Scientific) were transitioned to Matrigel (Corning) coated culture dishes in mTESR1 medium (StemCell Technologies). Transitioned cells were passaged every 4–5 days using 1mg/ml dispase (Thermo Fisher Scientific). Differentiation was initiated through embryoid body (EB) formation as previously described [25]. Briefly, EBs were generated on ultra-low adhesion plates and transitioned from mTESR1 to neural induction medium (NIM - DMEM/F12 (1:1), 1% N2 supplement, 1% non-essential amino acids, 1% Glutamax (Thermo Fisher Scientific), 2 µg/ml heparin (Sigma) and

0.2% Primocin (Invivogen)) over a three day time period. EBs were maintained free-floating in NIM until day 7, at which time they were induced to adhere to tissue culture-treated plates overnight in NIM supplemented with 25% fetal bovine serum (FBS). Media was replaced with NIM minus FBS on day 8 and the adherent EBs were fed with NIM every other day until day 16. On day 16, the entire EB outgrowth was mechanically lifted using a cell scraper and transferred to retinal differentiation medium (RDM - DMEM/F12 (3:1), 2% B27 supplement, 1% non-essential amino acids, 1% Glutamax and 0.2% Primocin). Three-dimensional aggregates maintained in RDM give rise to both retinal organoids and non-retinal neurospheres that can be isolated based on their morphological appearances. Retinal organoids were isolated and dissociated at 5–6 weeks using Accutase (StemCell Technologies) and cells were subsequently plated onto laminin (Sigma) coated tissue culture plates. Cells were maintained in RDM and collected at a series of time points for RNA analysis.

2.6. Reverse Transcription PCR

Total RNA was extracted from cells using either the NucleoSpin RNA extraction kit (Machery-Nagel) or TRIzol (Thermo Fisher Scientific) following the manufacturer's protocol. cDNA was generated with the High Capacity cDNA Reverse Transcription Kit (Applied Biosystems) using 200 ng of RNA template. *NR2E3* transcript was amplified using BIOLASE DNA polymerase (Bioline) and *NR2E3* specific primers (Table S1). PCR products were separated on an agarose gel and bands were excised, purified using the QIAquick Gel Extraction Kit (Qiagen) and subcloned using the PCR2.1 TOPO TA cloning kit (Invitrogen). Colonies were subsequently picked and Sanger sequenced using M13(-20)F or M13R primers.

3. Results

3.1. Testing CRISPR-Cas9 Guide Cleavage in HEK293T Cells and iPSCs

The goal of this study was to develop a CRISPR-Cas9 homology-directed repair strategy suitable for the correction of disease-causing mutations in iPSCs generated from two independent patients with molecularly confirmed *NR2E3*-associated enhanced S-cone syndrome (Figure 1A,B). As enhanced S-cone syndrome has a recessive mode of inheritance (such that correction of only one allele would be expected to mitigate the disease phenotype) and the p.(Arg73Ser) mutation on the paternal allele of Patient 2 is within 100 bps of the c.119-2A>C mutations in Patient 1, we hypothesized that a single CRISPR-Cas9 HDR cassette would be sufficient for the correction of iPSCs generated from both individuals. We began by designing and testing 5 different sgRNAs that utilized the spCas9 PAM sites. To determine the efficiency of cleavage, we evaluated nonhomologous end joining (NHEJ) using T7E1 assays in HEK293T cells transfected with each sgRNA and spCas9. While no cleavage was detected in controls (i.e., untransfected cells), all 5 guides induced cleavage and indel formation with similar efficiencies in the transfected cells (Figure 1C). The ability of all 5 guides to direct specific DNA cleavage was subsequently evaluated in iPSCs generated from a normal non-diseased individual. As with HEK293T cells, all 5 guides induced DNA cleavage and indel formation; however, more robust cleavage was detected in cells that received sg2 and sg4 (Figure 1D). As the PAM sequence used by sg4 could be readily modified with a synonymous mutation in the HDR cassette that would prevent re-cleavage events without altering the predicted amino acid sequence, this guide was chosen for all subsequent patient-specific genome repair experiments.

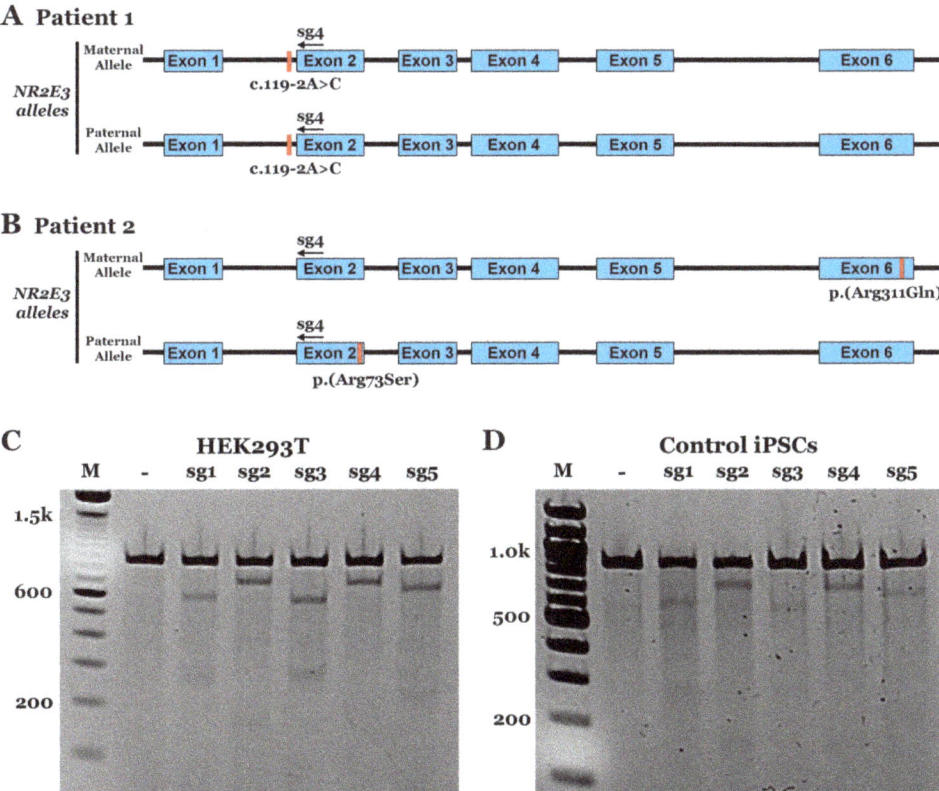

Figure 1. Analysis of CRISPR-Cas9 sgRNA mediated cleavage efficiency. **A,B**: Schematics depicting genomic disease-causing mutations in Patient 1—homozygous c.119-2A>C mutations (**A**) and Patient 2—compound heterozygous p.(Arg73Ser) and p.(Arg311Gln) mutations (**B**). **C,D**: Representative gel images of T7E1 assays in HEK293T (**C**) and control induced pluripotent stem cells (iPSCs) (**D**) for 5 different sgRNAs. No transfection control: (-).

3.2. CRISPR Correction of the NR2E3 c.119-2A>C mutation in Patient-Specific iPSCs using Homology-Directed Repair (HDR)

To correct the c.119-2A>C and p.(Arg73Ser) variants in iPSCs generated from the patients described in Figure 1, we designed an HDR donor cassette with ~500 bps of homologous sequence upstream and downstream of the sg4 cleavage site (Figure 2A). As indicated above, to prevent re-cleavage events, we included a synonymous variant in the sg4 PAM site (CGG>CGA). To select for cells that incorporated the HDR sequence, a puromycin resistance cassette under the control of the mPGK promoter was added to intron 1 as previously described [16,18]. In addition, the stop codon in the puromycin resistance sequence was replaced with a porcine 2A peptide (P2A) coding sequence, followed by the Herpes Simplex Virus type 1 thymidine kinase (vTK) gene (thymidine kinase phosphorylates ganciclovir, a nucleoside analog, which disrupts DNA synthesis and induces cell death) and a downstream polyadenylation sequence (PA) [16]. The entire cassette, mPGK-PuroR-vTK-PA, was flanked by loxP sites that enabled removal of the cassette via Cre recombinase [16]. Following Cre recombinase transfection, treatment of cells with ganciclovir allowed for the selection of cells that had lost the cassette [16]. Patient 1 iPSCs were transfected with sg4NR2E3-spCas9 and the HDR construct via lipofection. Puromycin selection was subsequently performed as described in the methods section. Following selection, cells were clonally expanded and screened for incorporation of the HDR sequence via PCR using a forward primer in the PA sequence (Figure 2A,F1) and a reverse primer outside the HDR cassette (Figure 2A,R1). Eighteen of the 25 screened clones amplified the expected PCR product, indicating incorporation of the HDR cassette (Figure S1). We chose 2 clones, clone 16 and clone 17, to confirm genomic correction. PCR was performed using primers that spanned the mutation (Figure 2A,F2,R2) and the PCR product was TA cloned. Sequencing demonstrated that all products from clone 17 still had the disease-causing c.119-2A>C mutation. However, 5 of the 12 clones from the clone 16 PCR product showed a normal sequence, indicating a monoallelic correction of the c.119-2A>C variant (Figure S2). Clone 16 was subsequently transfected with Cre recombinase to remove the floxed PuroR-vTK cassette. After a second transfection with Cre recombinase, some cells containing the PuroR-vTK cassette still remained (Figure 2C). To select for cells that lacked the PuroR-vTK cassette, cultures were treated with ganciclovir, which resulted in the removal of the PuroR-vTK containing cells (Figure 2C). PCR products using primers outside the PuroR-vTK cassette (Figure 2D,F2) and homology arm (Figure 2D,R2) demonstrated equal amounts of genomic DNA. To evaluate off-target cutting events, the top 10 off-target sites and 2 additional exonic loci selected from the top 24 off-target sites, each predicted via Benchling, were analyzed. T7E1 assays were performed with genomic DNA from unmodified control and CRISPR-corrected cells. We observed no evidence of off-target events at any of the genomic loci evaluated; that is, we observed no cleavage products that were specific to the corrected cells (Figure S3).

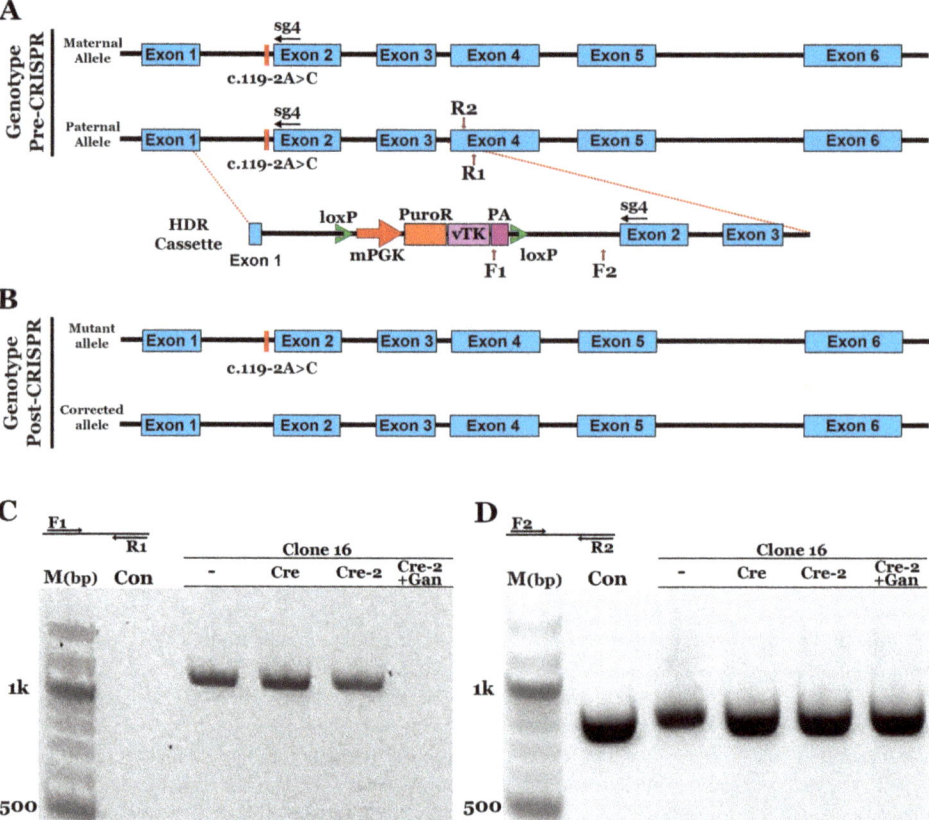

Figure 2. CRISPR-based homology-directed repair of the c.119-2A>C mutation in patient-derived iPSCs. (**A**): Schematic diagram depicting the genotype pre-CRISPR correction and the homology-directed repair (HDR) cassette designed to repair the c.119-2A>C mutation: Homologous sequence upstream

and downstream of the loxP flanked puromycin resistance (PuroR), viral thymidine kinase (vTK), and SV40 polyadenylation (PA). (**B**): Schematic depicting the genotype following CRISPR-based repair: Monoallelic correction results in a cell line that contains one corrected allele and one mutant allele. (**C**): Representative gel image of the genomic PCR confirming incorporation of HDR cassette in clone 16 and cassette removal following transfection of Cre recombinase and selection with ganciclovir (Cre-2, +Gan). (**D**): Representative gel image of genomic PCR from the same samples presented in panel C to demonstrate similar amounts of DNA. PCR products were also used for sequencing to confirm the correction of clone 16.

3.3. CRISPR Correction of the NR2E3 p.(Arg73Ser) Mutation in Patient-Specific iPSCs using HDR

As indicated above, the p.(Arg73Ser) mutation in Patient 2 is located 100 bps away from the c.119-2A>C mutations in Patient 1. We therefore wanted to determine if the same HDR cassette and genome editing strategy used to correct Patient 1's iPSCs could be used to correct iPSCs generated from this individual (Figure 3A). The same plasmids were delivered; however, instead of Lipofectamine Stem, electroporation was used to determine if a different delivery method could also be used to achieve robust correction. We observed a similar efficiency with electroporation; specifically, 20 of 24 clones screened had a PCR product that indicated incorporation of the HDR cassette (Figure S4,F1,R1 primers). Patient 2 is a compound heterozygote, and only the p.(Arg73Ser) mutation was targeted using this HDR cassette. As a result, extra screening was needed to identify clones that had the HDR sequence specifically incorporated into the p.(Arg73Ser)-containing paternal allele as opposed to the maternal allele, which is wild-type at this location (Figure 3A). To identify patient-derived iPSCs that had the paternal p.(Arg73Ser) allele corrected, PCR products obtained from 6 clonally expanded iPSC lines were sequenced using the F2/R2 primer pair. Following this analysis, clone 6 was found to be corrected. None of the 18 sequencing reactions performed on DNA obtained from clone 6 contained the p.(Arg73Ser) variant (Figure S5). Not surprisingly, the p.(Arg311Gln) mutation in exon 6, which lies outside of the region of homology covered by the HDR cassette, was still present (Figure S5). A single transfection with Cre recombinase and subsequent selection with ganciclovir resulted in the removal of cells containing the PuroR-vTK cassette (Figure 3C, Cre+Gan). PCR products using both sequencing primer sets F2/R2 and F3/R3 revealed equal amounts of genomic DNA (Figure 3D,E). Using the same strategy described for Patient 1 above, Patient 2 iPSCs were evaluated for off-target cleavage events. As shown in Figure S6, indel formation was identified in OT7. However, as OT7 is located within the middle of an intronic region of a non-retinal gene, it would not be predicted to affect retinal cell development, health, and/or function. Collectively, the above-described findings indicate that a single HDR cassette can be used to successfully correct iPSCs obtained from two independent patients with separate disease-causing mutations in the gene *NR2E3*.

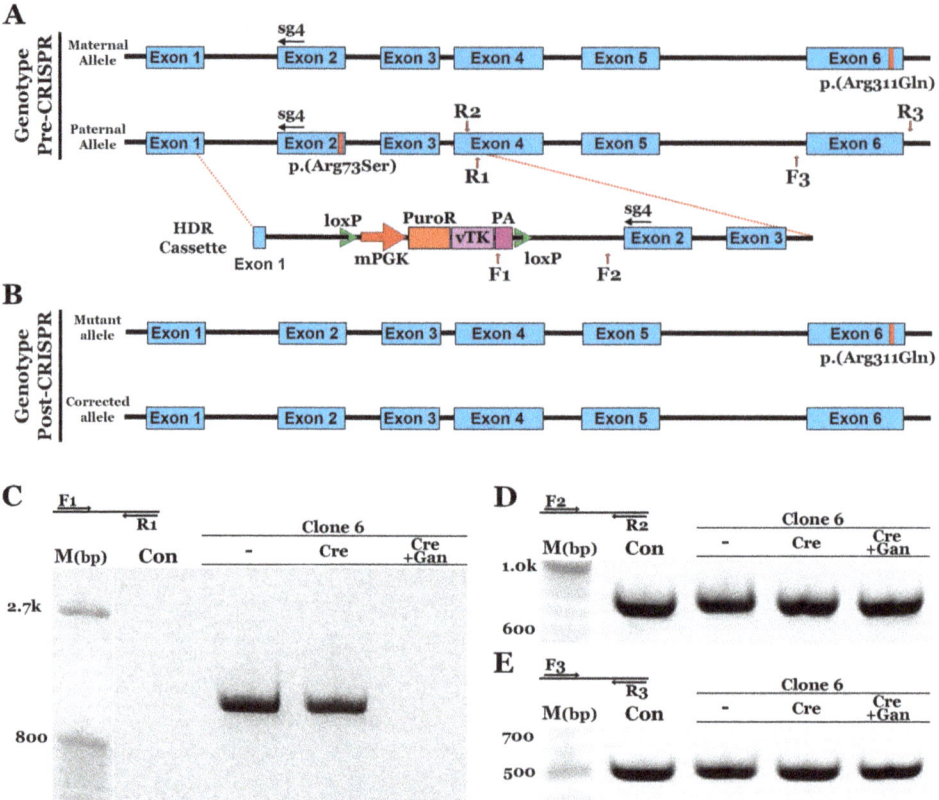

Figure 3. CRISPR-based homology-directed repair of the p.(Arg73Ser) mutation in patient-derived iPSCs. (**A**): Schematic diagram depicting the genotype pre-CRISPR correction and the HDR cassette used to repair the p.(Arg73Ser) mutation: Homologous sequence upstream and downstream of the loxP flanked puromycin resistance (PuroR), viral thymidine kinase (vTK), and SV40 polyadenylation (PA). (**B**): Schematic depicting the genotype following CRISPR-based repair: One corrected allele and one mutant allele harboring the p.(Arg311Gln) mutation. (**C**): Representative gel image of the genomic PCR confirming incorporation of the HDR cassette in clone 6 and cassette removal following transfection of Cre recombinase and selection with ganciclovir (Cre, +Gan). **D,E:** Representative gel images of the genomic PCR using the same samples in panel C to demonstrate similar amounts of DNA. PCR products were also used for sequencing to confirm the correction of clone 6 in one allele (**D**) and the presence of the p.(Arg311Gln) mutation in the other allele (**E**).

3.4. CRISPR-based Restoration of the NR2E3 Transcript in Patient-derived Retinal Cells

NR2E3 is a nuclear transcription factor that is required for rod photoreceptor cell genesis; thus, to confirm that CRISPR-based genomic correction restores expression of NR2E3 transcript, iPSCs (Figure 4A–C) were differentiated toward a retinal cell fate. The iPSCs generated from Patient 1, who is homozygous for the c.119-2A>C splice site mutation, were predicted to have the most overt molecular phenotype. Thus, Patient 1's cells were chosen for the transcriptional analysis. As shown in Figure 4, at 5–6 weeks post-differentiation, three-dimensional optic vesicles generated from control (D), affected patient (E), and CRISPR-corrected (F) iPSCs appear to develop normally. To evaluate the normal kinetics of NR2E3 expression, control iPSC-derived retinal cells were harvested at 6–20 weeks following initiation of differentiation. NR2E3 expression is first detected after approximately 10 weeks of differentiation and is strongly expressed between weeks 13–20 (Figure 4G). After 9 weeks of differentiation, the wild-type *NR2E3* transcript was detectable in CRISPR-corrected as opposed to non-corrected iPSC-derived retinal progenitor cells (Figure 4G). By week 14, the robust expression of wild-type *NR2E3* transcript could be detected in CRISPR-corrected retinal cells (Figure 4G). Interestingly, at this timepoint, a second larger transcript could also be detected in both corrected and uncorrected cells (Figure 4G). Following gel purification and sequencing, we found that the upper band actually contained two novel transcripts that differ by only 32 bps (which explains why they appear as a single product on a 2% agarose gel). The larger transcript included 143 bps of intron 1 followed by exon 2, and the smaller contained 111 bps of intron 1 followed by exon 2. In both cases, the inclusion of this intronic sequence resulted in a frame shift and the creation of a premature stop codon just 47 bps downstream of the canonical exon 1 boundary (Figure S7). In summary, monoallelic genomic correction of the c.119-2A>C variant in patient-derived iPSCs restores the cells ability to make wild-type *NR2E3* transcript during retinal cell differentiation.

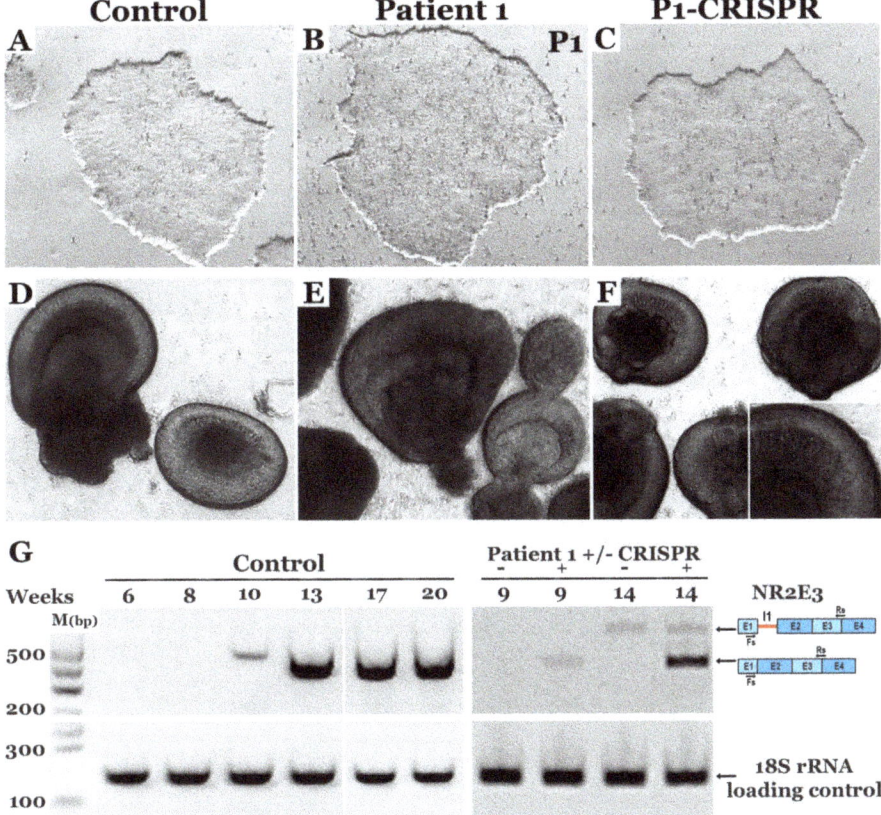

Figure 4. Correction of c.119-2A>C restores expression of normal *NR2E3* transcript in patient-derived retinal cells. **A–C**: Bright-field images of control (**A**), Patient 1 (**B**) and CRISPR-corrected Patient 1 (**C**) iPSCs. **D–F**: Bright-field images of control (**D**), Patient 1 (**E**) and CRISPR-corrected Patient 1 (**F**) optic vesicles at 5 weeks following initiation of differentiation. **G**: *NR2E3* transcript analysis by semi-quantitative PCR in control and Patient 1 iPSC derived retinal cells before (-) and after (+) CRISPR correction at various time points following the initiation of differentiation; 18S rRNA was amplified as a loading control.

4. Discussion

The discovery of iPSCs, the creation of protocols for successful tissue-specific differentiation, and the development of CRISPR-based genome editing have collectively enabled scientists to study pathophysiology in human tissues like the retina that are usually inaccessible in living individuals. For example, our ability to generate photoreceptor cells from patients with molecularly-undiagnosed retinitis pigmentosa allowed us to demonstrate how a newly identified mutation in the gene male germ cell associated kinase (MAK) causes photoreceptor cell-specific disease [26]. Similarly, by generating retinal pigmented epithelial cells from a patient with suspected RPE65 associated Leber congenital amaurosis (LCA), we were able to demonstrate that a novel intronic variant in a child of Haitian ancestry, which could have easily been a non-disease causing ethnic polymorphism, altered splicing and normal transcript production [27]. In the burgeoning field of retinal gene therapy, where molecular confirmation of a patient's disease-causing genotype is required for enrollment in a clinical gene augmentation trial, the ability to use these approaches to demonstrate that a patient truly has the disease being targeted will be invaluable.

In addition to being useful for confirming a patient's disease-causing genotype, disease-specific phenotypes identified in patient-derived cells (which can be confirmed via CRISPR-based genomic correction) are proving to be helpful for the evaluation and development of novel therapeutics. For instance, we recently demonstrated how AAV-based replacement of *CLN3* and mitigation of the molecular phenotype in patient-derived photoreceptor cells was preferable for the demonstration of treatment efficacy to the use of an animal model that does not accurately recapitulate the disease [28]. In the current study, we demonstrate how patient-derived iPSCs and CRISPR-based genome editing can be used to evaluate the molecular phenotype associated with the rare disease, enhanced S-cone syndrome. As indicated in the introduction, enhanced S-cone syndrome is caused by mutations in the gene *NR2E3*, which disrupt rod photoreceptor cell development and result in overproduction of blue cones. By identifying how genetic alterations in *NR2E3* expression alter both disease progression and the percentage of cone and rod photoreceptor cells, we may be able to further refine our current retinal differentiation protocols.

From a photoreceptor cell replacement perspective, to restore high-acuity vision, transplantation of high-density cone photoreceptor cells will be required. There are a few promising strategies for isolating cones from retinal organoids, which depending on cell line and differentiation protocol used can have different percentages of rods vs. cones that result from using current retinal differentiation protocols (reviewed in References [29,30]); however, all of them require a large scale culture in order to obtain a sufficient number of cones following selection for retinal transplantation. A method for directing retinal differentiation along a cone selective path would be a valuable improvement. Typically, we and others have taken cues from developmental biology and designed experiments to vary the type, dosage, and timing of exogenous factor delivery as we attempt to accelerate or shift differentiation in one direction or another [31–35]. Although not a traditional approach, taking cues from naturally occurring genetic disease, where single base pair changes can drastically alter the phenotypic outcome, may also be useful. As we demonstrate in this manuscript, a single CRISPR-based HDR strategy can be used to correct a variety of different mutations spanning several exons of NR2E3. By comparing these changes to both in vitro phenotype and patient history, it may be possible to identify variants that selectively promote cone cell genesis with little or no associated retinal degeneration.

Although unexpected, one of the more interesting findings that we report in this study pertains to the molecular mechanism of the c.119-2A>C variant and is in opposition to a previous publication on this subject [14]. It is important to note that the previous study was performed prior to the widespread use of iPSCs and the development of CRISPR-based genome editing, and as a result, the authors elected to test the function of this variant by transiently transfecting COS7 cells (transformed green monkey kidney cells) with an expression plasmid that contained the *NR2E3* gene harboring the c.119-2A>C mutation. Transcriptional analysis in their system indicated that this mutation resulted in skipping of exon 2, which caused a frameshift and creation of a premature stop codon in exon 3 [14]. In our study, by focusing on endogenously expressed *NR2E3* in human patient-derived photoreceptor cells, we found that the c.119-2A>C mutation in fact generates an abnormal transcript that includes a segment of intron 1 followed by exon 2, which also causes a frameshift and the creation of a premature stop codon. Interestingly, analysis of the wild-type and mutant alleles using the ESEFinder 3.0 program (rulai.cshl.edu) revealed a difference in predicted splicing factor binding sites. An SRSF1 site was found to be present in the wild-type but absent in the mutant, and an SRSF6 site that is absent in wild-type was found to be present in the mutant. We suspect that the change in splice factor binding activated a cryptic splice acceptor site in intron 1 in the iPSC-derived retinal cells rather than a skipping of exon 2 as observed in the previous COS7 study. The reason that the cryptic splice site was not used in the COS7 system could simply be due to species and cell type-specific differences in the splicing machinery. That is, it is possible that the splicing machinery used by monkey kidney cells is somewhat different from that used by human photoreceptor cells. Regardless, this finding illustrates the importance of using the appropriate cell type, obtained from the species of interest, when making inferences about the function of different genetic variants. This will be especially true when attempting to determine the pathogenicity of newly identified genetic variants in the age of clinical molecular medicine.

Supplementary Materials: The following are available online at http://www.mdpi.com/2073-4425/10/4/278/s1, Figure S1: Identification of HDR cassette incorporation in Patient 1 iPSCs., Figure S2: Sequencing of Patient 1 iPSCs., Figure S3: Off-target analysis of sg4 in Patient 1 iPSCs., Figure S4: Identification of HDR cassette incorporation in Patient 2 iPSCs., Figure S5: Sequencing of Patient 2 iPSCs., Figure S6: Off-target analysis of sg4 in Patient 2 iPSCs., Figure S7: Analysis of *NR2E3* transcript expression.; Table S1. List of sgRNAs and primers used., Table S2. List of off-target sequences, PAM sites, off-target scores, chromosomal location of off-targets and primer sequences.

Author Contributions: Study conceptualization, L.R.B., L.A.W., R.F.M., E.M.S. and B.A.T.; methodology, L.R.B., L.A.W., E.R.B., J.A.C., J.C.G., K.R.A. and J.L.A.; data curation, L.R.B., L.A.W., E.R.B., J.A.C., J.C.G., K.R.A. and J.L.A.; writing—original draft preparation, L.R.B., R.F.M., E.M.S. and B.A.T.; writing—review and editing, L.R.B., L.A.W., E.R.B., J.A.C., J.L.A., R.F.M., E.M.S. and B.A.T.; supervision, R.F.M., E.M.S. and B.A.T.; funding acquisition, R.F.M., E.M.S. and B.A.T.

Funding: This research was funded by the National Institutes of Health, National Eye Institute, grant #'s P30-EY025580 & RO1-EY026008, and the University of Iowa, Institute for Vision Research.

Acknowledgments: We would like to thank the patients for donating skin biopsies from which the iPSCs used in this study were generated. We would like to thank the Carver Non-Profit Genetic Testing Laboratory for providing sequencing support and molecular confirmation of the patients' disease-causing genotype.

Conflicts of Interest: The authors declare no conflict of interest. The funders had no role in the design of the study; in the collection, analyses, or interpretation of data; in the writing of the manuscript, or in the decision to publish the results.

References

1. Haider, N.B.; Jacobson, S.G.; Cideciyan, A.V.; Swiderski, R.; Streb, L.M.; Searby, C.; Beck, G.; Hockey, R.; Hanna, D.B.; Gorman, S.; et al. Mutation of a nuclear receptor gene, NR2E3, causes enhanced S cone syndrome, a disorder of retinal cell fate. *Nat. Genet.* **2000**, *24*, 127–131. [CrossRef] [PubMed]
2. Haider, N.B.; Naggert, J.K.; Nishina, P.M. Excess cone cell proliferation due to lack of a functional NR2E3 causes retinal dysplasia and degeneration in rd7/rd7 mice. *Hum. Mol. Genet.* **2001**, *10*, 1619–1626. [CrossRef] [PubMed]
3. Haider, N.B.; Demarco, P.; Nystuen, A.M.; Huang, X.; Smith, R.S.; McCall, M.A.; Naggert, J.K.; Nishina, P.M. The transcription factor Nr2e3 functions in retinal progenitors to suppress cone cell generation. *Vis. Neurosci.* **2006**, *23*, 917–929. [CrossRef] [PubMed]
4. Haider, N.B.; Mollema, N.; Gaule, M.; Yuan, Y.; Sachs, A.J.; Nystuen, A.M.; Naggert, J.K.; Nishina, P.M. Nr2e3-directed transcriptional regulation of genes involved in photoreceptor development and cell-type specific phototransduction. *Exp. Eye Res.* **2009**, *89*, 365–372. [CrossRef] [PubMed]
5. Cheng, H.; Khan, N.W.; Roger, J.E.; Swaroop, A. Excess cones in the retinal degeneration rd7 mouse, caused by the loss of function of orphan nuclear receptor Nr2e3, originate from early-born photoreceptor precursors. *Hum. Mol. Genet.* **2011**, *20*, 4102–4115. [CrossRef] [PubMed]

6. Chen, J.; Rattner, A.; Nathans, J. The rod photoreceptor-specific nuclear receptor Nr2e3 represses transcription of multiple cone-specific genes. *J. Neurosci.* **2005**, *25*, 118–129. [CrossRef]
7. Marmor, M.F.; Jacobson, S.G.; Foerster, M.H.; Kellner, U.; Weleber, R.G. Diagnostic clinical findings of a new syndrome with night blindness, maculopathy, and enhanced S cone sensitivity. *Am. J. Ophthalmol.* **1990**, *110*, 124–134. [CrossRef]
8. Fishman, G.A.; Jampol, L.M.; Goldberg, M.F. Diagnostic features of the Favre-Goldmann syndrome. *Br. J. Ophthalmol* **1976**, *60*, 345–353. [CrossRef]
9. Garafalo, A.V.; Calzetti, G.; Cideciyan, A.V.; Roman, A.J.; Saxena, S.; Sumaroka, A.; Choi, W.; Wright, A.F.; Jacobson, S.G. Cone Vision Changes in the Enhanced S-Cone Syndrome Caused by NR2E3 Gene Mutations. *Invest. Ophthalmol. Vis. Sci.* **2018**, *59*, 3209–3219. [CrossRef]
10. Yzer, S.; Barbazetto, I.; Allikmets, R.; van Schooneveld, M.J.; Bergen, A.; Tsang, S.H.; Jacobson, S.G.; Yannuzzi, L.A. Expanded clinical spectrum of enhanced S-cone syndrome. *JAMA Ophthalmol* **2013**, *131*, 1324–1330. [CrossRef] [PubMed]
11. Schorderet, D.F.; Escher, P. NR2E3 mutations in enhanced S-cone sensitivity syndrome (ESCS), Goldmann-Favre syndrome (GFS), clumped pigmentary retinal degeneration (CPRD), and retinitis pigmentosa (RP). *Hum. Mutat.* **2009**, *30*, 1475–1485. [CrossRef] [PubMed]
12. Escher, P.; Gouras, P.; Roduit, R.; Tiab, L.; Bolay, S.; Delarive, T.; Chen, S.; Tsai, C.-C.; Hayashi, M.; Zernant, J.; et al. Mutations in NR2E3 can cause dominant or recessive retinal degenerations in the same family. *Hum. Mutat.* **2009**, *30*, 342–351. [CrossRef] [PubMed]
13. Stone, E.M.; Andorf, J.L.; Whitmore, S.S.; DeLuca, A.P.; Giacalone, J.C.; Streb, L.M.; Braun, T.A.; Mullins, R.F.; Scheetz, T.E.; Sheffield, V.C.; et al. Clinically Focused Molecular Investigation of 1000 Consecutive Families with Inherited Retinal Disease. *Ophthalmology* **2017**, *124*, 1314–1331. [CrossRef] [PubMed]
14. Bernal, S.; Solans, T.; Gamundi, M.J.; Hernan, I.; de Jorge, L.; Carballo, M.; Navarro, R.; Tizzano, E.; Ayuso, C.; Baiget, M. Analysis of the involvement of the NR2E3 gene in autosomal recessive retinal dystrophies. *Clin. Genet.* **2008**, *73*, 360–366. [CrossRef]
15. Burnight, E.R.; Giacalone, J.C.; Cooke, J.A.; Thompson, J.R.; Bohrer, L.R.; Chirco, K.R.; Drack, A.V.; Fingert, J.H.; Worthington, K.S.; Wiley, L.A.; et al. CRISPR-Cas9 genome engineering: Treating inherited retinal degeneration. *Prog Retin Eye Res.* **2018**, *65*, 28–49. [CrossRef] [PubMed]
16. Giacalone, J.C.; Sharma, T.P.; Burnight, E.R.; Fingert, J.F.; Mullins, R.F.; Stone, E.M.; Tucker, B.A. CRISPR-Cas9-Based Genome Editing of Human Induced Pluripotent Stem Cells. *Curr Protoc Stem Cell Biol* **2018**, *44*, 5B.7.1–5B.7.22. [PubMed]
17. Burnight, E.R.; Gupta, M.; Wiley, L.A.; Anfinson, K.R.; Tran, A.; Triboulet, R.; Hoffmann, J.M.; Klaahsen, D.L.; Andorf, J.L.; Jiao, C.; et al. Using CRISPR-Cas9 to Generate Gene-Corrected Autologous iPSCs for the Treatment of Inherited Retinal Degeneration. *Mol. Ther.* **2017**, *25*, 1999–2013. [CrossRef]
18. Burnight, E.R.; Bohrer, L.R.; Giacalone, J.C.; Klaahsen, D.L.; Daggett, H.T.; East, J.S.; Madumba, R.A.; Worthington, K.S.; Mullins, R.F.; Stone, E.M.; et al. CRISPR-Cas9-Mediated Correction of the 1.02 kb Common Deletion in CLN3 in Induced Pluripotent Stem Cells from Patients with Batten Disease. *The CRISPR Journal* **2018**, *1*, 75–87. [CrossRef]
19. Buskin, A.; Zhu, L.; Chichagova, V.; Basu, B.; Mozaffari-Jovin, S.; Dolan, D.; Droop, A.; Collin, J.; Bronstein, R.; Mehrotra, S.; et al. Disrupted alternative splicing for genes implicated in splicing and ciliogenesis causes PRPF31 retinitis pigmentosa. *Nat. Commun* **2018**, *9*, 4234. [CrossRef]
20. Steyer, B.; Bu, Q.; Cory, E.; Jiang, K.; Duong, S.; Sinha, D.; Steltzer, S.; Gamm, D.; Chang, Q.; Saha, K. Scarless Genome Editing of Human Pluripotent Stem Cells via Transient Puromycin Selection. *Stem Cell Reports* **2018**, *10*, 642–654. [CrossRef]
21. Deng, W.-L.; Gao, M.-L.; Lei, X.-L.; Lv, J.-N.; Zhao, H.; He, K.-W.; Xia, X.-X.; Li, L.-Y.; Chen, Y.-C.; Li, Y.-P.; et al. Gene Correction Reverses Ciliopathy and Photoreceptor Loss in iPSC-Derived Retinal Organoids from Retinitis Pigmentosa Patients. *Stem Cell Reports* **2018**, *10*, 1267–1281. [CrossRef]
22. Maeder, M.L.; Stefanidakis, M.; Wilson, C.J.; Baral, R.; Barrera, L.A.; Bounoutas, G.S.; Bumcrot, D.; Chao, H.; Ciulla, D.M.; DaSilva, J.A.; et al. Development of a gene-editing approach to restore vision loss in Leber congenital amaurosis type 10. *Nat. Med.* **2019**, *25*, 229–233. [CrossRef] [PubMed]
23. Wiley, L.A.; Anfinson, K.R.; Cranston, C.M.; Kaalberg, E.E.; Collins, M.M.; Mullins, R.F.; Stone, E.M.; Tucker, B.A. Generation of Xeno-Free, cGMP-Compliant Patient-Specific iPSCs from Skin Biopsy. *Curr Protoc Stem Cell Biol* **2017**, *42*, 4A.12.1–4A.12.14. [PubMed]

24. Wiley, L.A.; Burnight, E.R.; DeLuca, A.P.; Anfinson, K.R.; Cranston, C.M.; Kaalberg, E.E.; Penticoff, J.A.; Affatigato, L.M.; Mullins, R.F.; Stone, E.M.; et al. cGMP production of patient-specific iPSCs and photoreceptor precursor cells to treat retinal degenerative blindness. *Sci Rep.* **2016**, *6*, 30742. [CrossRef] [PubMed]
25. Ohlemacher, S.K.; Iglesias, C.L.; Sridhar, A.; Gamm, D.M.; Meyer, J.S. Generation of highly enriched populations of optic vesicle-like retinal cells from human pluripotent stem cells. *Curr Protoc Stem Cell Biol.* **2015**, *32*, 1H.8.1–1H.8.20. [PubMed]
26. Tucker, B.A.; Scheetz, T.E.; Mullins, R.F.; DeLuca, A.P.; Hoffmann, J.M.; Johnston, R.M.; Jacobson, S.G.; Sheffield, V.C.; Stone, E.M. Exome sequencing and analysis of induced pluripotent stem cells identify the cilia-related gene male germ cell-associated kinase (MAK) as a cause of retinitis pigmentosa. *Proc. Natl. Acad. Sci. USA* **2011**, *108*, E569–E576. [CrossRef] [PubMed]
27. Tucker, B.A.; Cranston, C.M.; Anfinson, K.A.; Shrestha, S.; Streb, L.M.; Leon, A.; Mullins, R.F.; Stone, E.M. Using patient-specific induced pluripotent stem cells to interrogate the pathogenicity of a novel retinal pigment epithelium-specific 65 kDa cryptic splice site mutation and confirm eligibility for enrollment into a clinical gene augmentation trial. *Transl Res.* **2015**, *166*, 740–749.e1. [CrossRef] [PubMed]
28. Wiley, L.A.; Burnight, E.R.; Drack, A.V.; Banach, B.B.; Ochoa, D.; Cranston, C.M.; Madumba, R.A.; East, J.S.; Mullins, R.F.; Stone, E.M.; et al. Using Patient-Specific Induced Pluripotent Stem Cells and Wild-Type Mice to Develop a Gene Augmentation-Based Strategy to Treat CLN3-Associated Retinal Degeneration. *Hum. Gene Ther.* **2016**, *27*, 835–846. [CrossRef] [PubMed]
29. Llonch, S.; Carido, M.; Ader, M. Organoid technology for retinal repair. *Dev. Biol.* **2018**, *433*, 132–143. [CrossRef]
30. Achberger, K.; Haderspeck, J.C.; Kleger, A.; Liebau, S. Stem cell-based retina models. *Adv. Drug Deliv. Rev.* **2018**. [CrossRef]
31. Tucker, B.A.; Park, I.-H.; Qi, S.D.; Klassen, H.J.; Jiang, C.; Yao, J.; Redenti, S.; Daley, G.Q.; Young, M.J. Transplantation of adult mouse iPS cell-derived photoreceptor precursors restores retinal structure and function in degenerative mice. *PLoS ONE* **2011**, *6*, e18992. [CrossRef] [PubMed]
32. Ueda, K.; Onishi, A.; Ito, S.-I.; Nakamura, M.; Takahashi, M. Generation of three-dimensional retinal organoids expressing rhodopsin and S- and M-cone opsins from mouse stem cells. *Biochem. Biophys. Res. Commun.* **2018**, *495*, 2595–2601. [CrossRef] [PubMed]
33. Riazifar, H.; Jia, Y.; Chen, J.; Lynch, G.; Huang, T. Chemically induced specification of retinal ganglion cells from human embryonic and induced pluripotent stem cells. *Stem Cells Transl Med.* **2014**, *3*, 424–432. [CrossRef] [PubMed]
34. Tucker, B.A.; Anfinson, K.R.; Mullins, R.F.; Stone, E.M.; Young, M.J. Use of a synthetic xeno-free culture substrate for induced pluripotent stem cell induction and retinal differentiation. *Stem Cells Transl Med.* **2013**, *2*, 16–24. [CrossRef] [PubMed]
35. Nelson, B.R.; Hartman, B.H.; Georgi, S.A.; Lan, M.S.; Reh, T.A. Transient inactivation of Notch signaling synchronizes differentiation of neural progenitor cells. *Dev. Biol.* **2007**, *304*, 479–498. [CrossRef] [PubMed]

© 2019 by the authors. Licensee MDPI, Basel, Switzerland. This article is an open access article distributed under the terms and conditions of the Creative Commons Attribution (CC BY) license (http://creativecommons.org/licenses/by/4.0/).

Article

Antisense Oligonucleotide-Based Downregulation of the G56R Pathogenic Variant Causing *NR2E3*-Associated Autosomal Dominant Retinitis Pigmentosa

Sarah Naessens [1], Laurien Ruysschaert [1], Steve Lefever [1,2,3], Frauke Coppieters [1,†] and Elfride De Baere [1,*,†]

1. Center for Medical Genetics Ghent, Ghent University and Ghent University Hospital, Corneel Heymanslaan 10, 9000 Ghent, Belgium; sarah.naessens@ugent.be (S.N.); laurien.ruysschaert@ugent.be (L.R.); steve.lefever@ugent.be (S.L.); frauke.coppieters@ugent.be (F.C.)
2. Cancer Research Institute Ghent (CRIG), Ghent University, 9000 Ghent, Belgium
3. Bioinformatics Institute Ghent (BIG), Ghent University, 9000 Ghent, Belgium
* Correspondence: Elfride.DeBaere@ugent.be; Tel.: +32-9-332-51-86
† These authors contributed equally to this work.

Received: 1 April 2019; Accepted: 6 May 2019; Published: 10 May 2019

Abstract: The recurrent missense variant in Nuclear Receptor Subfamily 2 Group E Member 3 (NR2E3), c.166G>A, p.(Gly56Arg) or G56R, underlies 1%–2% of cases with autosomal dominant retinitis pigmentosa (adRP), a frequent, genetically heterogeneous inherited retinal disease (IRD). The mutant NR2E3 protein has a presumed dominant negative effect (DNE) by competition for dimer formation with Cone-Rod Homeobox (CRX) but with abolishment of DNA binding, acting as a repressor in *trans*. Both the frequency and DNE of G56R make it an interesting target for allele-specific knock-down of the mutant allele using antisense oligonucleotides (AONs), an emerging therapeutic strategy for IRD. Here, we designed gapmer AONs with or without a locked nucleic acid modification at the site of the mutation, which were analyzed for potential off-target effects. Next, we overexpressed wild type (WT) or mutant *NR2E3* in RPE-1 cells, followed by AON treatment. Transcript and protein levels of WT and mutant NR2E3 were detected by reverse transcription quantitative polymerase chain reaction (RT-qPCR) and Western blot respectively. All AONs showed a general knock-down of mutant and WT NR2E3 on RNA and protein level, showing the accessibility of the region for AON-induced knockdown. Further modifications are needed however to increase allele-specificity. In conclusion, we propose the first proof-of-concept for AON-mediated silencing of a single nucleotide variation with a dominant negative effect as a therapeutic approach for *NR2E3*-associated adRP.

Keywords: retinitis pigmentosa; autosomal dominant; *NR2E3*; G56R; putative dominant negative effect; gapmer antisense oligonucleotides; allele-specific knockdown

1. Introduction

Retinitis pigmentosa (RP, MIM 268000) encompasses a group of progressive inherited retinal diseases (IRDs) characterized by the loss of peripheral vision with the development of tunnel vison and subsequent loss of central vision [1]. Thirty to forty percent of all RP cases show autosomal dominant inheritance and currently 30 genes underlying autosomal dominant RP (adRP) have been identified [2,3]. One of them is the Nuclear Receptor Subfamily 2 Group E Member 3 (*NR2E3*, MIM 604485) gene, encoding a photoreceptor-specific nuclear receptor [4]. NR2E3 is part of a multi-protein complex with Neural Retina Leucine Zipper (NRL, MIM 162080) and Cone-Rod Homeobox (CRX, MIM 602225). This complex has a dual role in the development and function of rod photoreceptors by co-occupying the promoter and/or enhancer regions of photoreceptor-specific genes in the rod cells. In this way, NR2E3 suppresses cone gene expression and activates the expression of rod genes [5–7]. Mutations in *NR2E3* have been linked with autosomal recessive IRDs such as Enhanced S-cone syndrome (ESCS, MIM 268100) and Goldmann-Favre syndrome (GFS, MIM 268100). Furthermore, one specific founder variant in the DNA-binding domain of NR2E3, c.166G>A, p.(Gly56Arg) known as G56R has been found to cause 1%–2% of all adRP cases, being enriched in European populations and North American families of European descent [8–11]. This pathogenic variant is unique because of its presumed dominant negative effect (DNE) characterized by competition for dimer formation with CRX but loss of the necessary DNA-binding, which is caused by disruption of the α-helical DNA-binding motif [12,13] (Figure 1).

This DNE and the recurrence of the G56R mutation make it an interesting target for modulation with antisense oligonucleotides (AONs). AONs can bind their target RNA and recruit the RNAse-H1 enzyme, which degrades the RNA part of the formed RNA:DNA duplex and subsequently downregulates the target of interest [14]. Allele-specific knock-down using AONs or RNA interference has already been tested for various targets that exert a gain of function or dominant negative effect, such as *TMC1* (MIM 606706) for autosomal dominant hearing loss (MIM 606705) [15], *COL6A2* (MIM 120240), and *COL6A3* (MIM 120250) for Ullrich myopathy (MIM 254090) [16–18], *DNM2* (MIM 602378) for autosomal dominant centronuclear myopathy (MIM 160150) [19], *RHO* (MIM 180380) for adRP [20], *GCAP1* (MIM 600364) for adRP, and cone-rod dystrophy (MIM 602093) [21] and *HTT* (MIM 613004) for Huntington disease (MIM 143100) [22,23].

Recently, significant advances in AON-mediated therapy have been made in the field of IRD. For example, a recent clinical trial assessed intravitreal injections of an AON to restore correct splicing in ten patients with Leber Congenital Amaurosis (MIM 611755) due to a frequent deep-intronic mutation c.2991+1655A>G in *CEP290* (MIM 610142) [24]. This has a potential impact on other subtypes of IRD and other AON-mediated approaches are currently being investigated [25–30].

Here, we aimed to design and test the capacity of AONs to knock down the adRP-associated G56R mutation in an allele-specific manner, being one of the first studies employing allele-specific AONs to target a single nucleotide variation in IRD.

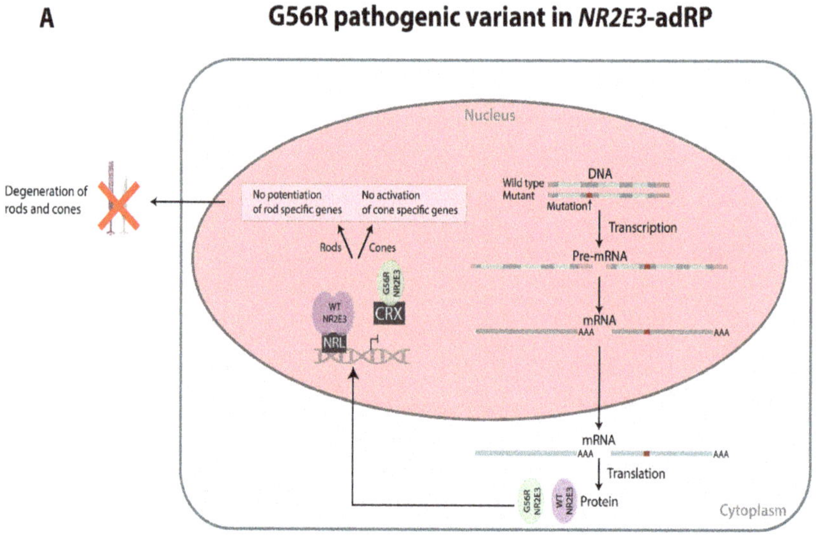

Figure 1. *Cont.*

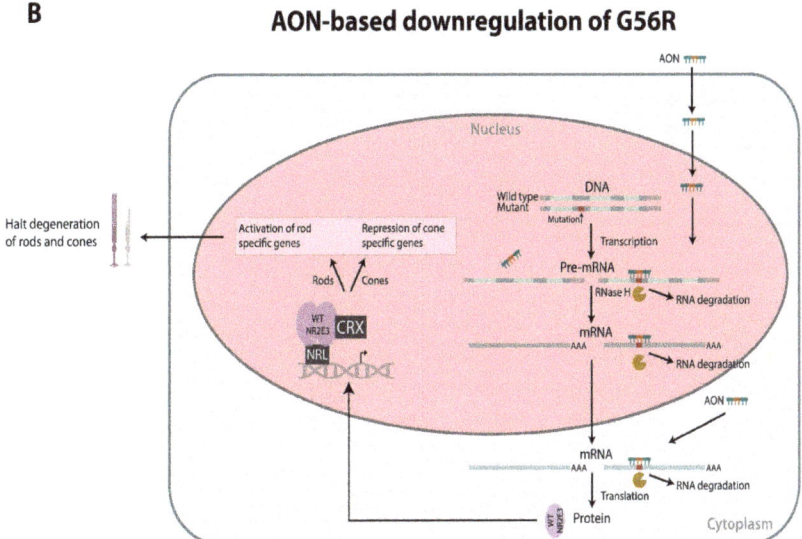

Figure 1. Schematic overview of the dominant negative effect of G56R Nuclear Receptor Subfamily 2 Group E Member 3 (NR2E3) (**A**) and allele-specific silencing of G56R using antisense oligonucleotides (AONs) (**B**). (**A**) Both wild type (WT) and mutant alleles are transcribed and translated. The wild type protein is able to form homo-dimers and bind the DNA, in complex with Neural Retina Leucine Zipper (NRL). The mutant protein is competing for binding with Cone-Rod Homeobox (CRX) and this complex is no longer able to bind the DNA, which leads to a failure of both potentiation of rod specific genes and activation of cone specific genes. (**B**) Using AONs, the mutant allele can be selectively downregulated, whereby the WT protein is binding the DNA in complex with both NRL and CRX. This complex is able to properly activate the rod specific genes and repress the cone specific genes, which would halt degeneration of the photoreceptors. Adapted from [18].

2. Materials and Methods

2.1. AON Design

A region of 150 bp around the c.166G>A mutation (Ensembl release 85) at the mRNA level was analyzed using Mfold software (version 3.6). Partially open or closed regions were identified using the ss-count tool. This led to the design of nine gapmer AONs overlapping with c.166G>A, differentiating in length of the DNA gap region, length of the RNA flanks, and the position of the mutation in the gap. Furthermore, we included the same nine gapmer AONs containing a locked nucleic acid (LNA) at the site of the mutation. Final AON sequences were analyzed using the OligoAnalyzer Tool (Integrated DNA Technologies, Coralville, IA, USA) to ensure that the GC content ranged between 40% and 60% and that the self-complementarity of the AON is above −9 kcal/mol. All nine AON pairs were analyzed for off-targets using Bowtie and Bowtie2 (Ensembl release 85), allowing a maximum of two mismatches.

All AONs were chemically modified by adding a phosphorothioate (PS) backbone to the complete AON sequence and 2-*O*-Methyl sugar modifications to the RNA flanks. AONs were generated by Eurogentec (Seraing, Belgium) and were dissolved in sterile TE-buffer to a final concentration of 100 μM.

2.2. Generation of Mutant c.166G>A Expression Construct

A wild type (WT) *NR2E3* (NM_014249) complementary DNA (cDNA) expression construct (OriGene, Rockville, MD, USA, TC308926) was used as a basis for mutagenesis. The c.166G>A mutation was inserted using the Q5 site-directed mutagenesis kit (New England Biolabs, Ipswich, MA, USA), and mutation-specific primers were designed with the NEBaseChanger software (version 1.2.8, New England Biolabs, Ipswich, MA, USA) (Supplementary Table S1). Mutagenized plasmids were transformed in One Shot TOP10 competent cells (Invitrogen, Life Technologies, Carlsbad, CA, USA) and DNA was subsequently isolated with the NucleoBond Xtra Midi/Maxi kit (Macherey-Nagel, Düren, Germany). The entire *NR2E3* insert was sequenced and selected plasmids were grown to obtain larger quantities. Sequencing primers can be found in Supplementary Table S1.

2.3. Cell Culture and AON Transfection Experiments

hTERT RPE-1 cells (ATCC, Manassas, VA, USA, CRL-4000™) were cultured in DMEM:F12 medium (ATCC, Manassas, VA, USA) supplemented with 10% fetal calf serum, 1% penicillin-streptomycin, 1% MEM non-essential amino acids, and 0.01 mg/mL hygromycin B. RPE-1 cells were seeded in six well plates at 1.5×10^5 cells/well. After 24 h, cells were co-transfected in duplicate with 2 µg of WT or mutant *NR2E3* plasmid or an empty control vector and 0.25 µM of AON, using DharmaFECT kb DNA transfection reagent (Dharmacon, Lafayette, CO, USA) according to manufacturer's instructions. Cells were grown for 48 h until confluence.

2.4. RNA Isolation and Reverse Transcription Quantitative Polymerase Chain Reaction (RT-qPCR)

Total RNA was extracted using the RNeasy mini kit (Qiagen, Hilden, Germany) with on-column DNase digestion (Qiagen, Hilden, Germany) according to manufacturer's instructions. A second DNase treatment was done using the Heat&Run genomic DNA (gDNA) removal kit (ArcticZymes, Tromsø, Norway). cDNA was synthesized with the iScript cDNA synthesis kit (Bio-Rad Laboratories, Hercules, CA, USA) using 1 µg of messenger RNA (mRNA).

Reference genes that are stably expressed in RPE-1 cells were first determined using a GeNorm analysis, integrating the M and V analysis. The average pairwise variation M of a particular gene with all other control genes was determined as the standard deviation of the logarithmically transformed expression ratios. In addition, the systemic variation V was calculated as the pairwise variation for repeated RT-qPCR experiments on the same gene (qbase+, Biogazelle, Ghent, Belgium) [31]. The following reference genes were tested for stability: *HMBS*, *SDHA*, *HPRT1*, *PPIA*, *GUSB*, and *TBP*. Primer sequences are listed in Supplementary Table S1.

Next, the expression level of *NR2E3* was determined using intron-spanning primers (Primer3Plus, version 2.0). Data analysis was done using the qbase+ software (Biogazelle, Ghent, Belgium) with following reference genes for normalization: *HMBS*, *SDHA*, and *TBP*. Primer sequences are listed in Supplementary Table S1. Transfection and RT-qPCR were performed twice.

2.5. Western Blot Analysis

Cell lysates were collected in Leammli lysis buffer supplemented with complete protease inhibitor cocktail (Sigma-Aldrich, St. Louis, MO, USA) and phosphatase inhibitors (Sigma-Aldrich, St. Louis, MO, USA). Protein concentrations were measured using the Pierce BCA protein assay kit (Thermo Scientific, Waltham, MA, USA). A total of 25 µg of protein sample was reduced by incubation at 98 °C with 1M DTT. SDS-PAGE was performed using NuPAGE™ 4%–12% Bis-Tris protein gels (Invitrogen, Life Technologies, Carlsbad, CA, USA). Subsequently, proteins were transferred to a nitrocellulose membrane using the iBlot®2 System (Life Technologies, Carlsbad, CA, USA). Membranes were incubated in 2% membrane blocking agent (GE Healthcare Life Sciences, Chicage, IL, USA) in 1x tris-buffered saline with Tween-20 (TBST) for 2 h at room temperature and immunolabeled with a primary antibody (anti-NR2E3, #AB2299, Millipore, Burlington, MA, USA) diluted 1:1000 in blocking buffer for 16 h at 4 °C. Membranes were probed with a secondary antibody (anti-rabbit IgG, HRP-linked antibody #7074, Cell Signaling Technologies, Danvers, MA, USA) diluted 1:2500 in blocking buffer for 2 h at room temperature. Membranes were developed using the SuperSignal® West Dura Extended Duration Substrate kit (Thermo Scientific, Life Technologies, Waltham, MA, USA) and scanned with the ChemiDoc-It® 500 Imaging System (UVP, Upland, CA, USA). Subsequently, membranes were stripped using the Restore PLUS Western Blot Stripping Buffer (Life Technologies, Carlsbad, CA, USA) and probed with a β-tubulin primary antibody (ab6046, Abcam, Cambridge, UK) as an internal loading control. The antibody was diluted 1:2000 in blocking buffer and incubated for 1 h at room temperature. Membranes were subsequently probed with a secondary antibody (anti-rabbit IgG, HRP-linked antibody, Cell Signaling Technologies, Danvers, MA, USA) diluted 1:2500 in blocking buffer for 1 h at room temperature. The development was done as described above. Relative densities of NR2E3 were measured on three independent Western blots using Image J (version 1.8.0_112) and normalized against β-tubulin. Statistical analysis was done using an unpaired *t*-test.

3. Results

3.1. AON Design

We designed nine gapmer AONs targeting the c.166G>A mutation but shifted the oligonucleotides each time a few bps, as it is known that only a few bps difference can lead to a complete abolishment of inhibitory activity of AONs due to secondary or tertiary structures that restrict binding possibilities of the AON [32]. Furthermore, LNA modifications increase the difference in melting temperature between duplexes formed with a perfectly matched target versus a mismatched target and are thus possibly increasing the allelic-discrimination potency of AONs [33,34]. Hence, we included nine gapmer AONs containing a LNA modification at the site of the mutation. An overview of gapmer AONs around the site of the mutation, differentiating in length of the gap region, length of RNA flanks, and position of the mutation can be found in Table 1. Three pairs of gapmer AONs were finally selected that contain no complete match between the AON sequence and the full human gDNA sequence, and are further referred to as AON1–6 (Table 1). All three pairs have a 5-10-5 composition containing a DNA-gap region with 10 PS modified nucleotides, which is needed to allow cleavage of the RNAse-H1 enzyme. The gap region is flanked on both sides by 5 2'-O-Methyl PS RNA nucleotides.

3.2. NR2E3 mRNA Expression Analysis

All AONs were transfected in RPE-1 cells together with either the WT or mutant *NR2E3* cDNA expression construct to test whether the AONs induce selective silencing of the mutant NR2E3 mRNA and protein. For normalization of RT-qPCR expression data, we first determined reference genes that are stably expressed in RPE-1 cells using a GeNorm M and V analysis [31] testing following genes: *HMBS*, *SDHA*, *HPRT1*, *PPIA*, *GUSB*, and *TBP* (Supplementary Figure S1). *HMBS*, *TBP*, and *SDHA* are the most stably expressed in RPE-1 cells (V < 0.15, lowest M values) and will be used in further experiments.

Next, relative quantities of WT and mutant *NR2E3* were determined using RT-qPCR of the harvested mRNA. All AONs show a non-selective knock-down of both WT and mutant *NR2E3* (Figure 2). However, when calculating the residual expression percentage after treatment relative to the non-treated sample, samples treated with AON2, 4, and 6 show lower remaining expression in the mutant versus the WT sample (Table 2). Interestingly, these AONs contain the LNA modification at the site of the mutation, possibly increasing the discrimination capacity of the AON [33].

Table 1. Antisense oligonucleotide (AON) sequences and potential off targets. Underlined AONs were selected, as they do not have predicted off targets at the genomic DNA (gDNA) level. cDNA = complementary DNA, M = 2-O-Methyl modification, L = locked nucleic acid modification, * = phosphodiesterase bond. The site of the mutation is indicated with a capital letter.

Gapmers	Sequence (5′→3′)	Complete Match Bowtie	Complete Match Bowtie2
AON1	Mg*Mu*Mg*Mc*Mu*t*t*c*c*T*g*c*t*g*c*t*t*g*Mc*Mu*Mg*Mu	gDNA: no cDNA: SLC29A4P1	gDNA: no cDNA: no
AON2	Mg*Mu*Mg*Mc*Mu*t*t*c*c*LT*g*c*t*g*c*t*t*g*Mc*Mu*Mg*Mu		
	Mg*Mc*Mu*t*c*c*T*g*c*t*g*c*t*Mg*Mc*Mu	gDNA: ICOS cDNA: GPR27	gDNA: CACNA2D3 cDNA: PCDHAC2
	Mg*Mc*Mu*t*c*c*LT*g*c*t*g*c*t*Mg*Mc*Mu		
	Mg*Mu*Mg*Mc*Mu*t*c*c*T*g*c*t*g*Mc*Mu*Mg*Mc*Mu	gDNA: intergenicc DNA: HCG9P5	gDNA: intergenic DNA: PRDM8
	Mg*Mu*Mg*Mc*Mu*t*c*c*LT*g*c*t*g*Mc*Mu*Mg*Mc*Mu		
AON3	Mc*Ma*Mu*Ma*Mg*t*g*c*t*t*c*c*T*g*c*Mu*Mg*Mc*Mu*Mg	gDNA: no cDNA: no	gDNA: no cDNA: no
AON4	Mc*Ma*Mu*Ma*Mg*t*g*c*t*t*c*c*LT*g*c*Mu*Mg*Mc*Mu*Mg		
	Mu*Ma*Mg*t*g*c*t*t*c*c*T*g*c*Mu*Mg*Mc	gDNA: intergenicc DNA: HCG9P5	gDNA: TANGO6 cDNA: HCG9P5
	Mu*Ma*Mg*t*g*c*t*t*c*c*LT*g*c*Mu*Mg*Mc		
	Ma*Mu*Ma*Mg*Mu*g*c*t*t*c*c*T*g*Mc*Mu*Mg*Mc*Mu	gDNA: AC007908.1 cDNA: no	gDNA: no cDNA: HCG9P5
	Ma*Mu*Ma*Mg*Mu*g*c*t*t*c*c*LT*g*Mc*Mu*Mg*Mc*Mu		
AON5	Mc*Mu*Mu*Mc*Mc*T*g*c*t*g*c*t*t*g*c*t*Mg*Mu*Mc*Mu*Mc	gDNA: no cDNA: PCDHAC2	gDNA: no cDNA: ACVR2B
AON6	Mc*Mu*Mu*Mc*Mc*LT*g*c*t*g*c*t*t*g*c*t*Mg*Mu*Mc*Mu*Mc		
	Mu*Mu*Mc*c*T*g*c*t*t*g*c*t*t*g*c*Mu*Mg*Mu	gDNA: EIF3H cDNA: LMAN2	gDNA: PDCD1LG2 cDNA: DYRK1A
	Mu*Mu*Mc*c*LT*g*c*t*t*g*c*t*t*g*c*Mu*Mg*Mu		
	Mc*Mu*Mu*Mc*Mc*T*g*c*t*t*g*c*t*t*g*Mc*Mu*Mg*Mu*Mc	gDNA: SEMA5A cDNA: LY6H	gDNA: SEMA5A cDNA: PLXNB3
	Mc*Mu*Mu*Mc*Mc*LT*g*c*t*t*g*c*t*t*g*Mc*Mu*Mg*Mu*Mc		

Table 2. Relative expression values of messenger RNA (mRNA) from wild type (WT) or mutant (MT) *NR2E3* overexpressed in RPE-1 cells and subsequently treated with AON1–6. Residual expression after AON treatment was calculated relative to the non-treated (NT) sample (=100%). SEM = standard error of relative expression values.

AON	Expression WT *NR2E3* (%)	SEM (%)	Expression MT *NR2E3* (%)	SEM (%)
NT	100.00	3.84	100.00	4.01
AON1	33.22	4.06	37.37	2.86
AON2	59.55	6.12	46.15	9.65
AON3	27.98	5.98	38.04	3.51
AON4	33.76	2.94	30.15	4.89
AON5	30.10	4.95	38.16	3.87
AON6	31.81	4.94	29.89	4.26

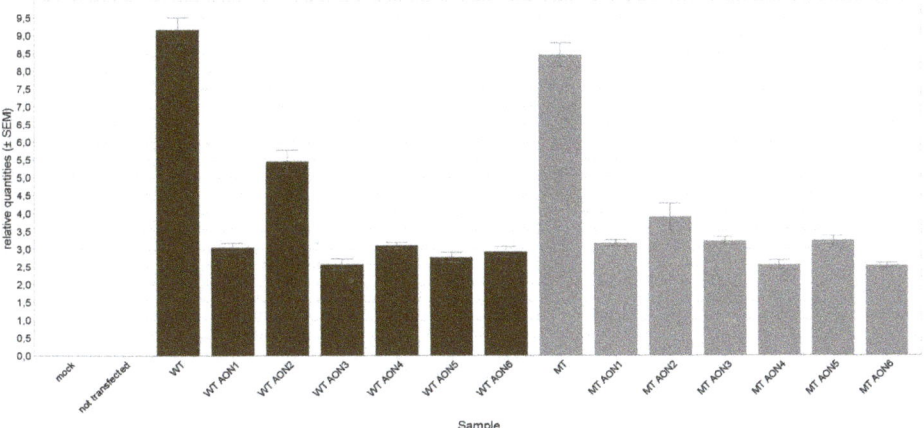

Figure 2. Quantitative polymerase chain reaction (qPCR)-based expression analysis of messenger RNA (mRNA) from wild type (WT) or mutant (MT) *NR2E3* overexpressed in RPE-1 cells and subsequently treated with AON1–6. All AONs lead to a partial knockdown of WT or MT *NR2E3* mRNA expression. Error bars represent the standard error of the relative quantities. Mock transfected cells were transfected with an empty vector and show no *NR2E3* expression.

3.3. NR2E3 Protein Expression Analysis

In parallel to mRNA expression analysis, Western blot analysis was performed to investigate whether the effects seen on mRNA level could be recapitulated on the protein level. A direct comparison of all conditions on the same gel was not possible, as the number of samples was too high. Therefore, a comparison of treated versus non-treated, and mutant versus WT samples was made per AON on the same gel. Three independent Western blots showed a clear partial knock-down of WT and mutant NR2E3 protein for all AONs (Figure 3A). Relative densities were calculated using β-tubulin for normalization. Unpaired *t*-tests between the non-treated sample and the treated samples revealed *p*-values between <0.0001 and 0.0328 (except for WT *NR2E3* treated with AON4, *p*-value: 0.058) (Figure 3B). Transformation of these relative densities into percentages showed no clear difference in allele-specificity between AONs with or without LNA at the site of the mutation, as was seen for the mRNA expression. Instead, all AONs, except for AON2, seem to preferentially downregulate the mutant NR2E3, with AON5 being the most specific one (Table 3).

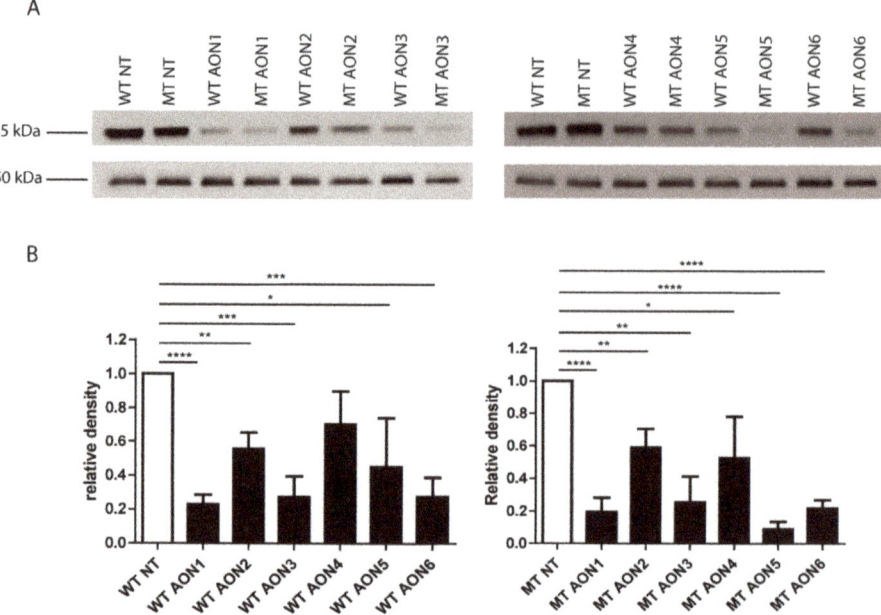

Figure 3. Western blot analysis. Wild type (WT) or mutant (MT) NR2E3 was overexpressed in RPE-1 cells and subsequently treated with AON1–6. (**A**). Upper images represent NR2E3 protein visualization, lower images represent β-tubulin visualization. (**B**). Densitometric analysis for three independent Western blots. Left panel represents WT samples, right panel represents MT samples. All AONs lead to a partial knock-down of WT and MT NR2E3 protein (p-values between <0.0001 and 0.0328). Error bars represent standard deviation between relative densities.

Table 3. Relative protein expression values from wild type (WT) or mutant (MT) NR2E3 overexpressed in RPE-1 cells and subsequently treated with AON1–6. Average residual protein expression after treatment with AON1–6 was calculated from three independent blots relative to the non-treated (NT) sample (=100%).

AON	Expression WT NR2E3 (%)	Expression MT NR2E3 (%)
NT	100.00	100.00
AON1	22.87	19.33
AON2	55.55	58.85
AON3	27.22	25.45
AON4	70.24	52.47
AON5	45.08	8.88
AON6	27.52	21.7

4. Discussion

We aimed to investigate if the adRP-associated NR2E3 mutation G56R with a dominant negative effect would be amenable to allele-specific knock-down using AONs. As other *NR2E3* mutations that have been found in autosomal recessive IRDs, such as enhanced S-cone syndrome (ESCS, MIM 268100), have a loss-of-function effect, we hypothesized that the c.166G>A allele could function as a therapeutic target for selective suppression [35] (Figure 1). Effective allele-selective approaches employing AONs have already been described for dominant mutations in *COL6A2* [18], *RHO* [20], and

HTT [22]. However, gapmer AONs targeting a single nucleotide variation have not yet been described for IRD.

As *NR2E3* expression is mainly limited to the photoreceptors, we co-transfected WT or mutant expression constructs in RPE-1 cells, together with each of the six AONs targeting the c.166G>A allele. A general decrease in NR2E3 expression could be seen for all AONs both on the mRNA and protein level, but not limited to the mutant NR2E3. However, on the mRNA level, a subtle mutant-specific preference could be seen for AON2, 4, and 6. Interestingly, these contain the LNA modification at the site of the mutation. On the protein level, a preferential mutant-specific knock-down could be observed for all AONs except for AON2 in three independent experiments. Apart from the fact that Western blot is a semi-quantitative technique, the observed mRNA-protein differences may be attributed by other factors, e.g., different gapmer AON activities in the nucleus versus cytoplasm [18].

The six evaluated AONs downregulate NR2E3 expression to 28%–60% at the mRNA level and to 9%–70% at the protein level. Importantly, in the context of the dominant negative *NR2E3* mutation, a complete AON-induced knock-down of the mutant allele is not required. Morphological or cellular improvements resulting from moderate reductions in mutant protein while preserving the WT protein [20] or from shifting the WT-mutant protein ratio [16,17] have been described respectively. Gualandi et al. showed that AON-targeting of a common single nucleotide polymorphism (SNP) caused a global suppression of *COL6A2* mRNA, albeit preferentially involving the mutated allele (10% difference in mutant versus WT allele ratio). Overall, this led to a significant improvement of the severe cellular phenotype in patient fibroblasts [16].

In order to increase the allele-specificity of the AONs targeting *NR2E3* mutation G56R, both the cellular system and AON sequences could be modified. As we had no access to patient-derived induced pluripotent stem cells (iPSCs) differentiated to photoreceptor precursor cells (PPCs) at the start of the study, we used an overexpression cellular system either for mutant or WT *NR2E3*. This is not representing the true biological situation however, in which both mutant and WT NR2E3 are expressed, exerting a dominant negative effect. In *NR2E3* expressing patient-derived cells, competition for AON binding might lead to a stronger allele-specificity of the AON. In this respect, iPSCs have recently been reprogrammed from patient fibroblasts with the c.166G>A mutation [36]. These cells will further be differentiated to PPCs [37], which will represent a relevant cellular model for further AON development.

Apart from using a different cellular system, several modifications to the AONs could be made to obtain a more selective knock-down of the mutant allele. A first potential modification could be shifting the AONs a few bps. Already three positions of AONs targeting the mutation have been investigated here, but several studies showed that even a change of one bp can have a substantial influence on allelic discrimination [38,39]. Next, reducing the length of the AONs could have positive effects on the discrimination capacity. The AONs used in this study have a 5-10-5 conformation. However, it has been shown that a long AON sequence can reduce the allele-specificity [18]. Shortening the AONs to 16 nucleotides could increase specificity on the one hand [39,40], but lead to an increase of possible off-target effects on the other hand (see Table 1). Finally, it has been suggested that the discrimination of single nucleotides between RNA alleles can be improved by introducing certain arrangements of mismatches between the RNA/AON duplexes, as the presence of non-canonical bps decreases the thermodynamic stability of the duplexes. In case of a G>A transition, it has been shown that the presence of G-dT in the WT RNA duplex instead of A-dT does not disturb the duplex structure. However, introducing tandem purine mismatches at the 5' end of the DNA gap strongly diminishes thermodynamic stability. This, combined with the third mismatch at the site of the mutation, has been shown to reduce the cleavage efficiency of the WT RNA [41].

In conclusion, we have designed and investigated gapmer AONs to elicit allele-specific silencing of a recurrent dominant negative mutation in the *NR2E3* gene implicated in 1%–2% of cases with adRP. We showed that the region of interest is accessible to AON-induced RNAse-H1 cleavage and that AON-targeting of G56R caused a global suppression of NR2E3 mRNA and protein, with limited mutation-specificity. Further studies will evaluate different modifications to AONs, and will validate gapmer AONs in a relevant patient-derived cellular model. Finally, our findings provide the first proof-of-concept for AON-mediated silencing of a single nucleotide variation with a dominant negative effect as a therapeutic approach for dominant IRD.

Supplementary Materials: The following are available online at http://www.mdpi.com/2073-4425/10/5/363/s1, Figure S1: GeNorm analysis to determine the number and most stable reference genes. Table S1: PCR primers.

Author Contributions: Conceptualization, S.N., F.C. and E.D.B.; Methodology, S.N. and F.C.; Software, S.L.; Validation, S.N.; Formal Analysis, S.N. and L.R.; Investigation, S.N. and L.R.; Resources, E.D.B.; Data Curation, S.N.; Writing–Original Draft Preparation, S.N.; Writing–Review & Editing, F.C. and E.D.B.; Visualization, S.N.; Supervision, F.C. and E.D.B.; Project Administration, E.D.B.; Funding Acquisition, E.D.B.

Funding: This work was supported by the institute for Innovation by Science and Technology (IWT), integrated in the FWO (FWO-SB) (S.N. 1S60616N). E.D.B. is Senior Clinical Investigator of the FWO (1802215N). This study was supported by the Ghent University Special Research Fund (BOF15/GOA/011) to E.D.B., Hercules Foundation AUGE/13/023 to E.D.B., by the Ghent University Hospital Innovation Fund NucleUZ (E.D.B. and F.C.).

Conflicts of Interest: The authors declare no conflict of interest.

References

1. Den Hollander, A.I.; Black, A.; Bennett, J.; Cremers, F.P. Lighting a candle in the dark: Advances in genetics and gene therapy of recessive retinal dystrophies. *J. Clin. Inverstigation* **2010**, *120*, 3042–3053. [CrossRef] [PubMed]
2. Hartong, D.T.; Berson, E.L.; Dryja, T.P. Retinitis pigmentosa. *Lancet* **2006**, *368*, 1795–1809. [CrossRef]
3. Farrar, G.J.; Carrigan, M.; Dockery, A.; Millington-Ward, S.; Palfi, A.; Chadderton, N.; Humphries, M.; Kiang, A.S.; Kenna, P.F.; Humphries, P. Toward an elucidation of the molecular genetics of inherited retinal degenerations. *Hum. Mol. Genet.* **2017**, *26*, R2–R11. [CrossRef] [PubMed]
4. Kobayashi, M.; Takezawa, S.; Hara, K.; Yu, R.T.; Umesono, Y.; Agata, K.; Taniwaki, M.; Yasuda, K.; Umesono, K. Identification of a photoreceptor cell-specific nuclear receptor. *Proc. Natl. Acad. Sci. USA* **1999**, *96*, 4814–4819. [CrossRef]
5. Peng, G.H.; Ahmad, O.; Ahmad, F.; Liu, J.; Chen, S. The photoreceptor-specific nuclear receptor Nr2e3 interacts with Crx and exerts opposing effects on the transcription of rod versus cone genes. *Hum. Mol. Genet.* **2005**, *14*, 747–764. [CrossRef]
6. Chen, J.; Rattner, A.; Nathans, J. The Rod Photoreceptor-Specific Nuclear Receptor Nr2e3 Represses Transcription of Multiple Cone-Specific Genes. *J. Neurosci.* **2005**, *25*, 118–129. [CrossRef] [PubMed]
7. Cheng, H.; Aleman, T.S.; Cideciyan, A.V.; Khanna, R.; Samuel, G.; Swaroop, A. In vivo function of the orphan nuclear receptor NR2E3 in establishing photoreceptor identity during mammalian retinal development. *Hum. Mol. Genet.* **2006**, *15*, 2588–2602. [CrossRef]
8. Coppieters, F.; Leroy, B.P.; Beysen, D.; Hellemans, J.; De Bosscher, K.; Haegeman, G.; Robberecht, K.; Wuyts, W.; Coucke, P.J.; Baere, E. De Recurrent Mutation in the First Zinc Finger of the Orphan Nuclear Receptor NR2E3 Causes Autosomal Dominant Retinitis Pigmentosa. *Am. J. Hum. Genet.* **2007**, *81*, 147–157. [CrossRef]
9. Van Cauwenbergh, C.; Coppieters, F.; Roels, D.; De Jaegere, S.; Flipts, H.; De Zaeytijd, J.; Walraedt, S.; Claes, C.; Fransen, E.; Van Camp, G.; et al. Mutations in splicing factor genes are a major cause of autosomal dominant retinitis pigmentosa in belgian families. *PLoS ONE* **2017**, *12*, 1–18. [CrossRef]
10. Gire, A.I.; Sullivan, L.S.; Bowne, S.J.; Birch, D.G.; Hughbanks-wheaton, D.; John, R.; Daiger, S.P. The Gly56Arg mutation in NR2E3 accounts for 1–2% of autosomal dominant retinitis pigmentosa. *Mol. Vis.* **2007**, *13*, 1970–1975.
11. Blanco-Kelly, F.; García Hoyos, M.; Lopez Martinez, M.A.; Lopez-Molina, M.I.; Riveiro-Alvarez, R.; Fernandez-San Jose, P.; Avila-Fernandez, A.; Corton, M.; Millan, J.M.; García Sandoval, B.; et al. Dominant retinitis pigmentosa, p.Gly56Arg mutation in NR2E3: Phenotype in a large cohort of 24 cases. *PLoS ONE* **2016**, *11*, 1–13. [CrossRef]
12. Escher, P.; Gouras, P.; Roduit, R.; Tiab, L.; Bolay, S.; Delarive, T.; Chen, S.; Tsai, C.C.; Hayashi, M.; Zernant, J.; et al. Mutations in NR2E3 Can Cause Dominant or Recessive Retinal Degenerations in the Same Family. *Hum. Mutat.* **2009**, *30*, 342–351. [CrossRef]

13. Roduit, R.; Escher, P.; Schorderet, D.F. Mutations in the DNA-Binding Domain of NR2E3 Affect In Vivo Dimerization and Interaction with CRX. *PLoS ONE* **2009**, *4*, 1–12. [CrossRef]
14. Levin, A.A. Treating Disease at the RNA Level with Oligonucleotides. *N. Engl. J. Med.* **2019**, *380*, 57–70. [CrossRef]
15. Shibata, S.B.; Ranum, P.T.; Moteki, H.; Pan, B.; Goodwin, A.T.; Goodman, S.S.; Abbas, P.J.; Holt, J.R.; Smith, R.J.H. RNA Interference Prevents Autosomal-Dominant Hearing Loss. *Am. J. Hum. Genet.* **2016**, *98*, 1101–1113. [CrossRef]
16. Gualandi, F.; Manzati, E.; Sabatelli, P.; Passarelli, C.; Bovolenta, M.; Pellegrini, C.; Perrone, D.; Squarzoni, S.; Pegoraro, E.; Bonaldo, P.; et al. Antisense-Induced Messenger Depletion Corrects a COL6A2 Dominant Mutation in Ullrich Myopathy. *Hum. Gene Ther.* **2012**, *23*, 1313–1318. [CrossRef]
17. Bolduc, V.; Zou, Y.; Ko, D.; Bönnemann, C.G. siRNA-mediated Allele-specific Silencing of a COL6A3 Mutation in a Cellular Model of Dominant Ullrich Muscular Dystrophy. *Mol. Ther. Nucleic Acids* **2014**, *3*, e147. [CrossRef]
18. Marrosu, E.; Ala, P.; Muntoni, F.; Zhou, H. Gapmer Antisense Oligonucleotides Suppress the Mutant Allele of COL6A3 and Restore Functional Protein in Ullrich Muscular Dystrophy. *Mol. Ther. Nucleic Acids* **2017**, *8*, 416–427. [CrossRef]
19. Trochet, D.; Prudhon, B.; Beuvin, M.; Peccate, C.; Lorain, S.; Julien, L.; Benkhelifa-Ziyyat, S.; Rabai, A.; Mamchaoui, K.; Ferry, A.; et al. Allele-specific silencing therapy for Dynamin 2-related dominant centronuclear myopathy. *EMBO Mol. Med.* **2017**, *10*, 239–253. [CrossRef]
20. Murray, S.F.; Jazayeri, A.; Matthes, M.T.; Yasumura, D.; Yang, H.; Peralta, R.; Watt, A.; Freier, S.; Hung, G.; Adamson, P.S.; et al. Allele-specific inhibition of rhodopsin with an antisense oligonucleotide slows photoreceptor cell degeneration. *Investig. Ophthalmol. Vis. Sci.* **2015**, *56*, 6362–6375. [CrossRef]
21. Jiang, L.; Frederick, J.M.; Baehr, W. RNA interference gene therapy in dominant retinitis pigmentosa and cone-rod dystrophy mouse models caused by GCAP1 mutations. *Front. Mol. Neurosci.* **2014**, *7*, 25. [CrossRef] [PubMed]
22. Østergaard, M.E.; Southwell, A.L.; Kordasiewicz, H.; Watt, A.T.; Skotte, N.H.; Doty, C.N.; Vaid, K.; Villanueva, E.B.; Swayze, E.E.; Bennett, C.F.; et al. Rational design of antisense oligonucleotides targeting single nucleotide polymorphisms for potent and allele selective suppression of mutant Huntingtin in the CNS. *Nucleic Acids Res.* **2013**, *41*, 9634–9650. [CrossRef] [PubMed]
23. Southwell, A.L.; Skotte, N.H.; Kordasiewicz, H.B.; Østergaard, M.E.; Watt, A.T.; Carroll, J.B.; Doty, C.N.; Villanueva, E.B.; Petoukhov, E.; Vaid, K.; et al. In Vivo Evaluation of Candidate Allele-specific Mutant Huntingtin Gene Silencing Antisense Oligonucleotides. *Mol. Ther. Am. Soc. Gene Cell Ther.* **2014**, *22*, 2093–2106. [CrossRef]
24. Cideciyan, A.V.; Jacobson, S.G.; Drack, A.V.; Ho, A.C.; Charng, J.; Garafalo, A.V.; Roman, A.J.; Sumaroka, A.; Han, I.C.; Hochstedler, M.D.; et al. Effect of an intravitreal antisense oligonucleotide on vision in Leber congenital amaurosis due to a photoreceptor cilium defect. *Nat. Med.* **2018**, *25*, 225–228. [CrossRef]
25. Slijkerman, R.W.; Vaché, C.; Dona, M.; García-García, G.; Claustres, M.; Hetterschijt, L.; Peters, T.A.; Hartel, B.P.; Pennings, R.J.; Millan, J.M.; et al. Antisense Oligonucleotide-based Splice Correction for USH2A-associated Retinal Degeneration Caused by a Frequent Deep-intronic Mutation. *Mol. Ther. Acids* **2016**, *5*, e381. [CrossRef] [PubMed]
26. Slijkerman, R.W.; Goloborodko, A.; Broekman, S.; de Vrieze, E.; Hetterschijt, L.; Peters, T.A.; Gerits, M.; Kremer, H.; Van Wijk, E. Poor Splice-Site Recognition in a Humanized Zebrafish Knockin Model for the Recurrent Deep-Intronic c.7595-2144A>G Mutation in USH2A. *Zebrafish* **2018**, *15*, 597–609. [CrossRef] [PubMed]
27. Albert, S.; Garanto, A.; Sangermano, R.; Khan, M.; Bax, N.M.; Hoyng, C.B.; Zernant, J.; Lee, W.; Allikmets, R.; Collin, R.W.J.; et al. Identification and Rescue of Splice Defects Caused by Two Neighboring Deep-Intronic ABCA4 Mutations Underlying Stargardt Disease. *Am. J. Hum. Genet.* **2018**, *102*, 517–527. [CrossRef]
28. Garanto, A.; van der Velde-Visser, S.D.; Cremers, F.P.M.; Collin, R.W.J. Antisense Oligonucleotide-Based Splice Correction of a Deep-Intronic Mutation in CHM Underlying Choroideremia. In *Retinal Degenerative Diseases. Advances in Experimental Medicine and Biology*; Springer: Cham, Switzerland, 2018; pp. 83–89.
29. Sangermano, R.; Garanto, A.; Khan, M.; Runhart, E.; Bauwens, M.; Bax, N.; Van den Born, I.; Verheij, J.; Pott, J.-W.; Thiadens, A.; et al. Deep-intronic ABCA4 mutations explain missing heritability in Stargardt disease and allow correction of splice defects by antisense oligonucleotides. *Genet. Med.* **2019**. [CrossRef]

30. Bauwens, M.; Garanto, A.; Sangermano, R.; Naessens, S.; Weisschuh, N.; De Zaeytijd, J.; Khan, M.; Sadler, F.; Balikova, I.; Van Cauwenbergh, C.; et al. ABCA4-associated disease as a model for missing heritability in autosomal recessive disorders: Novel non-coding splice, cis- regulatory, structural and recurrent hypomorphic variants. *Genet. Med.* **2019**. [CrossRef]
31. Vandesompele, J.; De Preter, K.; Pattyn, F.; Poppe, B.; Van Roy, N.; De Paepe, A.; Speleman, F. Accurate normalization of real-time quantitative RT-PCR data by geometric averaging of multiple internal control genes. *Genome Biol.* **2002**, *3*, 1–12. [CrossRef]
32. Schneier, A.J.; Fulton, A.B. The hermansky-pudlak syndrome: Clinical features and imperatives from an ophthalmic perspective. *Semin. Ophthalmol.* **2013**, *28*, 387–391. [CrossRef] [PubMed]
33. Grünweller, A.; Hartmann, R.K. Locked Nucleic Acid Oligonucleotides: The next generation of antisense agents? *BioDrugs* **2007**, *21*, 235–243. [CrossRef] [PubMed]
34. Jacobsen, N.; Bentzen, J.; Meldgaard, M.; Jakobsen, M.H.; Fenger, M.; Kauppinen, S.; Skouv, J. LNA-enhanced detection of single nucleotide polymorphisms in the apolipoprotein E. *Nucleic Acids Res.* **2002**, *30*, e100. [CrossRef] [PubMed]
35. Schorderet, D.F.; Escher, P. NR2E3 mutations in enhanced S-cone sensitivity syndrome (ESCS), Goldmann-Favre syndrome (GFS), clumped pigmentary retinal degeneration (CPRD), and retinitis pigmentosa (RP). *Hum. Mutat.* **2009**, *30*, 1475–1485. [CrossRef] [PubMed]
36. Terray, A.; Slembrouck, A.; Nanteau, C.; Chondroyer, C.; Zeitz, C.; Sahel, J.-A.; Audo, I.; Reichman, S.; Goureau, O. Generation of an induced pluripotent stem cell (iPSC) line from a patient with autosomal dominant retinitis pigmentosa due to a mutation in the NR2E3 gene. *Stem Cell Res.* **2017**, *24*, 1–4. [CrossRef]
37. Tucker, B.; Mullins, R.F.; Streb, L.M.; Anfinson, K.; Eyestone, M.E.; Kaalberg, E.; Riker, M.J.; Drack, A.V.; Braun, T.; Stone, E.M. Patient-specific iPSC-derived photoreceptor precursor cells as a means to investigate retinitis pigmentosa. *Elife* **2013**, *2*, e00824. [CrossRef]
38. Jepsen, J.S.; Pfundheller, H.M.; Lykkesfeldt, A.E. Downregulation of p21(WAF1/CIP1) and Estrogen Receptor? in MCF-7 Cells by Antisense Oligonucleotides Containing Locked Nucleic Acid (LNA). *Oligonucleotides* **2004**, *14*, 147–156. [CrossRef]
39. Ten Asbroek, A.L.; Fluiter, K.; van Groenigen, M.; Nooij, M.; Baas, F. Polymorphisms in the large subunit of human RNA polymerase II as target for allele-specific inhibition. *Nucleic Acids Res.* **2000**, *28*, 1133–1138. [CrossRef]
40. Monia, B.P.; Johnston, J.F.; Ecker, D.J.; Zounes, M.A.; Lima, W.F.; Freier, S.M. Selective inhibition of mutant Ha-ras mRNA expression by antisense oligonucleotides. *J. Biol. Chem.* **1992**, *267*, 19954–19962.
41. Magner, D.; Biala, E.; Lisowiec-Wachnicka, J.; Kierzek, R. Influence of mismatched and bulged nucleotides on SNP-preferential RNase H cleavage of RNA-antisense gapmer heteroduplexes. *Sci. Rep.* **2017**, *7*, 1–16. [CrossRef]

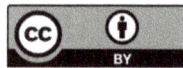

© 2019 by the authors. Licensee MDPI, Basel, Switzerland. This article is an open access article distributed under the terms and conditions of the Creative Commons Attribution (CC BY) license (http://creativecommons.org/licenses/by/4.0/).

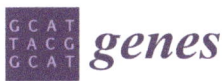

Review

Retinal miRNA Functions in Health and Disease

Marta Zuzic [1], Jesus Eduardo Rojo Arias [1], Stefanie Gabriele Wohl [2] and Volker Busskamp [1,*]

1. Center for Regenerative Therapies Dresden (CRTD), Technische Universität Dresden, 01307 Dresden, Germany; marta.zuzic@tu-dresden.de (M.Z.); Jesus_Eduardo.Rojo_Arias@tu-dresden.de (J.E.R.A.)
2. Department of Biological and Vision Sciences, The State University of New York, College of Optometry, New York, NY 10036, USA; swohl@sunyopt.edu
* Correspondence: volker.busskamp@tu-dresden.de

Received: 1 April 2019; Accepted: 15 May 2019; Published: 17 May 2019

Abstract: The health and function of our visual system relies on accurate gene expression. While many genetic mutations are associated with visual impairment and blindness, we are just beginning to understand the complex interplay between gene regulation and retinal pathologies. MicroRNAs (miRNAs), a class of non-coding RNAs, are important regulators of gene expression that exert their function through post-transcriptional silencing of complementary mRNA targets. According to recent transcriptomic analyses, certain miRNA species are expressed in all retinal cell types, while others are cell type-specific. As miRNAs play important roles in homeostasis, cellular function, and survival of differentiated retinal cell types, their dysregulation is associated with retinal degenerative diseases. Thus, advancing our understanding of the genetic networks modulated by miRNAs is central to harnessing their potential as therapeutic agents to overcome visual impairment. In this review, we summarize the role of distinct miRNAs in specific retinal cell types, the current knowledge on their implication in inherited retinal disorders, and their potential as therapeutic agents.

Keywords: microRNA; retina; photoreceptors; rods; cones; bipolar cells; Müller glia; retinal inherited disorders; retinitis pigmentosa; retinal degeneration

1. miRNA Biogenesis and Function

MicroRNAs (miRNAs) are a class of highly conserved ~22 nucleotide (nt)-long non-coding RNAs that have a repressive impact on gene expression in a sequence-specific manner (Figure 1). These miRNAs are derived from partially complementary primary RNA transcripts (pri-miRNA) produced mainly by RNA polymerase II, but also by RNA polymerase III. Pri-miRNAs self-anneal to form hairpin or stem–loop structures, which are subsequently cleaved 11 base pairs (bp) from the base of the hairpin stem by the miRNA-processing complex, a protein ensemble that contains the Drosha ribonuclease and the DiGeorge Critical Region 8 (Dgcr8) protein [1]. The resulting 70 nt-long sequence is known as precursor miRNA (pre-miRNA) and is characterized by a 5' phosphate and a 2-nt overhang at the 3' end [2]. Alternatively, miRNAs also result from splicing events independently of Drosha and Dgcr8 [3]. Pre-miRNAs are subsequently exported out of the nucleus for the next processing step in which the Dicer endoribonuclease creates a cut ~22 nt away from the cleaving site of the miRNA-processing complex. Thereby, an additional 5' phosphate and a new 2-nt 3' overhang are generated at the opposite end of the double-stranded RNA [4]. The final miRNA structure is thus a duplex formed by partially complementary 22 nt-long RNA sequences with 5' phosphates and 2-nt 3' overhangs at both ends. In the last processing step, these duplexes are incorporated into the Argonaute protein, which is a member of the RNA-induced silencing complex (RISC), where one of the strands is removed. The strand that remains bound to Argonaute coordinates the search of, and pairing to, partially complementary target mRNA transcripts [1,5]. Upon binding their mRNA targets, miRNAs either induce their degradation, promote their deadenylation, or reduce their translational efficacy [6]. As individual miRNAs can have thousands of mRNA targets, they represent potent regulators of gene expression at the systems level [7,8]. To date, there are 1917 annotated human miRNA sequences (miRbase v22, access date 2019-05-13) [9].

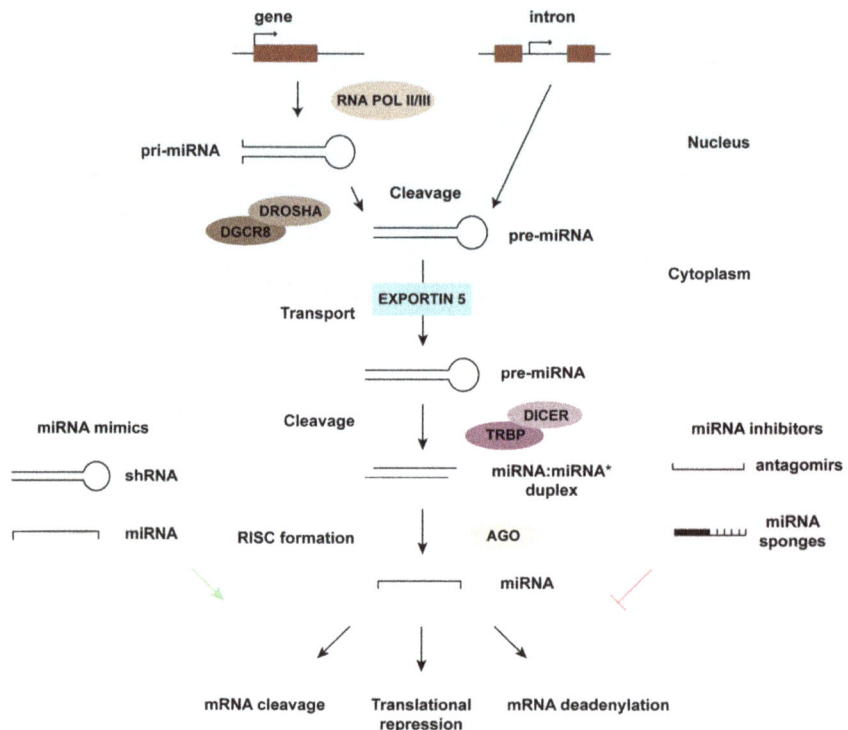

Figure 1. MicroRNA (miRNA) pathway. miRNA biogenesis starts in the nucleus where partially self-complementary RNA polymerase II or III transcripts from a miRNA gene or from an intronic region assemble into a hairpin-like structure known as primary (pri)-miRNA. Pri-miRNAs are cleaved by the DiGeorge Critical Region 8 (Dgcr8)/Drosha complex and transported to the cytoplasm via Exportin 5. In the cytoplasm, pre-miRNAs are cleaved by the Dicer/HIV-1 TAR RNA binding protein (TRBP) nuclease complex, thereby giving rise to a miRNA duplex. This duplex is then loaded onto the Argonaute (AGO) protein, a component of the RNA-induced silencing complex (RISC), where one of the two strands is discarded while the other serves to search complementary transcripts. Targets bound by miRNAs exhibit reduced translational efficiency, mainly as a consequence of mRNA cleavage or deadenylation. The miRNA pathway can be modulated by introducing miRNA mimics (green) or miRNA inhibitors (red). shRNA is small hairpin RNA.

Dysregulated miRNA expression during development can lead to severe defects and is connected to many pathological conditions such as cancer, neurodegenerative diseases, heart failure, diabetes, and inherited genetic disorders [10]. In mature organs and tissues, miRNAs support the robustness of gene networks and buffer against the fluctuations in gene expression often resulting from stochastic modulation and environmental stress [11]. As their metabolic activity is considerably high and they are often exposed to high levels of external stress, photoreceptors are highly vulnerable to cell death in retinal degenerative diseases. In this context, miRNAs play an important role in photoreceptor survival and function [12]. Moreover, as not all retinal disease phenotypes have been linked to specific genes, altered miRNA expression may underlie the emergence and progression of certain retinal disorders. Thus, exploring the function and gene regulatory networks of these and other non-coding RNAs is of the utmost importance. A dominant mutation in miR-204, for instance, is the genetic cause of retinal degeneration associated with ocular coloboma, a genetic developmental disorder characterized by keyhole-shaped defects in various eye structures [13]. It is thus tempting to speculate that miR-204 is not the sole case of a miRNA giving rise to an ocular disease, and that altered expression of non-coding RNAs might lead to other retinal disorders. Here, we discuss some of the known functions of miRNAs in the adult retina.

2. Controlling Cellular miRNA Expression

The deliberate modulation of gene expression through the use of non-coding RNAs, commonly referred to as RNA interference [14], has been extensively utilized in basic and biomedical research. Small hairpin RNAs (shRNAs), for instance, are artificial RNA molecules with a hairpin region processed by the same machinery as miRNAs and effectively acting as miRNA mimics [15,16]. Normally, shRNAs are designed to match the sequence of specific RNA molecules, which they target and downregulate upon delivery. The production of such shRNA molecules is driven by regular promoter elements within a plasmid or a viral vector. Standard gene delivery techniques can be applied to express the shRNA of interest in target cells. This system can also be used to overexpress specific miRNAs [17]. Alternatively, the consequences of miRNA overexpression can be studied by inserting them within artificial intron systems. In general, shRNA vectors are particularly interesting for silencing dominant disease-causing transcripts and their use in retinal cell types was established already over a decade ago [18].

Vice versa, for downregulating or silencing miRNAs, commonly used techniques include "antagomirs" [19] and so-called miRNA "sponges" [20]. Whereas antagomirs are chemically engineered oligonucleotides, miRNA sponges are RNAs with artificial tandem binding site arrays for specific miRNAs. Hence, these sponge sequences compete with physiological targets for miRNA binding, which ultimately leads to reduced silencing of primary mRNA targets. Sponge cassettes can be delivered to retinal cell types by adeno-associated viruses (AAV) [21], which are powerful clinically approved vectors for ocular gene transfer [22,23]. Thus, the therapeutic use of non-coding RNAs is presently growing at an accelerated pace due to increased knowledge of miRNA functions and the wide adoption of technologies that facilitate control of their expression levels in distinct retinal cell types.

3. Photoreceptor–miRNAs as Cell Maintenance and Survival Regulators

Rod photoreceptors are sensory neurons essential to night vision. To investigate the impact of miRNA deficiency in these cells, rod photoreceptor-specific Dicer conditional knock-out (cKO) mice have been generated. As mentioned above, Dicer is the endoribonuclease responsible for the second cleavage step in the canonical miRNA biosynthesis pathway. These mice were generated by crossing a $Dicer1^{fl/fl}$ line with mice expressing Cre recombinase exclusively in mature rods. Loss of $Dicer1$ at postnatal day 28 (P28), a time-point at which rods are mature and postmitotic, was reported to lead to outer segment disorganization in eight-week-old mice, followed by robust retinal degeneration and loss of visual function by 14 weeks. Notably, cKO mice did not exhibit significant defects in either phototransduction or the visual cycle before the onset of retinal degeneration, suggesting that the main role of miRNAs in rods is to support photoreceptor survival [24].

Additional studies have aimed at revealing the functions of miRNAs in cone photoreceptors, which are essential for high-acuity and daylight vision. Cone photoreceptor-specific miRNA-deficient mice have been generated by crossing $Dgcr8^{fl/fl}$ animals with mice expressing Cre recombinase solely in differentiated cones. In these mice, the Dgcr8 protein was only gradually depleted over time as a consequence of its prolonged half-life. Thus, loss of miRNA processing was first detected at P30 and was complete only by P60. The lack of miRNAs in these animals resulted in the progressive loss of cone outer segments, and therefore in low sensitivity to high light levels. However, cones without outer segments did not degenerate in spite of their severely altered gene expression profiles. The latter suggests a crucial role for miRNAs in regulating genetic pathways essential to cone outer segment maintenance and function, but not to cone survival [17]. On the other hand, a recent study reported that the conditional knockout of Dicer in cones results not only in outer segment loss but also in a more severe phenotype with enhanced cone cell death [25]. For proper phenotype interpretation, the targeted miRNA biogenesis proteins, Dgcr8 versus Dicer, are of importance as Dgcr8 knockouts may have residual miRNA expression from splicing products. Although these reports also differed in the cone-specific Cre driver lines used and in the onset of miRNA loss, together they provide strong evidence for the importance of miRNAs on photoreceptor homeostasis, function, and survival.

4. The Impact of the miR-183/96/182 Cluster on Photoreceptors

The miRNAs of the miR-183/96/182 cluster play important functional roles in multiple sensory tissues, as evidenced by their expression not only in the retina [26,27], but also in the inner ear [28], the olfactory and gustatory epithelium [27], and in dorsal root ganglia mechanosensory neurons [29]. miR-183, -96, and -182 are expressed as a single polycistronic transcript and exhibit significant sequence similarity in their seed regions. Thereby, they possess shared targets and can partially substitute each other's function. This overlap in function explains why targeted deletion of only one of these three miRNAs, i.e., miR-182, results in no visible alterations in retinal development [30]. More importantly, although these three miRNAs possess distinct targets, the majority of such targets are involved in identical pathways [31]. In the retina, the miR-183/96/182 cluster is enriched in rod and cone photoreceptors with transcript levels reduced in dark and increased in light conditions (Figure 2). Such dynamic changes in expression levels are the consequences of rapid miRNA decay and of increased transcription, respectively. The latter suggests that miRNA metabolism, in general, is higher in neurons than in other cell types, possibly due to neuronal activity [21].

The function of the miR-183/96/182 cluster was examined in a transgenic mouse line expressing a miRNA sponge for all three cluster miRNAs exclusively in mature rods [32]. Retinae from these mice displayed no detectable morphological or functional changes, likely because the sponge activity was insufficient to capture all mature miRNA molecules of such a highly expressed cluster. Nonetheless, after 30 min exposure to high light intensities (10,000 lux), transgenic mice but not wild type animals showed severe retinal degeneration, indicating that reduced levels of cluster miRNAs have an impact on rod function and survival. More severe retinal defects and retinal degeneration were observed in a miR-183/96/182 cluster knockout mouse model [33], although the miRNAs of the cluster were also missing during photoreceptor development, when cluster expression is tightly controlled [34]. Hence, in this case it is impossible to distinguish the functions of the miR-183/96/182 cluster in development from those in adulthood. Nevertheless, together these knockdown and knockout studies suggest that this cluster plays a neuroprotective role in the retina. Remarkably, re-introducing miR-182 and -183 in Dgcr8 cKO cones, i.e., cones depleted of all other miRNAs, has been reported to prevent the loss of cone outer segments [17]. Considering that miR-182 and -183 constitutes around 70% of all cone miRNA content, it is likely that these play major roles in cone functionality, including in the modulation of outer segment maintenance. Furthermore, overexpression of the miR-183/96/182 cluster in embryonic stem cell-derived retinal organoids induces the formation of light-responsive short outer segments [17], while in human RPE cells in vitro it triggers their reprogramming to neurons [35]. In this sense, a number of the cluster's targets have been validated, including pro-apoptotic genes, like *Casp2* [32], genes important for survival such as *Rac1* coding for the small GTP-binding protein [36], and neurotransmitter transporters like the voltage-dependent glutamate transporter *Slc1a1* [21] as well as the sodium- and chloride-dependent glycine transporter *Slc6a9* [36]. The latter, together with the neurogenic effects of overexpressing the miRNAs within this cluster in different cell types, suggests that the miR-183/96/182 cluster is central to photoreceptor homeostasis and serves as a pro-survival factor in stress conditions.

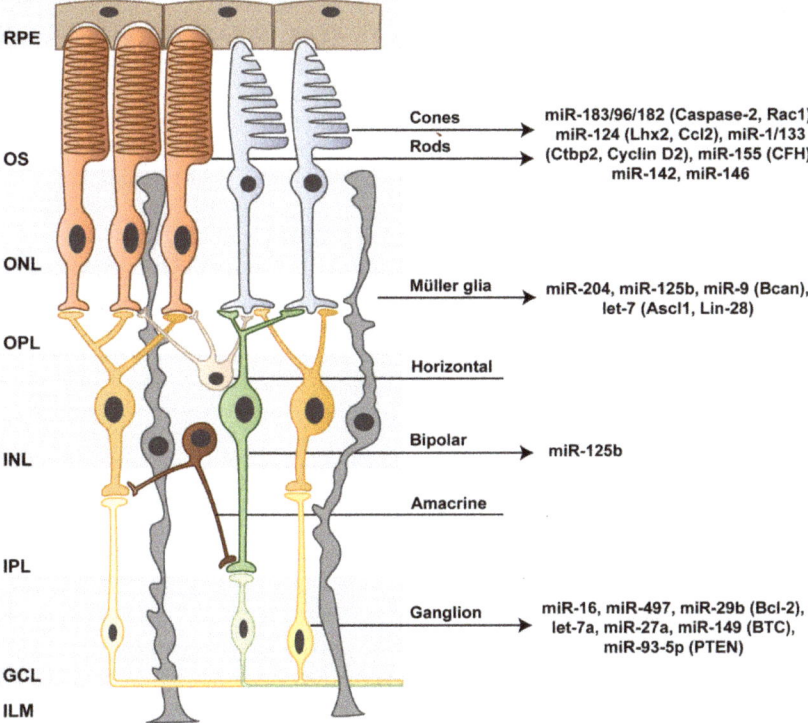

Figure 2. MiRNAs acting as modulators of retinal cell behavior. In the vertebrate eye, the retinal pigment epithelium (RPE) separates the retina from the subretinal space. Within the outermost layer of the retina, rod and cone photoreceptors sense light with their outer segments (OS). Photoreceptor bodies reside within the outer nuclear layer (ONL), and their axons protrude into the outer plexiform layer (OPL), where they synapse with excitatory bipolar cells and inhibitory horizontal cells. The bodies of these cells, as well as of amacrine cells, which create inhibitory synapses with the axons of bipolar cells, reside in turn within the inner nuclear layer (INL). The electrochemical signal produced by photoreceptors during phototransduction is transmitted through bipolar cells to ganglion cells via synaptic connections in the inner plexiform layer (IPL). In a final step, ganglion cells send this information to higher brain areas through their axons, which bundle up to form the optic nerve. An additional cell type within the retina is Müller glia. These cells play key roles in the support of neuronal functions and in mediating the reaction to a number of physiological signals, including immune responses. Müller glia feet form the outer limiting membrane (OLM), which separates photoreceptor OS from their somata. Within the retina, miRNAs play central roles in health and disease. Recognized miRNA species associated to the functionality of specific retinal cell types are shown with validated targets between parentheses. GCL, ganglion cell layer; ILM, inner limiting membrane.

5. miR-124 Protects Photoreceptors from Apoptosis

MiR-124 is enriched in neurons of the central nervous system [37,38] including the retina [39], and is one of the most well studied miRNA species. In the retina, miR-124 is expressed in all neuronal cell layers, but most prominently in photoreceptor outer (OS) and inner segments (IS). As both humans and mice possess three miR-124 loci, the generation of a complete miR-124 knockout model has been challenging. Recently, a full miR-124 KO (i.e., all six genomic copies) was achieved in a human induced pluripotent stem cell model of neurogenesis [8]. Neurons generated from KO cells displayed altered morphological and functional features and decreased long-term viability, pointing to the importance of miR-124 in neuronal survival. Of note, among the three miR-124 paralogs (a-1, a-2, and a-3), miR-124a-1 has been previously identified by in situ hybridization as the predominant form expressed in the developing mouse retina, with miR-124a-2 being detected at very low levels and miR-124a-3 expression being almost negligible [40]. In agreement with this, knocking out the miR-124a-1 host gene, i.e., the retinal non-coding RNA 3 (*Rncr3*), abolishes miR-124 expression almost entirely in the mouse cone photoreceptor layer. Additional consequences of miR-124a-1 KO included cone mislocalization and apoptosis, decreased expression of cone-specific genes, and reduced light-responsiveness [40].

A validated target of miR-124a in the retina is *Lhx2*. Indeed, the miR-124a-mediated downregulation of *Lhx2* mRNA levels is necessary for cone survival [40]. As depletion of Dgcr8 in adult cones does not cause cone degeneration, it is very likely that miR-124 is effective in these cells early during development but that after differentiation they remain unaffected by miR-124 deletion. In agreement, neurogenesis is hindered neither in the complete miR-124 KO in vitro model nor in miR-124a-1 KO mice, although increased apoptosis was observed over time in both cases. Moreover, as cones but no other retinal neurons degenerate in miR-124a-1 KO mice, it is possible for the compensatory effects of the other two miR-124 paralogs to be insufficient in these photoreceptors but more potent in other retinal cell types.

In the retina, miR-124 is expressed not only in photoreceptors but also in neurons within the inner nuclear layer and the ganglion cell layer. An altered distribution of miR-124 expression from primarily the outer nuclear layer to the inner nuclear layer has been reported to occur in age-related macular degeneration (AMD) patients and mouse models of retinal degeneration [41], with such changes being followed by miR-124 depletion at later degeneration stages. Moreover, environmental stress factors, such as high light intensities, are speculated to induce the translocation of this miRNA from photoreceptors to Müller glia (MG) cells, where it targets the CC-chemokine ligand 2 (*Ccl2*). Ccl2 is a pro-inflammatory chemokine that attracts microglia/macrophages and that is produced and released by MG cells in response to retinal damage [42]. Further, this chemokine is upregulated in both neovascular and atrophic forms of AMD [43] and in retinitis pigmentosa [44]. By downregulating *Ccl2*, miR-124 translocation would thus dampen the inflammatory cascade and promote photoreceptor survival. After prolonged stress, on the other hand, miR-124 depletion results in highly pro-inflammatory environments and thereby in subsequent photoreceptor degeneration. Supporting these observations, *Ccl2* downregulation has been shown to reduce photoreceptor cell death in animal models of retinal degeneration [44–46]. Notably, intravitreal administration of miR-124 mimics decreases retinal inflammation and photoreceptor cell death, while preserving retinal function [41]. The latter might be a consequence, at least partially, of increased *Ccl2* targeting.

6. miRNA Functions in Inner Retinal Neurons

For the maintenance and survival of retinal cell types other than photoreceptors, miRNAs are also remarkably important. For example, miR-125b has been described as a regulator of neuritogenesis during remodeling in rod bipolar cells after retinal degeneration [47]. Similarly, in retinal ganglion cells (RGCs), miRNA expression profiles and functions have been investigated. RGCs are responsible for sending the visual information collected by photoreceptors to higher brain areas via the optic nerve, and their damage is a hallmark of glaucoma. In retinae of a glaucoma mouse model, nine miRNAs (out of 17 tested) were identified as differentially expressed relative to controls. Among those nine miRNAs, the pro-apoptotic miR-16, -497, -29b, and let-7a were downregulated, while the anti-apoptotic miR-27a was upregulated. Whereas let-7a exerts its apoptotic function by inducing neurodegeneration via Toll-like receptor signaling, miR-16, -29b, and -497 negatively regulate the apoptosis regulator Bcl-2. These alterations in miRNA expression profiles suggest a shift towards a protective anti-apoptotic phenotype [48]. In a different mouse model of glaucoma, downregulation of miR-149 led to an increased RGC number and minimized ultrastructural RGC alterations [49]. In this study, betacellulin (*Btc*) was also identified as a miR-149 target. BTC is a mitogen influencing the activation of the PI3K/AKT signaling pathway, which mediates RGC protection via its pro-survival and anti-apoptotic effects. Further, in the N-methyl-D-aspartate (NMDA)-induced glaucoma mouse model, significant reductions in RGC viability were accompanied by miR-93-5p downregulation [50]. Reduced miR-93-5p levels in these mice, in turn, resulted in the elevated presence of its target phosphatase and tensin homolog (PTEN), which promotes autophagy of RGCs via the AKT/mTOR pathway. Confirming the central role of miR-93-5p in this context, the reduced viability of RGCs isolated from retinae of NMDA-induced glaucoma animals was counteracted either by overexpressing this miRNA species or by transfection with a miR-93-5p mimic.

In mouse models of optic nerve injury, increased expression of specific miRNAs has also been detected. miR-21 expression, for instance, correlated with reactive MG gliosis. Whereas activated MGs are neuroprotective after injury in the acute response phase, they later acquire a pro-inflammatory and pro-apoptotic phenotype. Modulating MG gliosis in both the acute and chronic post-injury phases in these mice resulted in enhanced RGC survival and functionality and led to improvements in retinal structural integrity [51]. Often, however, the protective roles of distinct miRNAs in RGCs have been assessed in vitro. In rat RGC-5 cells, for instance, overexpression of miR-187 was reported to suppress apoptosis and promote proliferation by targeting *Smad7* [52]. Similarly, upregulation of miR-211 was shown to downregulate *Frs2* and to decrease the extent of cell death in RGC-5 cells subjected to a high-pressure challenge [53]. These results hint at a protective effect of miR-187 and miR-211 on RGCs. On the other hand, lentivirus-mediated down-regulation of miR-100 has been described to reduce hydrogen peroxide-induced RGC apoptosis and to enhance neurite growth by activating the AKT/ERK and TRKB pathways through phosphorylation [54]. In a similar experimental approach, hydrogen peroxide-induced apoptosis of RGC was described to decrease upon miR-134 downregulation. In this case, a luciferase reporter assay confirmed that miR-134 directly interacts with the cyclic AMP-response element-binding protein (*Creb*), a transcription factor with central roles in neuronal protection that modulates the expression of the anti-apoptotic proteins BDNF and Bcl-2. Thus, inhibiting miR-134 effectively reduces apoptosis levels by allowing the enhanced translation of CREB and, consequently, the upregulation of its downstream targets BDNF and Bcl-2 [55].

7. The role of miRNAs in Müller Glia Development and Function

MiRNAs play an important role in retinal development as described in several studies using Dicer conditional knockouts [56–58] (summarized in [59]). One study in particular reported that the blockade of miRNA genesis in an αPax6-Cre mouse model prevented the development of late retinal progenitors and their progenies, including MG [60]. Specifically, three miRNAs have been identified as key regulators of the early to late developmental transition in retinal progenitors, namely let-7, miR-125, and miR-9 [61,62]. Thus, miRNAs may be involved in MG differentiation. As mentioned above, the miRNA expression of whole retinae has been previously profiled [63,64]. Since the vast majority of retinal cells are rod photoreceptors and MG account for only around 2% of them [65], the profiling and identification of MG-specific miRNAs requires FACS-purification or primary cultures. Two independent studies have so far aimed at identifying these miRNAs. The authors of the first study isolated MG from P8 retinae and cultured the cells before miRNA profiling. The culture period, however, was not clarified. In this study, miR-143, miR-145, miR-214, miR-199a, miR-199b*, and miR-29a were identified as highly expressed [66]. In the second study, miR-204, miR-125b, and miR-9 were identified as MG-specific miRNAs (mGliomiRs) in reporter-labelled (RlbpCreERT-dtTomato) FACS-purified P11/P12 murine MG [67]. These three miRNAs had high expression levels in MG, with increasing levels from P11 to adulthood. Moreover, besides these MG-specific miRNAs, a distinct set of miRNAs had similar expression levels in both neurons and glia (termed shared miRNAs). This set includes most members of the let-7 family and miR-29a. Thus, it is conceivable that miR-125, miR-9, and let-7 are not only key regulators in the early to late progenitor transition [61], but that they are also important for MG maturation and function.

A remaining question was whether miRNAs are required for proper MG function. This was addressed in a Dicer cKO study using a MG-specific Rlbp-CreERT:tdTomato:Dicer$^{fl/fl}$ reporter mouse [68]. Dicer deletion was induced in these mice by tamoxifen administration at P12, when MG are differentiated, as well as in one-month old animals. Over a period of 6–12 months, glia aggregated abnormally, leading in turn to massive structural disturbances. Although MG usually do not express the *Bcan* gene, which encodes a chondroitin sulfate proteoglycan, RNA-Seq showed this to be the most highly upregulated gene in these cells. Notably, this phenotype was primarily the consequence of miR-9 loss. miR-9 targets the 3'UTR of *Bcan*, and its administration in vitro or ex vivo prevented abnormal glia development and/or partially restored overall retinal structure. Although in these mice miRNAs were only deleted in MG and not in neurons, a massive loss of photoreceptors was also observed. More importantly, retinal remodeling also subsequently ensued. Remodeling generally occurs as a result of photoreceptor degeneration [69]. Interestingly, MG from human retinitis pigmentosa tissue displayed similar cell aggregation and were positive for Brevican (the protein encoded by *Bcan*). This suggests that not only loss of or disturbances in neuronal miRNAs, but also dysregulation of the glial miRNA biogenesis machinery could be causative of retinal diseases [68]. This hypothesis is further supported by MG ablation studies showing that the dysfunction of this cell population plays an important role in retinal diseases [70–73].

8. miRNAs in Müller Glia De-Differentiation and Their Potential Regeneration Capacity

Although there are miRNAs specific to retinal progenitors, neurons, and MG, and despite many of these miRNAs playing important roles in cell fate decisions, their capacity to alter the fate of mature, fully-differentiated cells remains controversial. In contrast to mammalian retinae, the fish retina can regenerate completely after injury. Remarkably, MG are the cells that mediate the regeneration process. MG de-differentiate to progenitors, proliferate, migrate, and differentiate de novo into all retinal cell types, including RGCs and photoreceptors. Key regulators in this regenerative process are the Acheate-scute family bHLH transcription factor 1 (*Ascl1*) and the RNA-binding protein Lin-28, which are both regulated by the miRNA let-7 [74,75]. Additional factors discovered to be involved in this process include Wnt [76] and Shh [77], which are regulated by the miRNA let-7 in fish and mouse. Notwithstanding, the mechanisms of MG reprogramming in mice, especially at adult ages, are more intricate and involve epigenetic alterations [78].

The brain-enriched miR-124 is known to regulate neurogenesis [39,41,67,79]. Accordingly, overexpression of miR-124 in MG-derived mouse progenitors in vitro results in twice as many βIII-Tubulin-positive cells as in wild-type control cells [66]. This indicates that this neuronal miRNA can be used to direct retinal progenitor like-cells towards a neuronal fate, as it has previously been observed on neural stem cells [80,81]. Moreover, when miR-124 alone or in combination with miR-9/9* was overexpressed in P12 mouse MG in vitro, MG de-differentiated into *Ascl1*-expressing progenitor-like cells that later on expressed mature neuronal markers including *Map2*, Calbindin, and Calretinin. The underlying mechanism for this process is known to require the RE1-silencing transcription factor (Rest) pathway [67], an evolutionarily conserved transcriptional regulator that inhibits neuronal gene expression in non-neuronal cells such as glia or fibroblasts [82–84], and whose inhibition by miR-124 enhances the expression of neuronal genes [85–87]. In addition, miR-124 has recently been described to promote axon growth in RGCs differentiated from young rat retinal stem cell-derived MG by silencing the REST complex [88]. Besides miR-124, miR-28 has also been reported to potentially play a role in photoreceptor differentiation. MG-derived progenitors treated with anti-miR-28 exhibited *Crx* and Rhodopsin expression while miR-28 overexpression did not [89]. In this case, however, the underlying mechanisms remain elusive.

9. Global miRNA Alterations in Retinal Diseases

Retinitis pigmentosa (RP) is a complex inherited retinal disease that emerges from a heterogeneous pool of mutations [90]. Yet, irrespective of the underlying mutation, clinical manifestations are often similar and include progressive photoreceptor loss and visual impairment. To determine if miRNA dysregulation is involved in the pathophysiology of RP, miRNA expression levels have been interrogated in multiple mouse models of retinal degeneration. One study examined the miRNA expression profile of two rhodopsin (*Rho*) mutants (recessive rho–/– knockout and dominant P347S-Rhodopsin, also known as R347) and two RDS/Peripherin mutants (recessive rds–/– null mutant and dominant Δ307-rds) [91]. The authors reported all four mouse models to exhibit miR-96, -182, and -183 downregulation, and miR-1, -133, and -142 upregulation. The dysregulated miRNA signature of isolated rods as well as of whole retinae of R347 and Δ307-rds mice were similar. These findings suggest that altered miRNA profiles are indeed associated with RP, irrespective of the causative mutation or of its dominant or recessive nature. However, the miR-183/96/182 cluster is highly expressed in photoreceptors and therefore its downregulation might be a consequence of the massive rod photoreceptor degeneration rather than causative of RP. In a follow-up study, C-terminal Binding Protein 2 (*Ctbp2*) was validated as a miR-1 target, with *Slc6a9* and *Rac1* being recognized by miR-9, -182, and -183 [36]. CTBP2, a major component of specialized synapses, was shown to be co-expressed with the miR-1/133 cluster in photoreceptors, and its levels were reported to decrease in photoreceptor synaptic regions of R347 retinae. The latter suggests that miR-1/133 may play a role in regulating synaptic remodeling at photoreceptor synapses by targeting *Ctbp2*. In contrast, *Slc6a9*, which encodes one of the two main transporters involved in removing glycine from the synaptic cleft, was co-expressed with miR-1/133 exclusively in cone photoreceptors.

The retinal degeneration 10 (rd10) mouse is a commonly used model of autosomal recessive retinitis pigmentosa and has been utilized to study miRNA expression patterns in early retinal degeneration [92]. In these mice, a spontaneous mutation in the rod phosphodiesterase (*Pde*) gene leads to photoreceptor death from post-natal day 16 on as a result of calcium dysregulation [93]. By using microarrays to profile the expression of over 1900 miRNAs in rd10 retinae, 152 differentially expressed miRNAs have been identified after (P17, P19, and P22), but also shortly before (P15) the initiation of photoreceptor apoptosis [92]. The miRNAs identified as differentially expressed prior to the onset of apoptosis include miR-6240, miR-6937-5p, miR-3473b, and miR-7035-5p, which are likely involved in the disease etiology. On the other hand, miR-155-5p, miR-142-5p, and miR-146a-5p were differentially expressed after the onset of apoptosis. Thus, it remains unclear whether these miRNAs counteract or enhance disease progression. By comparing differentially expressed miRNAs with inversely correlated mRNAs and performing gene ontology and biological pathway analyses, a large number of miRNA targets were revealed to encode factors involved in apoptosis, the inflammatory response, calcium signaling, visual perception, and phototransduction.

The differential expression of miRNAs in the context of retinal degenerative diseases has also been studied in canine models. Notably, the early onset retinal degeneration models Xlpra2 (RPGRORF15-microdeletion), Rcd1 (PDE6B-mutation), and Erd (STK38L-mutation), as well as the slowly progressing Prcd (PRCD-mutation) model, have been reported to exhibit similar miRNA expression profiles as healthy control dogs both prior to and at the peak of photoreceptor cell death [94]. Divergences were reported to arise only during the chronic cell death stage, with anti-apoptotic miRNAs such as miR-9, -19a, -20, -21, -29b, -146a, -155, and -221 being upregulated and pro-apoptotic miR-122 and miR-129 being downregulated. Although the miRNA species differentially expressed in canine and murine models of retinal degeneration are not identical, available reports hint at miRNAs playing a role in counteracting the degenerative processes characteristic of diseased retinae by delaying photoreceptor cell death.

A number of additional studies have interrogated the retinal miRNA expression profile in response to injury. Inducing photoreceptor death by ablating MG, for instance, leads to the differential expression of 16 miRNAs, with miR-142, miR-146, and the miR-1/133 cluster in particular exhibiting increased expression levels [95]. In this study, increased miR-133 expression was mainly detected within the outer nuclear layer, where it targets the anti-apoptotic gene cyclin D2. In fact, the cyclin D2 family has been reported to play a neuroprotective role in retinal degeneration [96]. Unexpectedly, a positive correlation between miR-133 and cyclin D2 was also reported, suggesting that miR-133 up-regulates the expression levels of its own target. Further, in models of light-induced photoreceptor death, 37 miRNAs have been described to increase in expression upon light damage, including seven that regulate the inflammatory response (miR-125, -155, -207, -347, -449, -351, -542). Among the latter, miR-155 is of particular interest as it is linked to the progression of the inflammatory response through the targeting of complement factor H (*Cfh*) [97], a major inhibitor of the alternative complement pathway [98]. Moreover, upregulation of miR-155 has been detected in both mouse and canine models of inherited retinal diseases [92,94], suggesting that the roles of certain miRNAs are conserved across species and, more notably, shared in different injury response contexts.

The miRNA profile of human retinae has been recently investigated via high-throughput sequencing [99]. The assessment of miRNA expression levels in 16 retinae from healthy donors led to the detection of 480 miRNA species with more than 3000 variants. Of note, the five most highly expressed miRNAs accounted for 70% and the top 20 miRNAs for almost 90% of the entire retinal miRNA profile. Moreover, the miRNAs miR-182 and miR-183 were the most prevalent miRNA species in retinal neurons and miR-204 was the most abundant miRNA in retinal pigment epithelium (RPE) cells. Some of these highly expressed human miRNAs coincide with those previously identified in murine retinae by microarray analyses and RNA in situ hybridization experiments [27,64,100,101], pointing to their potentially conserved retinal functions across mammalian species [102]. It is known from animal models that miRNA expression patterns change over the course of retinal development [64,101] and that such dynamic miRNA expression profiles are crucial to retinal cell differentiation (reviewed in [59]). Altogether, it is very likely that the impact miRNAs have in animal models is transferable to human retinal cell types in health and disease. This further implies that particular miRNAs may be used as disease biomarkers and, additionally, that the precise modulation of their expression levels might represent a valuable therapeutic strategy for the treatment of diverse retinal inherited disorders.

10. Conclusions

We are in the process of understanding the complex functions of miRNAs in retinal health and disease. Further studies are required to obtain coherent pictures of gene expression regulators in order to harness their potential use not only as biomarkers but also to treat and counteract retinal diseases. As individual miRNA species have the potential to orchestrate entire genetic programs, the possibility to use them as master regulators to stabilize or reset the cellular state of neurons and glial cells in the retina is highly promising.

Author Contributions: Conceptualization, M.Z. and V.B.; writing—original draft preparation, writing—review and editing, M.Z., J.E.R.A., S.G.W., and V.B.; visualization, M.Z.; funding acquisition, S.G.W. and V.B.

Funding: M.Z. and J.E.R.A. were supported by the Dresden International Graduate School for Biomedicine and Bioengineering (DIGS-BB) and the Graduate Academy of TU Dresden. S.G.W. is supported by the New York State Empire Innovator Program. V.B. acknowledges financial support by the Volkswagen Foundation (Freigeist Fellowship-A110720), the European Research Council (ERC starting grant-678071-ProNeurons), and the Deutsche Forschungsgemeinschaft (DFG, SPP 2127 and EXC-2068-390729961-Cluster of Excellence-Physics of Life).

Acknowledgments: The authors would like to thank Sylvia J. Gasparini for critical feedback on the manuscript.

Conflicts of Interest: The authors declare no conflict of interest, except for V.B., who is an inventor of a patent application that is related to some aspects of this manuscript filed by Friedrich Miescher Institute for Biomedical Research, Basel, Switzerland.

References

1. Ha, M.; Kim, V.N. Regulation of microRNA biogenesis. *Nat. Rev. Mol. Cell Biol.* **2014**, *15*, 509–524. [CrossRef]
2. Han, J.; Lee, Y.; Yeom, K.H.; Kim, Y.K.; Jin, H.; Kim, V.N. The Drosha-DGCR8 complex in primary microRNA processing. *Genes Dev.* **2004**, *18*, 3016–3027. [CrossRef]

3. Westholm, J.O.; Lai, E.C. Mirtrons: microRNA biogenesis via splicing. *Biochimie* **2011**, *93*, 1897–1904. [CrossRef]
4. Chiang, H.R.; Schoenfeld, L.W.; Ruby, J.G.; Auyeung, V.C.; Spies, N.; Baek, D.; Johnston, W.K.; Russ, C.; Luo, S.; Babiarz, J.E.; et al. Mammalian microRNAs: Experimental evaluation of novel and previously annotated genes. *Genes Dev.* **2010**, *24*, 992–1009. [CrossRef]
5. Bartel, D.P. MicroRNAs: Target recognition and regulatory functions. *Cell* **2009**, *136*, 215–233. [CrossRef]
6. Krol, J.; Loedige, I.; Filipowicz, W. The widespread regulation of microRNA biogenesis, function and decay. *Nat. Rev. Genet.* **2010**, *11*, 597–610. [CrossRef]
7. Tan, C.L.; Plotkin, J.L.; Veno, M.T.; von Schimmelmann, M.; Feinberg, P.; Mann, S.; Handler, A.; Kjems, J.; Surmeier, D.J.; O'Carroll, D.; et al. MicroRNA-128 governs neuronal excitability and motor behavior in mice. *Sci. (N.Y.)* **2013**, *342*, 1254–1258. [CrossRef] [PubMed]
8. Kutsche, L.K.; Gysi, D.M.; Fallmann, J.; Lenk, K.; Petri, R.; Swiersy, A.; Klapper, S.D.; Pircs, K.; Khattak, S.; Stadler, P.F.; et al. Combined Experimental and System-Level Analyses Reveal the Complex Regulatory Network of miR-124 during Human Neurogenesis. *Cell Syst.* **2018**, *7*, 438–452 e438. [CrossRef]
9. Kozomara, A.; Griffiths-Jones, S. miRBase: Annotating high confidence microRNAs using deep sequencing data. *Nucleic Acids Res.* **2014**, *42*, D68–D73. [CrossRef]
10. Ha, T.-Y. MicroRNAs in human diseases: From cancer to cardiovascular disease. *Immune. Netw.* **2011**, *11*, 135–154. [CrossRef]
11. Ebert, M.S.; Sharp, P.A. Roles for microRNAs in conferring robustness to biological processes. *Cell* **2012**, *149*, 515–524. [CrossRef]
12. Sundermeier, T.R.; Palczewski, K. The impact of microRNA gene regulation on the survival and function of mature cell types in the eye. *FASEB J.* **2016**, *30*, 23–33. [CrossRef]
13. Conte, I.; Hadfield, K.D.; Barbato, S.; Carrella, S.; Pizzo, M.; Bhat, R.S.; Carissimo, A.; Karali, M.; Porter, L.F.; Urquhart, J.; et al. MiR-204 is responsible for inherited retinal dystrophy associated with ocular coloboma. *Proc. Natl. Acad. Sci. USA* **2015**, *112*, E3236–E3245. [CrossRef]
14. Fire, A.; Xu, S.; Montgomery, M.K.; Kostas, S.A.; Driver, S.E.; Mello, C.C. Potent and specific genetic interference by double-stranded RNA in Caenorhabditis elegans. *Nature* **1998**, *391*, 806–811. [CrossRef]
15. Paddison, P.J.; Caudy, A.A.; Bernstein, E.; Hannon, G.J.; Conklin, D.S. Short hairpin RNAs (shRNAs) induce sequence-specific silencing in mammalian cells. *Genes Dev.* **2002**, *16*, 948–958. [CrossRef] [PubMed]
16. Brummelkamp, T.R.; Bernards, R.; Agami, R. A system for stable expression of short interfering RNAs in mammalian cells. *Sci. (N.Y.)* **2002**, *296*, 550–553. [CrossRef] [PubMed]
17. Busskamp, V.; Krol, J.; Nelidova, D.; Daum, J.; Szikra, T.; Tsuda, B.; Juttner, J.; Farrow, K.; Scherf, B.G.; Alvarez, C.P.; et al. miRNAs 182 and 183 are necessary to maintain adult cone photoreceptor outer segments and visual function. *Neuron* **2014**, *83*, 586–600. [CrossRef]
18. Michel, U.; Malik, I.; Ebert, S.; Bahr, M.; Kugler, S. Long-term in vivo and in vitro AAV-2-mediated RNA interference in rat retinal ganglion cells and cultured primary neurons. *Biochem. Biophys. Res. Commun.* **2005**, *326*, 307–312. [CrossRef] [PubMed]
19. Krutzfeldt, J.; Rajewsky, N.; Braich, R.; Rajeev, K.G.; Tuschl, T.; Manoharan, M.; Stoffel, M. Silencing of microRNAs in vivo with 'antagomirs'. *Nature* **2005**, *438*, 685–689. [CrossRef]
20. Ebert, M.S.; Neilson, J.R.; Sharp, P.A. MicroRNA sponges: Competitive inhibitors of small RNAs in mammalian cells. *Nat. Methods* **2007**, *4*, 721–726. [CrossRef] [PubMed]
21. Krol, J.; Busskamp, V.; Markiewicz, I.; Stadler, M.B.; Ribi, S.; Richter, J.; Duebel, J.; Bicker, S.; Fehling, H.J.; Schubeler, D.; et al. Characterizing light-regulated retinal microRNAs reveals rapid turnover as a common property of neuronal microRNAs. *Cell* **2010**, *141*, 618–631. [CrossRef]
22. Trapani, I.; Auricchio, A. Seeing the Light after 25 Years of Retinal Gene Therapy. *Trends Mol. Med.* **2018**, *24*, 669–681. [CrossRef] [PubMed]
23. Hudry, E.; Vandenberghe, L.H. Therapeutic AAV Gene Transfer to the Nervous System: A Clinical Reality. *Neuron* **2019**, *101*, 839–862. [CrossRef]
24. Sundermeier, T.R.; Zhang, N.; Vinberg, F.; Mustafi, D.; Kohno, H.; Golczak, M.; Bai, X.; Maeda, A.; Kefalov, V.J.; Palczewski, K. DICER1 is essential for survival of postmitotic rod photoreceptor cells in mice. *FASEB J.* **2014**, *28*, 3780–3791. [CrossRef]

25. Aldunate, E.Z.; Di Foggia, V.; Di Marco, F.; Hervas, L.A.; Ribeiro, J.C.; Holder, D.L.; Patel, A.; Jannini, T.B.; Thompson, D.A.; Martinez-Barbera, J.P.; et al. Conditional Dicer1 depletion using Chrnb4-Cre leads to cone cell death and impaired photopic vision. *Sci. Rep.* **2019**, *9*, 2314. [CrossRef]
26. Lagos-Quintana, M. New microRNAs from mouse and human. *RNA* **2003**, *9*, 175–179. [CrossRef]
27. Xu, S.; Witmer, P.D.; Lumayag, S.; Kovacs, B.; Valle, D. MicroRNA (miRNA) transcriptome of mouse retina and identification of a sensory organ-specific miRNA cluster. *J. Biol. Chem.* **2007**, *282*, 25053–25066. [CrossRef]
28. Weston, M.D.; Pierce, M.L.; Rocha-Sanchez, S.; Beisel, K.W.; Soukup, G.A. MicroRNA gene expression in the mouse inner ear. *Brain Res.* **2006**, *1111*, 95–104. [CrossRef] [PubMed]
29. Aldrich, B.T.; Frakes, E.P.; Kasuya, J.; Hammond, D.L.; Kitamoto, T. Changes in expression of sensory organ-specific microRNAs in rat dorsal root ganglia in association with mechanical hypersensitivity induced by spinal nerve ligation. *Neuroscience* **2009**, *164*, 711–723. [CrossRef]
30. Jin, Z.B.; Hirokawa, G.; Gui, L.; Takahashi, R.; Osakada, F.; Hiura, Y.; Takahashi, M.; Yasuhara, O.; Iwai, N. Targeted deletion of miR-182, an abundant retinal microRNA. *Mol. Vis.* **2009**, *15*, 523–533.
31. Dambal, S.; Shah, M.; Mihelich, B.; Nonn, L. The microRNA-183 cluster: The family that plays together stays together. *Nucleic Acids Res.* **2015**, *43*, 7173–7188. [CrossRef]
32. Zhu, Q.; Sun, W.; Okano, K.; Chen, Y.; Zhang, N.; Maeda, T.; Palczewski, K. Sponge transgenic mouse model reveals important roles for the microRNA-183 (miR-183)/96/182 cluster in postmitotic photoreceptors of the retina. *J. Biol. Chem.* **2011**, *286*, 31749–31760. [CrossRef] [PubMed]
33. Lumayag, S.; Haldin, C.E.; Corbett, N.J.; Wahlin, K.J.; Cowan, C.; Turturro, S.; Larsen, P.E.; Kovacs, B.; Witmer, P.D.; Valle, D.; et al. Inactivation of the microRNA-183/96/182 cluster results in syndromic retinal degeneration. *Proc. Natl. Acad. Sci. USA* **2013**, *110*, E507–E516. [CrossRef]
34. Krol, J.; Krol, I.; Alvarez, C.P.; Fiscella, M.; Hierlemann, A.; Roska, B.; Filipowicz, W. A network comprising short and long noncoding RNAs and RNA helicase controls mouse retina architecture. *Nat. Commun.* **2015**, *6*, 7305. [CrossRef] [PubMed]
35. Davari, M.; Soheili, Z.S.; Samiei, S.; Sharifi, Z.; Pirmardan, E.R. Overexpression of miR-183/-96/-182 triggers neuronal cell fate in Human Retinal Pigment Epithelial (hRPE) cells in culture. *Biochem. Biophys. Res. Commun.* **2017**, *483*, 745–751. [CrossRef] [PubMed]
36. Palfi, A.; Hokamp, K.; Hauck, S.M.; Vencken, S.; Millington-Ward, S.; Chadderton, N.; Carrigan, M.; Kortvely, E.; Greene, C.M.; Kenna, P.F.; et al. microRNA regulatory circuits in a mouse model of inherited retinal degeneration. *Sci. Rep.* **2016**, *6*, 31431. [CrossRef] [PubMed]
37. Lagos-Quintana, M.; Rauhut, R.; Yalcin, A.; Meyer, J.; Lendeckel, W.; Tuschl, T. Identification of tissue-specific microRNAs from mouse. *Curr. Biol.: Cb.* **2002**, *12*, 735–739. [CrossRef]
38. Landgraf, P.; Rusu, M.; Sheridan, R.; Sewer, A.; Iovino, N.; Aravin, A.; Pfeffer, S.; Rice, A.; Kamphorst, A.O.; Landthaler, M.; et al. A mammalian microRNA expression atlas based on small RNA library sequencing. *Cell* **2007**, *129*, 1401–1414. [CrossRef]
39. Karali, M.; Peluso, I.; Marigo, V.; Banfi, S. Identification and characterization of microRNAs expressed in the mouse eye. *Invest. Ophthalmol. Vis. Sci.* **2007**, *48*, 509–515. [CrossRef] [PubMed]
40. Sanuki, R.; Onishi, A.; Koike, C.; Muramatsu, R.; Watanabe, S.; Muranishi, Y.; Irie, S.; Uneo, S.; Koyasu, T.; Matsui, R.; et al. miR-124a is required for hippocampal axogenesis and retinal cone survival through Lhx2 suppression. *Nat. Neurosci.* **2011**, *14*, 1125–1134. [CrossRef]
41. Chu-Tan, J.A.; Rutar, M.; Saxena, K.; Aggio-Bruce, R.; Essex, R.W.; Valter, K.; Jiao, H.; Fernando, N.; Wooff, Y.; Madigan, M.C.; et al. MicroRNA-124 Dysregulation is Associated With Retinal Inflammation and Photoreceptor Death in the Degenerating Retina. *Invest. Ophthalmol. Vis. Sci.* **2018**, *59*, 4094–4105. [CrossRef]
42. Rutar, M.; Natoli, R.; Valter, K.; Provis, J.M. Early focal expression of the chemokine Ccl2 by Muller cells during exposure to damage-inducing bright continuous light. *Invest. Ophthalmol. Vis. Sci.* **2011**, *52*, 2379–2388. [CrossRef]
43. Newman, A.M.; Gallo, N.B.; Hancox, L.S.; Miller, N.J.; Radeke, C.M.; Maloney, M.A.; Cooper, J.B.; Hageman, G.S.; Anderson, D.H.; Johnson, L.V.; et al. Systems-level analysis of age-related macular degeneration reveals global biomarkers and phenotype-specific functional networks. *Genome Med.* **2012**, *4*, 16. [CrossRef] [PubMed]
44. Guo, C.; Otani, A.; Oishi, A.; Kojima, H.; Makiyama, Y.; Nakagawa, S.; Yoshimura, N. Knockout of ccr2 alleviates photoreceptor cell death in a model of retinitis pigmentosa. *Exp. Eye Res.* **2012**, *104*, 39–47. [CrossRef] [PubMed]

45. Rutar, M.; Natoli, R.; Provis, J.M. Small interfering RNA-mediated suppression of Ccl2 in Muller cells attenuates microglial recruitment and photoreceptor death following retinal degeneration. *J. Neuroinflammation* **2012**, *9*, 221. [CrossRef] [PubMed]
46. Sennlaub, F.; Auvynet, C.; Calippe, B.; Lavalette, S.; Poupel, L.; Hu, S.J.; Dominguez, E.; Camelo, S.; Levy, O.; Guyon, E.; et al. CCR2(+) monocytes infiltrate atrophic lesions in age-related macular disease and mediate photoreceptor degeneration in experimental subretinal inflammation in Cx3cr1 deficient mice. *Embo. Mol. Med.* **2013**, *5*, 1775–1793. [CrossRef]
47. Fu, Y.; Hou, B.; Weng, C.; Liu, W.; Dai, J.; Zhao, C.; Yin, Z.Q. Functional ectopic neuritogenesis by retinal rod bipolar cells is regulated by miR-125b-5p during retinal remodeling in RCS rats. *Sci. Rep.* **2017**, *7*, 1011. [CrossRef]
48. Jayaram, H.; Cepurna, W.O.; Johnson, E.C.; Morrison, J.C. MicroRNA Expression in the Glaucomatous Retina. *Invest. Ophthalmol. Vis. Sci.* **2015**, *56*, 7971–7982. [CrossRef]
49. Nie, X.G.; Fan, D.S.; Huang, Y.X.; He, Y.Y.; Dong, B.L.; Gao, F. Downregulation of microRNA-149 in retinal ganglion cells suppresses apoptosis through activation of the PI3K/Akt signaling pathway in mice with glaucoma. *Am. J. Physiol. Cell Physiol.* **2018**, *315*, C839–C849. [CrossRef]
50. Li, R.; Jin, Y.; Li, Q.; Sun, X.; Zhu, H.; Cui, H. MiR-93-5p targeting PTEN regulates the NMDA-induced autophagy of retinal ganglion cells via AKT/mTOR pathway in glaucoma. *Biomed. Pharm.* **2018**, *100*, 1–7. [CrossRef]
51. Li, H.J.; Sun, Z.L.; Pan, Y.B.; Sun, Y.Y.; Xu, M.H.; Feng, D.F. Inhibition of miRNA-21 promotes retinal ganglion cell survival and visual function by modulating Muller cell gliosis after optic nerve crush. *Exp. Cell Res.* **2019**, *375*, 10–19. [CrossRef]
52. Zhang, Q.L.; Wang, W.; Li, J.; Tian, S.Y.; Zhang, T.Z. Decreased miR-187 induces retinal ganglion cell apoptosis through upregulating SMAD7 in glaucoma. *Biomed. Pharm.* **2015**, *75*, 19–25. [CrossRef] [PubMed]
53. Yang, J.; Wang, N.; Luo, X. Intraocular miR-211 exacerbates pressure-induced cell death in retinal ganglion cells via direct repression of FRS2 signaling. *Biochem. Biophys. Res. Commun.* **2018**, *503*, 2984–2992. [CrossRef]
54. Kong, N.; Lu, X.; Li, B. Downregulation of microRNA-100 protects apoptosis and promotes neuronal growth in retinal ganglion cells. *BMC Mol. Biol.* **2014**, *15*, 25. [CrossRef] [PubMed]
55. Shao, Y.; Yu, Y.; Zhou, Q.; Li, C.; Yang, L.; Pei, C.G. Inhibition of miR-134 Protects Against Hydrogen Peroxide-Induced Apoptosis in Retinal Ganglion Cells. *J. Mol. Neurosci.* **2015**, *56*, 461–471. [CrossRef]
56. Damiani, D.; Alexander, J.J.; O'Rourke, J.R.; McManus, M.; Jadhav, A.P.; Cepko, C.L.; Hauswirth, W.W.; Harfe, B.D.; Strettoi, E. Dicer inactivation leads to progressive functional and structural degeneration of the mouse retina. *J. Neurosci.* **2008**, *28*, 4878–4887. [CrossRef] [PubMed]
57. Pinter, R.; Hindges, R. Perturbations of microRNA function in mouse dicer mutants produce retinal defects and lead to aberrant axon pathfinding at the optic chiasm. *Plos ONE* **2010**, *5*, e10021. [CrossRef]
58. Iida, A.; Shinoe, T.; Baba, Y.; Mano, H.; Watanabe, S. Dicer plays essential roles for retinal development by regulation of survival and differentiation. *Invest. Ophthalmol. Vis. Sci* **2011**, *52*, 3008–3017. [CrossRef] [PubMed]
59. Reh, T.A.; Hindges, R. MicroRNAs in Retinal Development. *Annu. Rev. Vis. Sci.* **2018**, *4*, 25–44. [CrossRef]
60. Georgi, S.A.; Reh, T.A. Dicer is required for the transition from early to late progenitor state in the developing mouse retina. *J. Neurosci.* **2010**, *30*, 4048–4061. [CrossRef]
61. La Torre, A.; Georgi, S.; Reh, T.A. Conserved microRNA pathway regulates developmental timing of retinal neurogenesis. *Proc. Natl. Acad. Sci. USA* **2013**, *110*, E2362–E2370. [CrossRef] [PubMed]
62. Xia, X.; Ahmad, I. let-7 microRNA regulates neurogliogenesis in the mammalian retina through Hmga2. *Dev. Biol.* **2016**, *410*, 70–85. [CrossRef] [PubMed]
63. Karali, M.; Manfredi, A.; Puppo, A.; Marrocco, E.; Gargiulo, A.; Allocca, M.; Corte, M.D.; Rossi, S.; Giunti, M.; Bacci, M.L.; et al. MicroRNA-restricted transgene expression in the retina. *Plos ONE* **2011**, *6*, e22166. [CrossRef]
64. Hackler, L., Jr.; Wan, J.; Swaroop, A.; Qian, J.; Zack, D.J. MicroRNA profile of the developing mouse retina. *Invest. Ophthalmol. Vis. Sci.* **2010**, *51*, 1823–1831. [CrossRef]
65. Jeon, C.J.; Strettoi, E.; Masland, R.H. The major cell populations of the mouse retina. *J. Neurosci.* **1998**, *18*, 8936–8946. [CrossRef]
66. Quintero, H.; Gomez-Montalvo, A.I.; Lamas, M. MicroRNA changes through Muller glia dedifferentiation and early/late rod photoreceptor differentiation. *Neuroscience* **2016**, *316*, 109–121. [CrossRef]

67. Wohl, S.G.; Reh, T.A. The microRNA expression profile of mouse Muller glia in vivo and in vitro. *Sci. Rep.* **2016**, *6*, 35423. [CrossRef]
68. Wohl, S.G.; Jorstad, N.L.; Levine, E.M.; Reh, T.A. Muller glial microRNAs are required for the maintenance of glial homeostasis and retinal architecture. *Nat. Commun.* **2017**, *8*, 1603. [CrossRef]
69. Jones, B.W.; Watt, C.B.; Frederick, J.M.; Baehr, W.; Chen, C.K.; Levine, E.M.; Milam, A.H.; Lavail, M.M.; Marc, R.E. Retinal remodeling triggered by photoreceptor degenerations. *J. Comp. Neurol.* **2003**, *464*, 1–16. [CrossRef]
70. Chung, S.H.; Shen, W.; Jayawardana, K.; Wang, P.; Yang, J.; Shackel, N.; Gillies, M.C. Differential gene expression profiling after conditional Muller-cell ablation in a novel transgenic model. *Invest. Ophthalmol. Vis. Sci.* **2013**, *54*, 2142–2152. [CrossRef]
71. Chung, S.H.; Gillies, M.; Sugiyama, Y.; Zhu, L.; Lee, S.R.; Shen, W. Profiling of microRNAs involved in retinal degeneration caused by selective Muller cell ablation. *Plos ONE* **2015**, *10*, e0118949. [CrossRef] [PubMed]
72. Byrne, L.C.; Khalid, F.; Lee, T.; Zin, E.A.; Greenberg, K.P.; Visel, M.; Schaffer, D.V.; Flannery, J.G. AAV-mediated, optogenetic ablation of Muller Glia leads to structural and functional changes in the mouse retina. *Plos ONE* **2013**, *8*, e76075. [CrossRef] [PubMed]
73. Shen, W.; Lee, S.R.; Araujo, J.; Chung, S.H.; Zhu, L.; Gillies, M.C. Effect of glucocorticoids on neuronal and vascular pathology in a transgenic model of selective Muller cell ablation. *Glia* **2014**, *62*, 1110–1124. [CrossRef]
74. Ramachandran, R.; Fausett, B.V.; Goldman, D. Ascl1a regulates Muller glia dedifferentiation and retinal regeneration through a Lin-28-dependent, let-7 microRNA signalling pathway. *Nat. Cell Biol.* **2010**, *12*, 1101–1107. [CrossRef] [PubMed]
75. Goldman, D. Muller glial cell reprogramming and retina regeneration. *Nat. Rev. Neurosci.* **2014**, *15*, 431–442. [CrossRef]
76. Yao, K.; Qiu, S.; Tian, L.; Snider, W.D.; Flannery, J.G.; Schaffer, D.V.; Chen, B. Wnt Regulates Proliferation and Neurogenic Potential of Muller Glial Cells via a Lin28/let-7 miRNA-Dependent Pathway in Adult Mammalian Retinas. *Cell Rep.* **2016**, *17*, 165–178. [CrossRef] [PubMed]
77. Kaur, S.; Gupta, S.; Chaudhary, M.; Khursheed, M.A.; Mitra, S.; Kurup, A.J.; Ramachandran, R. let-7 MicroRNA-Mediated Regulation of Shh Signaling and the Gene Regulatory Network Is Essential for Retina Regeneration. *Cell Rep.* **2018**, *23*, 1409–1423. [CrossRef] [PubMed]
78. Jorstad, N.L.; Wilken, M.S.; Grimes, W.N.; Wohl, S.G.; VandenBosch, L.S.; Yoshimatsu, T.; Wong, R.O.; Rieke, F.; Reh, T.A. Stimulation of functional neuronal regeneration from Muller glia in adult mice. *Nature* **2017**, *548*, 103–107. [CrossRef]
79. Papagiannakopoulos, T.; Kosik, K.S. MicroRNA-124: Micromanager of neurogenesis. *Cell Stem Cell* **2009**, *4*, 375–376. [CrossRef]
80. Cheng, L.C.; Pastrana, E.; Tavazoie, M.; Doetsch, F. miR-124 regulates adult neurogenesis in the subventricular zone stem cell niche. *Nat. Neurosci.* **2009**, *12*, 399–408. [CrossRef]
81. Maiorano, N.A.; Mallamaci, A. Promotion of embryonic cortico-cerebral neuronogenesis by miR-124. *Neural Dev.* **2009**, *4*, 40. [CrossRef]
82. Masserdotti, G.; Gillotin, S.; Sutor, B.; Drechsel, D.; Irmler, M.; Jorgensen, H.F.; Sass, S.; Theis, F.J.; Beckers, J.; Berninger, B.; et al. Transcriptional Mechanisms of Proneural Factors and REST in Regulating Neuronal Reprogramming of Astrocytes. *Cell Stem Cell* **2015**, *17*, 74–88. [CrossRef]
83. Abrajano, J.J.; Qureshi, I.A.; Gokhan, S.; Zheng, D.; Bergman, A.; Mehler, M.F. REST and CoREST modulate neuronal subtype specification, maturation and maintenance. *Plos ONE* **2009**, *4*, e7936. [CrossRef]
84. Visvanathan, J.; Lee, S.; Lee, B.; Lee, J.W.; Lee, S.K. The microRNA miR-124 antagonizes the anti-neural REST/SCP1 pathway during embryonic CNS development. *Genes Dev.* **2007**, *21*, 744–749. [CrossRef] [PubMed]
85. Conaco, C.; Otto, S.; Han, J.J.; Mandel, G. Reciprocal actions of REST and a microRNA promote neuronal identity. *Proc. Natl. Acad. Sci. USA* **2006**, *103*, 2422–2427. [CrossRef]
86. Nesti, E.; Corson, G.M.; McCleskey, M.; Oyer, J.A.; Mandel, G. C-terminal domain small phosphatase 1 and MAP kinase reciprocally control REST stability and neuronal differentiation. *Proc. Natl. Acad. Sci. USA* **2014**, *111*, E3929–E3936. [CrossRef] [PubMed]
87. Yeo, M.; Lee, S.K.; Lee, B.; Ruiz, E.C.; Pfaff, S.L.; Gill, G.N. Small CTD phosphatases function in silencing neuronal gene expression. *Sci. (N.Y.)* **2005**, *307*, 596–600. [CrossRef] [PubMed]

88. He, Y.; Li, H.B.; Li, X.; Zhou, Y.; Xia, X.B.; Song, W.T. MiR-124 Promotes the Growth of Retinal Ganglion Cells Derived from Muller Cells. *Cell Physiol. Biochem.* **2018**, *45*, 973–983. [CrossRef]
89. Ji, H.P.; Xiong, Y.; Song, W.T.; Zhang, E.D.; Gao, Z.L.; Yao, F.; Su, T.; Zhou, R.R.; Xia, X.B. MicroRNA-28 potentially regulates the photoreceptor lineage commitment of Muller glia-derived progenitors. *Sci. Rep.* **2017**, *7*, 11374. [CrossRef]
90. Hartong, D.T.; Berson, E.L.; Dryja, T.P. Retinitis pigmentosa. *Lancet* **2006**, *368*, 1795–1809. [CrossRef]
91. Loscher, C.J.; Hokamp, K.; Wilson, J.H.; Li, T.; Humphries, P.; Farrar, G.J.; Palfi, A. A common microRNA signature in mouse models of retinal degeneration. *Exp. Eye Res.* **2008**, *87*, 529–534. [CrossRef]
92. Anasagasti, A.; Ezquerra-Inchausti, M.; Barandika, O.; Munoz-Culla, M.; Caffarel, M.M.; Otaegui, D.; Lopez de Munain, A.; Ruiz-Ederra, J. Expression Profiling Analysis Reveals Key MicroRNA-mRNA Interactions in Early Retinal Degeneration in Retinitis Pigmentosa. *Invest. Ophthalmol. Vis. Sci.* **2018**, *59*, 2381–2392. [CrossRef]
93. Chang, B.; Hawes, N.L.; Hurd, R.E.; Davisson, M.T.; Nusinowitz, S.; Heckenlively, J.R. Retinal degeneration mutants in the mouse. *Vis. Res.* **2002**, *42*, 517–525. [CrossRef]
94. Genini, S.; Guziewicz, K.E.; Beltran, W.A.; Aguirre, G.D. Altered miRNA expression in canine retinas during normal development and in models of retinal degeneration. *BMC Genom.* **2014**, *15*, 172. [CrossRef]
95. Vasudevan, S.; Tong, Y.; Steitz, J.A. Switching from repression to activation: microRNAs can up-regulate translation. *Sci. (N.Y.)* **2007**, *318*, 1931–1934. [CrossRef] [PubMed]
96. Ma, C.; Papermaster, D.; Cepko, C.L. A unique pattern of photoreceptor degeneration in cyclin D1 mutant mice. *Proc. Natl. Acad. Sci. USA* **1998**, *95*, 9938–9943. [CrossRef] [PubMed]
97. Kutty, R.K.; Nagineni, C.N.; Samuel, W.; Vijayasarathy, C.; Hooks, J.J.; Redmond, T.M. Inflammatory cytokines regulate microRNA-155 expression in human retinal pigment epithelial cells by activating JAK/STAT pathway. *Biochem. Biophys. Res. Commun.* **2010**, *402*, 390–395. [CrossRef]
98. Lukiw, W.J.; Surjyadipta, B.; Dua, P.; Alexandrov, P.N. Common micro RNAs (miRNAs) target complement factor H (CFH) regulation in Alzheimer's disease (AD) and in age-related macular degeneration (AMD). *Int. J. Biochem. Mol. Biol.* **2012**, *3*, 105–116.
99. Karali, M.; Persico, M.; Mutarelli, M.; Carissimo, A.; Pizzo, M.; Singh Marwah, V.; Ambrosio, C.; Pinelli, M.; Carrella, D.; Ferrari, S.; et al. High-resolution analysis of the human retina miRNome reveals isomiR variations and novel microRNAs. *Nucleic Acids Res* **2016**, *44*, 1525–1540. [CrossRef]
100. Ryan, D.G.; Oliveira-Fernandes, M.; Lavker, R.M. MicroRNAs of the mammalian eye display distinct and overlapping tissue specificity. *Mol. Vis.* **2006**, *12*, 1175–1184.
101. Karali, M.; Peluso, I.; Gennarino, V.A.; Bilio, M.; Verde, R.; Lago, G.; Dolle, P.; Banfi, S. miRNeye: A microRNA expression atlas of the mouse eye. *BMC Genom.* **2010**, *11*, 715. [CrossRef] [PubMed]
102. Berezikov, E. Evolution of microRNA diversity and regulation in animals. *Nat. Rev. Genet.* **2011**, *12*, 846–860. [CrossRef] [PubMed]

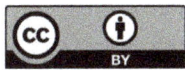

© 2019 by the authors. Licensee MDPI, Basel, Switzerland. This article is an open access article distributed under the terms and conditions of the Creative Commons Attribution (CC BY) license (http://creativecommons.org/licenses/by/4.0/).

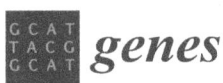

Article

AON-Mediated Exon Skipping to Bypass Protein Truncation in Retinal Dystrophies Due to the Recurrent *CEP290* c.4723A > T Mutation. Fact or Fiction?

Iris Barny [1], Isabelle Perrault [1], Christel Michel [1], Nicolas Goudin [2], Sabine Defoort-Dhellemmes [3], Imad Ghazi [4], Josseline Kaplan [1], Jean-Michel Rozet [1,*] and Xavier Gerard [1,5,*]

1. Laboratory of Genetics in Ophthalmology (LGO), INSERM UMR1163, Institute of Genetics Diseases, Imagine and Paris Descartes University, 75015 Paris, France; iris.barny@institutimagine.org (I.B.); isabelle.perrault@inserm.fr (I.P.); christel.michel@agroparistech.fr (C.M.); josseline.kaplan@inserm.fr (J.K.)
2. Cell Imaging Core Facility of the Structure Fédérative de Recherche Necker, INSERM US24/CNRS UMS3633, Imagine and Paris Descartes University, 75015 Paris, France; nicolas.goudin@inserm.fr
3. Service D'exploration de la Vision et Neuro-Ophtalmologie, Pôle D'imagerie et Explorations Fonctionnelles, CHRU de Lille, 59037 Lille, France; sabine.defoort@chru-lille.fr
4. Department of Ophthalmology, IHU Necker-Enfants Malades, 75015 Paris, France; imad.ghazi@aphp.fr
5. Unit of Retinal Degeneration and Regeneration, Department of Ophthalmology, University of Lausanne, Hôpital Ophtalmique Jules Gonin, Fondation Asile des Aveugles, 1004 Lausanne, Switzerland
* Correspondence: jean-michel.rozet@inserm.fr (J.-M.R.); xavier.gerard@fa2.ch (X.G.); Tel.: +33-1444-95156 (J.-M.R.); +41-2162-68321 (X.G.)

Received: 29 March 2019; Accepted: 9 May 2019; Published: 14 May 2019

Abstract: Mutations in *CEP290* encoding a centrosomal protein important to cilia formation cause a spectrum of diseases, from isolated retinal dystrophies to multivisceral and sometimes embryo–lethal ciliopathies. In recent years, endogenous and/or selective non-canonical exon skipping of mutant exons have been documented in attenuated retinal disease cases. This observation led us to consider targeted exon skipping to bypass protein truncation resulting from a recurrent mutation in exon 36 (c.4723A > T, p.Lys1575*) causing isolated retinal ciliopathy. Here, we report two unrelated individuals (P1 and P2), carrying the mutation in homozygosity but affected with early-onset severe retinal dystrophy and congenital blindness, respectively. Studying skin-derived fibroblasts, we observed basal skipping and nonsense associated–altered splicing of exon 36, producing low (P1) and very low (P2) levels of CEP290 products. Consistent with a more severe disease, fibroblasts from P2 exhibited reduced ciliation compared to P1 cells displaying normally abundant cilia; both lines presented however significantly elongated cilia, suggesting altered axonemal trafficking. Antisense oligonucleotides (AONs)-mediated skipping of exon 36 increased the abundance of the premature termination codon (PTC)-free mRNA and protein, reduced axonemal length and improved cilia formation in P2 but not in P1 expressing higher levels of skipped mRNA, questioning AON-mediated exon skipping to treat patients carrying the recurrent c.4723A > T mutation.

Keywords: Leber congenital amaurosis and allied retinal ciliopathies; *CEP290*; Flanders founder c.4723A > T nonsense mutation; Cilia elongation; spontaneous nonsense correction; AON-mediated exon skipping

1. Introduction

Leber congenital amaurosis (LCA, MIM204000) is a group of neonatal-onset and severe retinal dystrophies and a leading cause of incurable blindness in childhood (Frequency 1:30,000; 20% of children attending schools for the blind in western Europe) [1]. It typically occurs as a non-syndromic disease that displays large genetic, allelic and physio–pathological heterogeneity, challenging therapeutic developments [2]. Mutations in *CEP290* (MIM610142) encoding a widely expressed centrosomal protein involved in cilia formation and maintenance [3], are the leading cause of the disease, referred to as LCA type 10 (LCA10; MIM611755) [4,5]. Despite early-onset visual loss, LCA10 individuals display prolonged (>30 years) sparing of central photoreceptors with intact visual brain pathway, creating the conditions to develop therapies built on correcting genetic lesions [6]. A large number of LCA10-causing mutations are reported, including the highly prevalent c.2991 + 1655A > G (p.Cys998*) and c.4723A > T (p.1575Lys*) variants involved in 10% and 2.5% of all LCA cases, respectively [5,7]. The c.2991 + 1655A > G change activates a deep intronic cryptic splice site and introduces a frameshifting pseudo-exon in the mRNA [8–11]. Antisense oligonucleotides (AONs) have proven effective to redirect the splicing machinery towards the consensus splice sites and bypass protein truncation in primary fibroblasts, IPSC-derived 3D retinal organoids and humanized mice carrying the mutation [8,10,12]. Subsequently, a phase I/II clinical trial (NCT03140969) has been launched which demonstrated safety and clinical relevance (vision improvement) of intravitreal injections of splice-modulating oligonucleotide [13]. The c.4723A > T variant, like the vast majority of *CEP290* mutations, is predicted to truncate the protein and is amenable to gene augmentation therapy. However, this approach is challenging due to both the *CEP290* cDNA size (7.4 Kb) which over-exceed cargo capacities of AAV vectors (<5 Kb) preferred in the field of retinal diseases [14–16] and risk of overexpression toxicity [17,18]. Interestingly, consistent with an important role in cilia metabolism, *CEP290* mutations have been associated with additional human phenotypes, including oculo-renal Senior Loken syndrome (SLSN6, MIM610189), oculo-cerebro-renal Joubert syndrome (JBTS5, MIM610188) and embryo-lethal Meckel syndrome type 4 (MKS; MIM611134) [19]. Observation of endogenous basal exon-skipping producing low-levels of alternatively spliced coding *CEP290* mRNAs has inspired a model of pathogenesis according to which disease severity is a function of the amount of CEP290 a cell can produce from mutant alleles [20]. Consistently, low levels of premature termination codon (PTC)-free *CEP290* mRNA produced by endogenous basal alternative splicing and/or nonsense associated altered splicing have been identified in fibroblasts from individuals with biallelic *CEP290* truncating mutations but mild retinal phenotypes [21–23]. Lessening the disease through somatic frame-restoration mechanisms is reminiscent of genetic reversion in dystrophin-positive muscular fibers from individuals with Duchene muscular dystrophy which inspired AON-mediated exon skipping to bypass dystrophin truncation and switch the disease to attenuated Becker muscular dystrophy. Following this example, we considered AON-mediated skipping of *CEP290* exon 36 to bypass protein truncation resulting from the c.4723A > T nonsense mutation. Here, studying fibroblasts from two unrelated individuals homozygous for the mutation and controls, we show combination of endogenous and selective exon skipping producing a minimally shortened *CEP290* mRNA and a protein that localized at the centrosome. Cilia analysis revealed no major anomaly but a significant axonemal elongation. Using AON specific to the donor consensus splice-site of exon 36 in patient and control fibroblasts, we were able to increase the abundance of the alternatively spliced mRNA and shortened protein and to reduce axonemal length. However, fibroblasts with highest levels of alternatively spliced products displayed reduced ability to ciliate, questioning the relevance of AON-mediated exon skipping to treat patients carrying the recurrent c.4723A > T mutation.

2. Materials and Methods

2.1. Genetic Analysis

P1 and P2, two unrelated simplex cases born to apparently non-consanguineous parents originating from the transnational Flanders region were addressed to the Molecular Diagnosis Unit of our Genetic Department for molecular diagnosis of early-onset and severe retinal dystrophy. Patient DNAs were subjected to panel-based molecular testing of 199 genes involved in retinal dystrophies (Figure S1) and variant datasets were filtered using the Polydiag software of the Polyweb series developed in-house. Biallelism for apparently homozygous *CEP290* c.4723A > T variant was assessed by Sanger sequencing of parental DNA using primers specific to *CEP290* exon 36 (Supplementary Materials, Table S1). Written informed consents were obtained from all participating individuals and the study was approved by the Comité de Protection des Personnes "Ile-De-France II" (3 March 2015/DC 2014–2272).

2.2. In Silico Analysis of the Nonsense c.4723A > T (p.Lys1575*) Mutation on Splicing

The consequence of the c.4723A > T substitution on splicing was assessed using several prediction softwares, as previously described [21].

2.3. Cell Culture

Fibroblast cell lines were derived from skin biopsies of affected subjects (P1 and P2) and three healthy individuals (C1–C3). A table recapitulating their genetic and clinical features is presented in Table S2. Primary fibroblasts (<15 passages) were cultured as previously described [21].

2.4. AON and Transfection

AON specific to the donor splice site of *CEP290* exon 36 was identified using software prediction tools (m-fold and ESEfinder3.0 programs available online at http://mfold.rna.albany.edu/ and http://rulai.cshl.edu/cgi-bin/tools/ESE3/esefinder.cgi respectively) and following general recommendations [24].

The sequence of H36D (+98 −11) AON was as following: 5′-UAGAAUCUUACCCAAG CCGUUU-3′.

This AON was synthetized by Eurofins Genomics (St. Quentin Fallavier, France) and contains 2′-O-methyl RNA and full-length phosphorothioate backbone. Cells at 80% confluence were transfected with different concentrations of H36D AON, ranging from 20–300 nmol/L, in Opti-MEM supplemented with 10% fetal bovine serum using Lipofectamine2000 (Invitrogen, Carlsbad, CA, USA) according to the manufacturer's instruction. Cells were harvested for mRNA or protein analysis between 4 and 72 h.

2.5. RNA Analysis

RNA isolation from fibroblasts and wild-type human fetal retina (22 weeks) and cDNA synthesis were performed according to previously described methods [21].

Reverse transcription-PCR (RT-PCR) was performed using 2 μL of cDNA as described previously [21]. *CEP290* splicing isoforms were amplified using primer pairs specific to exons 35 and 37 (Figure S2 and Table S3) and PCR products were resolved in a 3% agarose gel.

For real-time quantitative PCR (RT-qPCR), cDNA (5 μL of a 1:25 dilution) were amplified using primers specific to the full-length and skipped isoforms, respectively (Figure S2 and Table S4), according to the protocol described in Barny et al. 2018. The human β-glucuronidase (*GUSB*, NM_000181.3) and P0 large ribosomal protein (*RPLP0*, NM_001002.3) mRNAs were used to normalize the data. The data were analyzed as described previously [8].

2.6. Protein Analysis

For Western blot analysis, total proteins from treated and untreated cells were extracted and quantified as described previously [21], and the relative abundance of CEP290 protein was estimated by densitometry using β-Actin as reference in each cell line.

For immunocytochemistry analysis, cells were grown for 24 h on coverslips in 12-well plates to reach 90–100% confluence and either transfected using the H36D (+98 −11) AON or left untreated. After 24 h, treated and untreated cells were serum-starved for 48 to 72 h before cold methanol fixation and immune-labeling of ARL13B, CEP290, CP110, IFT88, pericentrin, RAB8A, γ-Tubulin and/or acetylated α-Tubulin. Immunofluorescence images were acquired and processed to analyze cilia abundance, axonemal length, subcellular localization and/or staining intensities. All experimental procedures and analytical methods were described in Barny et al., 2018.

2.7. Statistics

All statistical analyses were run using the Prism6 software, and the significance was determined using one-way ANOVA with post hoc Tukey's test. The data obtained from C1–C3 were systematically pooled for immune-labelling analysis. Error bars reflect the standard errors for the mean (SEMs).

3. Results

3.1. Panel-Based Molecular Diagnosis Testing Identifies Homozygosity for the CEP290 c.4723A > T Founder Mutation in Two Individuals with Congenital Retinal Dystrophy of Variable Severity

We studied two apparently unrelated non-consanguineous sporadic cases of Belgian and/or French Flanders origin addressed for congenital retinal dystrophy with no extraocular involvement. The first individual (P1) presented at birth with nystagmus, photoaversion, hyperopia (+6 diopters LRE), absent cone-derived electroretinogram but present, yet highly hypovolted, rod-derived responses. He experienced spontaneous improvement of his visual capacities in the first decade of life. At the age of 20 years, he displayed a tubular visual field with a visual acuity (VA) of 20/67 (RE) and 20/50 (LE) and thin retinal vessels, optic nerve atrophy and peripheral pigmentary deposits at the fundus. While the initial symptoms suggested early-onset severe cone-rod dystrophy, this outcome is consistent with a rod-dominant LCA-like disease referred to as early-onset severe rod-cone dystrophy. The second individual (P2) presented with a typical LCA10-associated disease, i.e., a stationary congenital blindness with nystagmus, inability to follow lights or objects and flat cone- and rod-derived electroretinographic responses. Panel-based molecular diagnosis for inherited retinal dystrophies (199 genes) and Sanger-based familial segregation analysis identified homozygosity for the Flanders founder *CEP290* c.4723A > T (p.Lys1575*) mutation in the two cases.

3.2. In Silico Analysis Suggests That the CEP290 c.4723A > T Mutation Induced Nonsense-Associated Altered Splicing

We analyzed the effect of the c.4723A > T mutation on splicing by using prediction software solutions scrutinizing splice signals and exonic splicing silencer (ESS)/exonic splicing enhancer (ESE) binding sites. The mutation had no effect on the canonical splice sites of exon 36 (not shown), but it increased the exon 36 ESS/ESE ratio, thus elevating the susceptibility of skipping compared to the wild-type sequence (Table 1). The substitution of the c.4723 adenine into a guanine but not a cytosine is predicted to have the same effect.

Table 1. Impact of the c.4723A > T mutation on exonic splicing silencer (ESS) and exonic splicing enhancer (ESE) motifs within the *CEP290* exon 36.

	Nucleotide	EX-SKIP Predictions			HOT-SKIP Predictions			Skipping Predictions of Mutant Allele Compared to WT Allele
		ESS	ESE	ESS/ESE	ESS	ESE	ESS/ESE	
c.4723 (exon 36)	*A*	12	88	0.14	2	17	0.12	-
	T	19	75	**0.25**	9	4	**2.25**	**Higher chance**
	G	13	87	0.15	3	16	0.19	Higher chance
	C	11	82	0.13	1	11	0.09	Lower chance

Nucleotide change effect at position c.4723 on ESS and ESE motifs according to EX-SKIP and HOT-SKIP prediction programs. The wild-type (WT) and mutant alleles identified in this study are marked in italic and bold, respectively. ESS = Exonic splicing silencer; ESE = Exonic splicing enhancer.

3.3. mRNA Analysis Supports c.4723A > T-Mediated Nonsense-Associated Altered Splicing and Basal Endogenous Alternative Splicing of Exon 36

Agarose gel analysis and Sanger sequencing of RT-PCR products generated from P1 and P2 skin fibroblast mRNAs carrying the c.4723A > T variant in homozygosity using primers specific to *CEP290* exons 35 and 37 (Figure S2 and Table S3) detected the full-length mutant cDNA (*CEP290*) and a PTC-free alternatively spliced product lacking exon 36 (*CEP290*$^{\Delta 36}$). Control fibroblasts expressed the full-length wild-type cDNA but the *CEP290*$^{\Delta 36}$ product was undetectable, contrasting with human retina where both isoforms were identified. These observations indicate that *CEP290* exon 36 undergoes endogenous basal skipping in the retina and that, consistent with in silico analysis, the c.4723A > T variant induces nonsense-associated altered splicing (Figure 1A). Interestingly, RT-qPCR analysis using primers specific to the *CEP290*$^{\Delta 36}$ isoform (Figure S2 and Table S4) detected the product in control fibroblasts (Figure 1C). Consistent with expression below the threshold of agarose gel detection, the abundance of the *CEP290*$^{\Delta 36}$ mRNA in controls was approximately one-tenth that measured in patient cells (Figure 1C). This observation supports some contribution of endogenous basal exon skipping in *CEP290*-frame-restoration documented in P1 and P2 mutant fibroblasts. RT-qPCR analysis using primers specific to the full-length mutant/wild-type cDNA (Figure S2 and Table S4) showed reduced abundance of the mutant product in P1 and P2 cell lines compared to the wild-type counterpart in controls supporting nonsense-mediated RNA decay (NMD) of the mRNA carrying the nonsense c.4723A > T variant (Figure 1B).

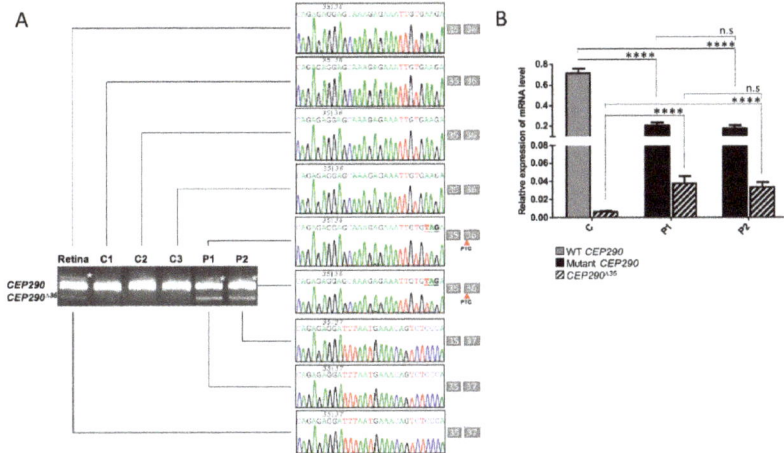

Figure 1. Naturally occurring exclusion of *CEP290* exon 36 encompassing premature stop codon. (**A**) Analysis of *CEP290* transcript extracted from wild-type human fetal retina (Retina), control (C1–C3) and patient (P1 and P2) cell lines. Image of agarose gel and Sanger sequencing electropherograms showing amplicons produced using primer pairs surrounding mutant exon 36 and corresponding sequences. The boxes close to electropherograms summarize the exonic organization and phasing of each reverse transcription (RT)-PCR fragment. White asterisks point to heteroduplex products. Red arrows show the position of the premature termination codon (PTC) within exon 36 *CEP290* isoform. (**B**) Relative expression levels of WT (grey bar) and mutant (black bars) full-length and skipped (*CEP290*$^{\Delta 36}$; hatched bars) *CEP290* mRNAs in control (C represents pooled values of C1–C3) and patient (P1 and P2) fibroblasts as determined by RT-qPCR. Bars correspond to the mean ± SEM derived from ten independent experiments. **** $p \leq 0.0001$, n.s = not significant.

3.4. Protein Analysis Detects Low Levels of a CEP290 Protein That Localizes at the Centrosome in Patient Fibroblasts Homozygous for the c.4723A > T Nonsense Mutation

Western blot analysis of protein extracts from serum-starved P1 and P2 fibroblasts detected minimal amounts of a CEP290 product around 290 KDa (Figures 2 and 3C) that localized at the centrosome upon immunocytochemistry analysis (Figure 3A,B). These results indicate that the PTC-free alternatively spliced product lacking exon 36 was translated into a stable protein that can be recruited at the centrosome as does the wild-type protein.

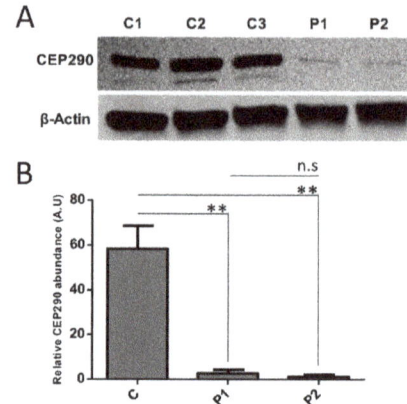

Figure 2. Effect of the natural exclusion of PTC-encoding exon 36 on CEP290 protein production. (**A**) Immune detection of the CEP290 and β-Actin in control cell lines (C1–C3) and mutant fibroblasts (P1 and P2). (**B**) Quantification of CEP290 abundance relative to β-Actin in control (C represents the pooled values of C1–C3) and patient fibroblasts. Bars correspond to the mean value ± SEM from four independent experiments. ** $p \leq 0.01$, n.s = not significant.

3.5. Cilia Analysis of Serum-Starved Patient Fibroblasts Shows Apparently Normal RAB8A Localization at the Centrosome but Elongated Axonemes

CEP290 exon 36 encodes 36 amino-acids contributing to the CEP290 domain that binds RAB8A, the recruitment of which at the centrosome leads to the release of the cilia formation-suppressor CP110, hence initiating ciliogenesis during transition of the cells from proliferation to quiescence [25–27]. Interestingly, RAB8A immune-labeling in quiescent fibroblasts showed comparable localization at the basal body in patient and control fibroblasts, suggesting that the absence of information encoded by exon 36 does not alter the recruitment of RAB8A at the centrosome (Figure 4A,B). Furthermore, we observed comparable CP110 abundance at the centrosome of control and P1 fibroblasts indicating correct release upon RAB8A recruitment (Figure 4C,D). In contrast, the amount of CP110 at the centrosome of P2 cells was significantly higher than in control and P1 cells ($p \leq 0.0001$; Figure 4C,D). Whether CP110 accumulation in P2 could be correlated to reduced abundance of CEP290$^{\Delta 36aa}$ protein compared to P1 is possible but remains hypothetic as the difference in CEP290$^{\Delta 36aa}$ amounts was not statistically significant between patient cell lines. Consistent with normal and impaired CP110 release, cilia abundance was in the normal range and reduced in P1 and P2 fibroblasts, respectively ($p \leq 0.001$; Figure 5A,B).

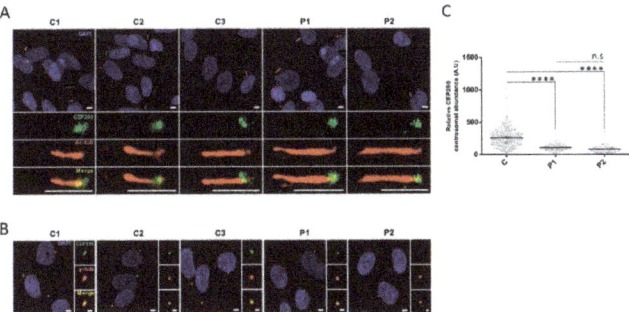

Figure 3. CEP290 expression assessment in quiescent cells. (**A**) Representative images of CEP290 (green) localization in quiescent control and mutant fibroblasts. Acetylated α-tubulin (Ac-tub; red) is used to stain the ciliary axoneme. As in control cell lines (C1–C3), CEP290 is correctly localized at the base of the cilia in patient (P1 and P2) fibroblasts. Scale bar, 5 µm. (**B**) Centrosomal localization of CEP290 (green) in control and mutant fibroblasts. The γ-tubulin (γ-tub; red) labeling is used as a centrosomal marker. Image scale bar, 5 µm and inset scale bar, 2 µm. (**C**) Quantification of the CEP290 immunofluorescence intensity at the basal body in each cell line (C represents the pooled values of C1–C3). Each dot depicts the labeling intensity of the protein in individual cells from six microscope fields (recorded automatically). The solid line indicates the mean. **** $p \leq 0.0001$, n.s = not significant. A.U. = arbitrary unit.

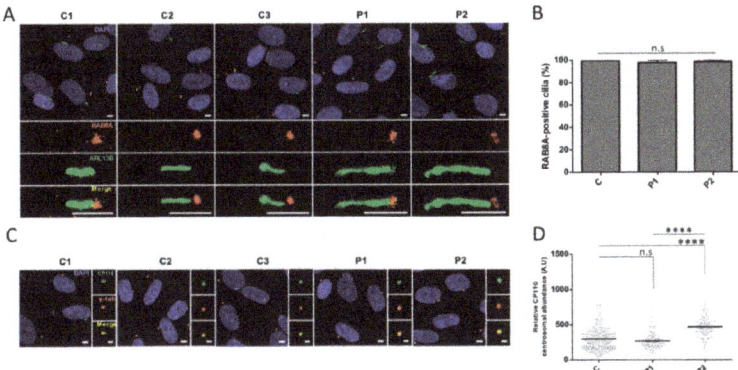

Figure 4. Localization and abundance of CEP290 centriolar satellite partners. (**A**) Representative images of RAB8A (red) localization in the cilia from control (C1–C3) and mutant (P1 and P2) fibroblasts induced to quiescence. ARL13B (green) labeling is used to mark the ciliary membrane. Scale bar, 5 µm. (**B**) Quantification of RAB8A-positive cilia in each cell line (C represents the pooled values of C1–C3). Bars correspond to the mean ± SEM ($n \geq 50$ cilia for each group). n.s = not significant. A.U. = arbitrary unit. (**C**) Representative images of CP110 (green) centrosomal staining in quiescent control and mutant fibroblasts. Centrosomes are stained by γ-tubulin (γ-tub.; red). Image scale bar, 5 µm and inset scale bar, 2 µm. (**D**) Quantification of CP110 immunofluorescence intensity at centrosomes in quiescent fibroblasts (C represents the pooled values of C1–C3). Each dot depicts the labeling intensity of the protein in individual cells from six microscope fields (recorded automatically). The solid line indicates the mean. **** $p \leq 0.0001$, n.s = not significant. A.U. = arbitrary unit.

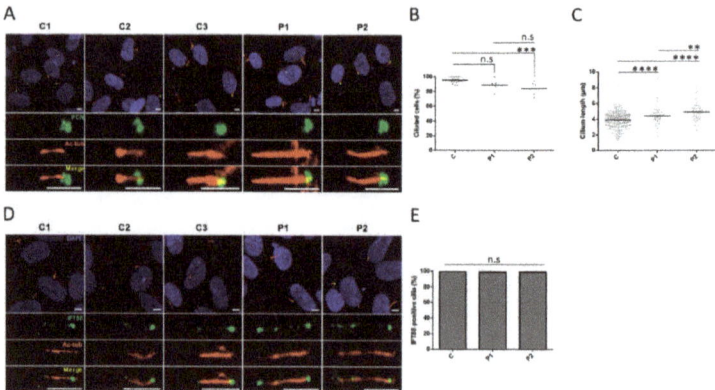

Figure 5. Ciliogenesis and axonemal trafficking. (**A**) Representative images of cilia in the quiescent control (C1–C3) and mutant (P1 and P2) fibroblasts. The cilium axoneme is labeled with acetylated α-tubulin (Ac-tub; red) and the basal body using pericentrin as a marker (PCN; green). Scale bar, 5 μm. (**B**) Percentage of ciliated cells and (**C**) length of cilia axonemes in control and patient fibroblasts. A minimum of 90 ciliated cells were considered for each cell lines. (**D**) Representative images of IFT88 (green) localization along the cilium in quiescent control (C1–C3) and mutant (P1 and P2) fibroblasts. Acetylated α-tubulin (Ac-tub; red) staining was used as a marker of the ciliary axoneme. Scale bar, 5 μm. (**E**) Quantification of IFT88-positive cilia. Bars represent the mean ± SEM ($n \geq 80$ cilia for each group). C regroups the values of C1–C3. ** $p \leq 0.01$, *** $p \leq 0.001$, **** $p \leq 0.0001$, n.s = not significant.

On another note, measuring cilia length, we observed statistically significant axonemal elongation in both patient cell lines compared to controls (mean axonemal sizes of 4.4 μm in P1 and 4.9 μm in P2 versus 3.9 μm in controls, $p \leq 0.0001$; Figure 5A,C). Cilia in P2 expressing lower amounts of the CEP290$^{\Delta 36aa}$ isoform at the centrosome displayed significantly longer axoneme than P1 counterparts ($p \leq 0.01$; Figure 5A,C), further supporting a possible correlation between the severity of cilia phenotype and the amount of minimally shortened CEP290 cells are able to produce from mutant alleles.

As observed in controls cells, IFT88 immune-labelling in patient fibroblasts revealed this intraflagellar trafficking (IFT) complex B protein all along the axoneme (Figure 5D,E), assuming that the abnormal cilia elongation in patient cells is not related to a defect of the anterograde trafficking driven by IFT88.

3.6. Targeting the Consensus Donor Splice Site Enables Dose- and Time-Dependent Skipping of CEP290 Exon 36

The RNA conformation around *CEP290* exon 36 and splicing regulatory elements were predicted in silico using m-fold and ESEfinder3.0 programs to design splice switching AON. We designed 2′-O-methyl-phosphorothioate (2′-OMePs) AON targeting the donor site (H36D (+98-11)) (Figure 6). The AON was delivered in patient and control fibroblasts at a final concentration of 150nM for 24h prior to mRNA analysis. Treatment with H36D (+98 − 11) AON elevated significantly the abundance of products lacking exon 36 and reduced by half the amount of full-length mutant and wild-type products in patient and control fibroblasts, respectively (Figure 7). Due to NMD, the abundance of the full-length mutant was significantly reduced in patient compared to control cells (Figure 7B). Consistent with a switch from a mRNA prone to NMD to a PTC-free isoform, the abundance of the alternatively spliced product lacking exon 36 in patient fibroblasts was comparable to that of controls upon treatment with the H36D (+98 − 11) AON. Treatment with the transfection reagent alone did not alter *CEP290* expression whatever the cell line (Figure 7).

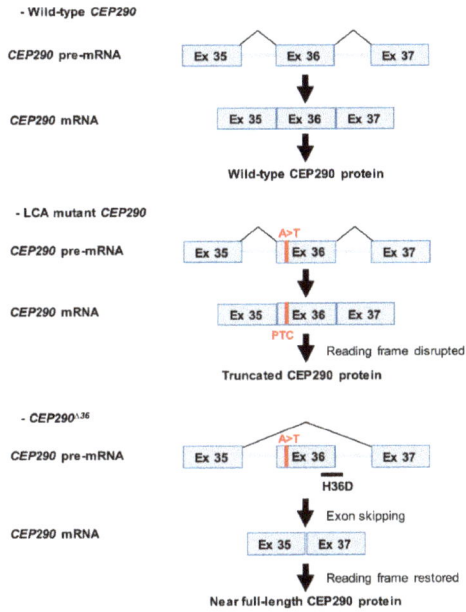

Figure 6. Antisense oligonucleotides (AONs)-mediated splicing alteration of *CEP290* pre-mRNA to bypass protein truncation. An exonic mutation in *CEP290* pre-mRNA (c.4723A > T, in red) introduces a PTC within exon 36 to *CEP290* mRNA. Administration of AON (in black), targeting the splice donor site (H36D), is predicted to alter splicing by blocking the recognition of exon 36. Exclusion of exon 36 (*CEP290*$^{\Delta 36}$) should allow bypassing protein truncation while maintaining the reading frame, and lead to the production of near full-length CEP290 protein.

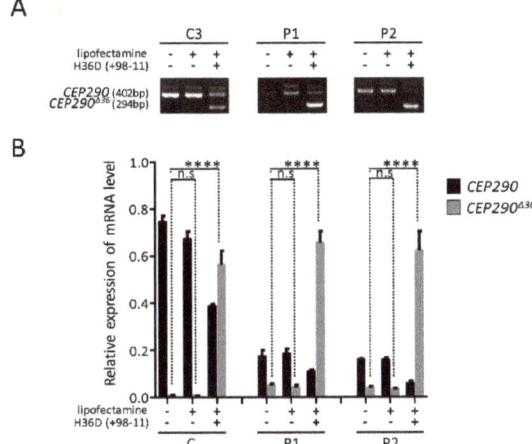

Figure 7. Effect of AON-mediated exon 36 skipping on *CEP290* mRNAs. (**A**) RT-PCR analysis of *CEP290* transcripts expressed in control (C3) and patient (P1 and P2) fibroblasts untreated or treated for 24h with lipofectamine alone or associated to H36D AON. Images of agarose gel showing amplicons produced using primer pairs surrounding mutant exon 36. (**B**) Relative expression levels of full-length (black bars) and exon 36-skipped (grey bars) *CEP290* mRNAs in control (C1–C3) and patient (P1 and P2) fibroblasts as determined by RT-qPCR. Bars show the mean ± SEM from three independent experiments. C represents the pooled values of C1–C3. **** $p \leq 0.0001$, n.s., not significant.

To assess dose-dependent skipping efficiency, patient and control fibroblasts were treated with increasing doses of H36D (+98 − 11) AON for 24 h, revealing that the amount of alternatively splice products lacking exon 36 reached a maximum in almost all cell lines at an AON concentration of 75 nmol/l (Figure 8A). At this concentration, we observed accumulation of alternatively splice products and CEP290 proteins with treatment time (Figure 8B–D).

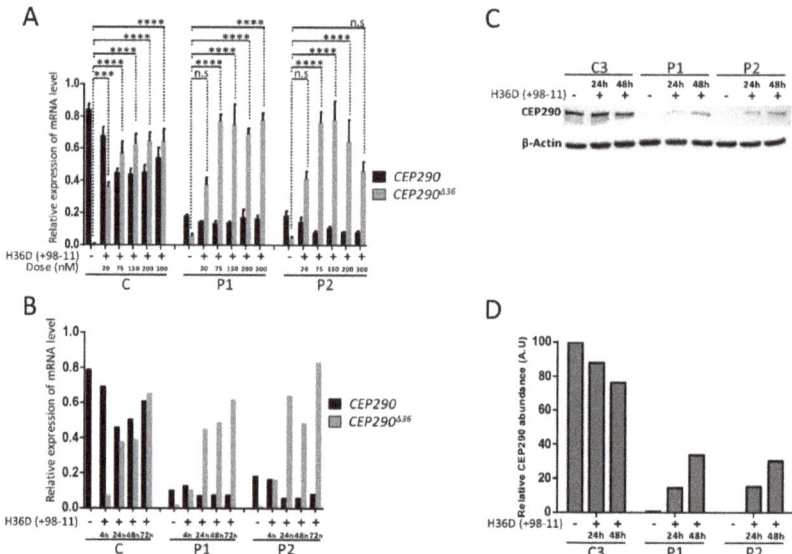

Figure 8. Optimization of transfection conditions. (**A**) RT-qPCR analysis of reverse transcribed *CEP290* mRNA extracted from control (C1–C3) and patient (P1 and P2) fibroblasts untreated or after transfection of increasing doses (20 nM to 300 nM) of H36D oligonucleotide. The graph shows the mean amounts (±SEM) of full-length (*CEP290*; black bars) and exon 36-skipped transcripts (*CEP290$^{\Delta 36}$*; grey bars) from three independent experiments. C regroups the values obtained for C1–C3. *** $p \leq 0.001$, **** $p \leq 0.0001$, n.s., not significant. (**B**) RT-qPCR analysis of reverse transcribed *CEP290* mRNA extracted from control (C1–C3) and patient (P1 and P2) fibroblasts untreated or treated during increasing times of treatment (4 h to 72 h) with 75nM of H36D oligonucleotide. The graph shows the amounts of full-length (*CEP290*; black bars) and exon 36-skipped transcripts (*CEP290$^{\Delta 36}$*; grey bars). C corresponds to C1–C3 pooled values. (**C**) CEP290 protein analysis in control (C3) and mutant (P1 and P2) cell lines untreated or treated with 75nM of H36D during 24 h or 48 h. (**D**) Relative quantification of CEP290 protein abundance depending on treatment time. β-Actin was used for normalization.

3.7. AON-Mediated Skipping Allows to Bypass Protein-Truncation but May Not Restore Full CEP290 Functions

The abundance of full length *CEP290* mRNA in control cells treated with 75nM of H36D (+98 − 11) AON for 48 h was around 60% that of untreated control cells, as determined by RT-qPCR (Figure 8B), indicating that approximately 40% of full length *CEP290* pre-mRNA underwent AON-mediated skipping of exon 36. The amount of CEP290 protein (full-length + Δ36aa) was comparable in treated and untreated cells (Figure 9A,B, left), suggesting that the CEP290$^{\Delta 36aa}$ isoform is stable. Yet, treated cells displayed a moderate diminution of CEP290 staining at the centrosome ($p \leq 0.05$, Figure 9C) with statistically significant, yet minimal, alteration of CP110 centrosomal staining ($p \leq 0.05$, Figure 9D). The abundance of ciliated cells tended to be slightly diminished (95.5% versus 92.5%, Figure 9F) as was the mean axonemal length (3.9 μm versus 3.6 μm, $p \leq 0.01$, Figure 9E). Together, these results suggest that the CEP290$^{\Delta 36aa}$ isoform interferes with the wild-type counterpart and can compromise ciliation, possibly through disorganization of centriolar satellites. The same treatment in P1 cells, allowed a highly significant increase in CEP290$^{\Delta 36aa}$ protein abundance, as determined by western blot and immunocytochemistry analyses (Figure 9A–C). Interestingly, the intensity of CEP290 staining at the centrosome reached that of treated control cells (Figure 9C). However, expressing increased levels of CEP290$^{\Delta 36aa}$ isoform in cells deprived of wild-type CEP290 altered the dynamics of centriolar satellites, as documented by increased dispersion of CP110-specific centrosomal staining ($p \leq 0.001$, Figure 9D). Consistently, the proportion of ciliated cells tended to diminish (89% versus 79.8%) upon AON treatment (Figure 9F), as did axonemal length (4.4 µm versus 3.5 µm, $p \leq 0.0001$, Figure 9E). In P2, AON treatment also led to a significant increase in the centrosomal abundance of the CEP290$^{\Delta 36aa}$ isoform ($p \leq 0.0001$, Figure 9C). However, the amount of this product was significantly reduced compared to the counterpart in treated P1 cells ($p \leq 0.001$). We observed a reduced impact of the treatment on centriolar satellites (Figure 9D) compared to P1, cilia abundance tended to minimally increase (Figure 9F) and cilia length significantly decreased ($p \leq 0.0001$, Figure 9E).

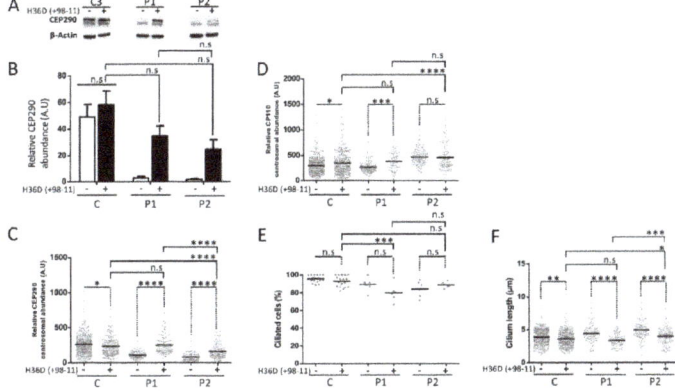

Figure 9. AON-treatment effect at protein level and impact on ciliation. (**A**) CEP290 protein analysis in control and mutant cell lines untreated or treated during 48 h with 75 nM of H36D. (**B**) Quantification of CEP290 protein abundance relative to β-Actin. Bars correspond to the mean value ± SEM from three independent experiments = not significant. A.U. = arbitrary unit. (**C**) Quantification of CEP290 immunofluorescence intensity at the basal body in each cell line. Each dot depicts the labeling intensity of the protein in individual cells recorded automatically from six microscope fields. The solid line indicates the mean. (**D**) Quantification of CP110 immunofluorescence intensity at centrosomes in quiescent fibroblasts. All automatic intensity measures were recorded from six fields. (**E**) Percentage of ciliated cells and (**F**) length of cilia axonemes in control and mutant fibroblasts. A minimum of 90 ciliated cells were considered for each cell lines. C corresponds to C1–C3 pooled values. * $p \leq 0.05$, ** $p \leq 0.01$, *** $p \leq 0.001$, **** $p \leq 0.0001$, n.s = not significant, A.U. = arbitrary unit.

4. Discussion

Targeted exon skipping is gaining a growing interest in rare hereditary diseases involving cell types as diverse as myocytes, keratinocytes or motor neurons. Recently, renal cells were added to this list with the report on AON-mediated rescue of Joubert phenotypes in patient-derived primary tubular cells and in a murine model with *CEP290* mutations [28]. Photoreceptors of these individuals and more generally of individuals carrying PTCs in skippable *CEP290* exons certainly deserve consideration. Here, we used skin-derived fibroblasts from two unrelated individuals carrying a *CEP290* nonsense founder mutation to implement AON-mediated frame-restoration to non-syndromic retinal diseases. CEP290 is expressed in the transition zone at the base of cilia of multiple cells systems. There, it bridges the cilia membrane and the axoneme by binding the cellular membrane to microtubules through sequences in the amino-terminal and myosin-tail homology domains, respectively [29]. The integrity of this bridge, known as the ciliary gate CEP290 [3], is essential to allow proper ciliation as demonstrated by reduced cilia formation and/or aberrant axonemal ultrastructure in cells from patients carrying *CEP290* mutations [8,19] and in cellular and in-vivo models of *Cep290* knockdown [10,30–32]. Studying the ciliation ability of fibroblasts from the two individuals carrying the c.4723A > T mutation, we observed normal to discreetly reduced abundance of ciliated cells upon serum starvation, suggesting the production of a CEP290 protein from mutant alleles. Accordingly, we observed expression of an alternatively spliced *CEP290* mRNA lacking exon 36 encompassing the PTC and low levels of CEP290 protein. The PTC-free mRNA product was detected both in patient and control cells, though with minimal amounts in controls. This observation indicates (*i*) that *CEP290* exon 36, like exons 6, 10, 18, 32, 41, 46, and 51 [20,21,33], undergoes endogenous non-canonical basal exon skipping in wild-type skin fibroblasts and (*ii*) that the A to T transversion at position c.4723 enhances skipping. In silico analysis which predicted that the variation lies within an ESE indicates that skipping augmentation is promoted through nonsense-associated altered splicing. Indeed, ESE sequences are usually purine- or A/C-rich [34,35]. Introducing a T into an artificial polypurine sequence mimicking a *DMD* ESE has been reported to reduce enhancer activity, in particular when it introduced a nonsense codon [36]. Accordingly, the introduction of a T at position c.4723 is predicted to reduce significantly the strength of ESE and increase the chance of exon skipping, whereas the introduction of a G and a C has a minimal and no effect, respectively (Table 1).

During the transition of cells from proliferation to quiescence, ciliation is initiated by CEP290-mediated recruitment of RAB8A at the centrosome, leading to the release of the cilia formation suppressor CP110 [25–27]. Preserved ability of P1 and P2 fibroblasts to ciliate upon serum starvation indicated that the *CEP290*$^{\Delta 36}$ mRNA was translated into a protein isoform able to recruit RAB8A despite the loss of 36 CEP290 residues involved in binding. Accordingly, immune-staining demonstrated the presence of CEP290 and RAB8A at the centrosome. The abundance of CEP290 in P1 and P2 cells were 40% and 30% of the wild-type levels in controls, respectively. Despite reduced CEP290 abundance, the intensity of CP110-specific staining at the centrosome of P1 cells was comparable to controls, indicating a normal release that was further supported by a normal abundance of ciliated cells. In contrast, P2 cells which tended to express slightly less *CEP290*$^{\Delta 36}$ mRNA and CEP290$^{\Delta 36aa}$ protein exhibited moderate, yet statistically significant, reduction in CP110 release and, accordingly, in cilia abundance. As to why P2 cells tend to express diminished amounts of *CEP290*$^{\Delta 36}$ isoform, the reduced abundance of full length mutant mRNA in P2 compared to P1 suggests a depletion of full length mutant pre-mRNA from which the skipped isoform arises. Whether this observation would result from increased NMD in P2, similar amounts of *CEP290*$^{\Delta 36}$ isoform should be measured in the two cell lines. Further studies using NMD inhibitors could help in addressing this interesting question. Whatever the mechanism, these results further support the predictive model of *CEP290*-associated pathogenesis and it would be tempting to correlate the severity of the retinal disease of P2 compared to P1 (congenital blindness vs. measurable VA of 20/67 (RE) and 20/50 (LE) at 20 years, respectively) to a reduced abundance of CEP290$^{\Delta 36aa}$ product in photoreceptor cells. Evidence of abundant endogenous basal skipping of exon 36 in human retina makes this hypothesis plausible. However, this cannot be demonstrated, in particular since the level of endogenous and selective (if any) skipping of exon 36 in the photoreceptors of affected individuals cannot be anticipated from the *CEP290* genotype as determined by sequencing of exon and intron boundaries only. Variants in other *CEP290* regions and/or in genes encoding proteins important to endogenous and/or selective exon skipping, the mechanisms of which are not or poorly known, could contribute to the individual *CEP290* pre-mRNA splicing variability. Along the same lines, it is worth mentioning that three individuals carrying the c.4723A > T mutation were reported to present with LCA and intellectual disability, autistic behavior or cerebro-renal anomalies consistent with Joubert syndrome [5,7,37]. Whether the extraocular expression in these individuals is due to reduced skipping of exon 36 in the brain and/or the kidney or to additional mutations is opened to debate. Further, consistent with a correlation between the abundance of centrosomal CEP290 and the cilia phenotype of fibroblasts, AON-mediated augmentation of the amount of CEP290$^{\Delta 36aa}$ at the centrosome of P2 fibroblasts improved the ciliary phenotype. However, a more important increase in P1 cells aggravated the cilia phenotype, supporting the view that the $CEP290^{\Delta 36}$ mRNA encodes an imperfectly functional protein, the expression of which might be preferable compared to knock-out, provided it is not too high. This indicates that exon 36 encodes an important functional region of CEP290. The centrosomal depletion of CEP290 in control cells expressing significant levels of $CEP290^{\Delta 36}$ mRNA (40% of total CEP290) upon AON treatment, suggests that the $CEP290^{\Delta 36aa}$ has reduced ability to associate to the centrosome, predicting a diminution of RAB8A recruitment, possibly aggravated by the loss of 36 amino-acid participating to the binding of RAB8A. The centrosomal retention of the CP110 cilia formation-suppressor along with the cilia defect, yet minor, we observed that controls on the AON treatment are consistent with this view.

Intriguingly, while the majority of fibroblasts from individuals homozygous for the c.4723A > T mutation were able to produce a primary cilium upon serum starvation, we observed a highly significant elongation of cilia. Axonemal elongation with normal or abnormal ultrastructure has been originally reported in kidney tissues, cultured kidney-derived cells and skin-derived fibroblasts from individuals or animal models with cystic kidney diseases involving *BBS4* (MIM600374), *NEK8* (MIM609799, NPHP9), *KIF7* (MIM611254, JBTS12), *TMEM67* (MIM609884, MKS3), *KIAA0556* (MIM616650, JBTS26) [38–44], and in fibroblasts from individuals affected with rod-cone dystrophy and hearing loss due to *CEP78* mutation [45]. Recently, *CEP290*-associated cilia elongation has been described in primary renal epithelial cells from three individuals affected with Joubert syndrome. Two of them were compound heterozygous siblings carrying the c.2817G > T (splice alteration and p.K939N) and c.2848insC (p.Q950Pfs*6) mutations in exon 25 and 26, respectively [46]. The skipping of either exon would preserve the reading frame, leading to the production of a minimally shortened protein that would lack part of the NPHP5 and/or CCD2D2A binding domains. Consistent with positive ciliation, hURECs derived from one of the two siblings expressed minimal amounts of a CEP290 product as determined by western blot analysis. But, the third individual was a sporadic case homozygous for the c.5668G > T (p.G1890*) mutation in exon 41. This in-frame exon has been reported to undergo endogenous basal exon skipping in fibroblasts [20], producing a minimal loss of the microtubule binding domain. Yet, consistent with tissue variability of *CEP290* pre-mRNA splicing [10,21,33,47], RT-PCR analysis of hURECs from the patient harboring elongated cilia showed no skipping of exon 41, Western blot analysis and immunocytochemistry detected no CEP290. Furthermore, siRNA-mediated knockdown of CEP290 led to elongated cilia [46].

To our knowledge, this is the first study showing elongated cilia in fibroblasts for individuals affected with non-syndromic retinal diseases rather than an impairment of cilia formation [8,10,12,21,32]. This observation in two unrelated individuals homozygous for the same mutation strongly supports genotype–phenotype correlation.

It has been proposed that the length of the axoneme which elongates from the basal body is regulated by the balance between the rates of anterograde and retrograde IFT [48]. Whether axonemal elongation in fibroblasts from patients carrying the c.4723A > T mutation is due to alteration of IFT certainly merits consideration. In particular, addressing this question might help in understanding the relation between the abundance of the $CEP290^{\Delta 36aa}$ protein isoform and ciliation and whether AON-mediated axonemal shortening of patient cell cilia may be regarded as a positive read-out of treatment efficiency.

In summary, here we report expression of a PTC-free *CEP290* mRNA resulting from endogenous and selective exclusion of exon 36 encompassing the founder *CEP290* c.4723A > T nonsense mutation in two apparently unrelated individuals. We show that a CEP290 isoform is produced that localizes to centrosomes and that cilia are produced upon serum starvation, yet improperly, as demonstrated by significant axonemal elongation. We demonstrate that increasing the quantity of the *CEP290* mRNA lacking exon 36 through the use of AON increased the abundance of the CEP290 product at the centrosome and allowed axonemal shortening. However, while a moderate quantity of CEP290 product ameliorated cilia formation, a high abundance compromised cilia formation. Whether this would occur in photoreceptor cell is an important question, especially knowing that mRNA metabolism is higher in the retina than in any other cell type [49], that *CEP290* transcripts are far more expressed in neural retina compared to other tissues and organs [19] and that *CEP290* pre-mRNA splicing in iPSC-derived 3D optic cups has been shown to differ significantly from that observed in fibroblasts [10]. AON-mediated skipping of exon 36 in iPSC-derived retinal organoids from individuals carrying the c.4723A > T mutation would certainly merit consideration to address this burning question.

Supplementary Materials: The following are available online at http://www.mdpi.com/2073-4425/10/5/368/s1, Figure S1: Panel of 199 genes involved in retinal dystrophies, Figure S2: Localization of primers used to amplify the full-length and *CEP290* mRNAs lacking exon 36, Table S1: Sequences and positions of sequencing primers, Table S2: Genetic and clinical features of individuals, Table S3: Sequences and positions of RT-PCR primers, Table S4: Sequences and positions of RT-qPCR primers.

Author Contributions: Conceptualization, J.-M.R. and X.G.; formal analysis, I.B. and X.G.; funding acquisition, I.B., I.P., J.K., J.-M.R. and X.G.; investigation, I.B., I.P., C.M. and X.G.; project administration, J.-M.R. and X.G.; resources, S.D.-D., I.G. and J.K.; software, N.G.; supervision, J.-M.R. and X.G.; validation, J.-M.R. and X.G.; visualization, I.B.; writing—original draft, J.-M.R. and X.G.; writing—review and editing, I.B., J.-M.R. and X.G.

Funding: This research was funded by grants from Retina France to I.P. and J.K., from the Fondation JED-Belgique to X.G., from UNADEV-AVIESAN/ITMO NNP (R16074KS) to I.P. and UNADEV-AVIESAN/ITMO NNP (R16073KS) to J.-M.R., and from the Fondation pour la recherche médicale (FRM FDT201904007931).

Acknowledgments: We gratefully acknowledge the patients who donated skin biopsies for this study.

Conflicts of Interest: The authors declare no conflict of interest.

References

1. Kaplan, J. Leber congenital amaurosis: From darkness to spotlight. *Ophthalmic Genet.* **2008**, *29*, 92–98. [CrossRef] [PubMed]
2. Hanein, S.; Perrault, I.; Gerber, S.; Tanguy, G.; Barbet, F.; Ducroq, D.; Calvas, P.; Dollfus, H.; Hamel, C.; Lopponen, T.; et al. Leber congenital amaurosis: Comprehensive survey of the genetic heterogeneity, refinement of the clinical definition, and genotype–phenotype correlations as a strategy for molecular diagnosis. *Hum. Mutat.* **2004**, *23*, 306–317. [CrossRef] [PubMed]
3. Craige, B.; Tsao, C.C.; Diener, D.R.; Hou, Y.; Lechtreck, K.F.; Rosenbaum, J.L.; Witman, G.B. CEP290 tethers flagellar transition zone microtubules to the membrane and regulates flagellar protein content. *J. Cell Biol.* **2010**, *190*, 927–940. [CrossRef]
4. Den Hollander, A.I.; Roepman, R.; Koenekoop, R.K.; Cremers, F.P.M. Leber congenital amaurosis: genes, proteins and disease mechanisms. *Prog. Retin. Eye Res.* **2008**, *27*, 391–419. [CrossRef]
5. Perrault, I.; Delphin, N.; Hanein, S.; Gerber, S.; Dufier, J.L.; Roche, O.; Defoort-Dhellemmes, S.; Dollfus, H.; Fazzi, E.; Munnich, A.; et al. Spectrum of NPHP6/CEP290 mutations in Leber congenital amaurosis and delineation of the associated phenotype. *Hum. Mutat.* **2007**, *28*, 416. [CrossRef] [PubMed]
6. Cideciyan, A.V.; Aleman, T.S.; Jacobson, S.G.; Khanna, H.; Sumaroka, A.; Aquirre, G.K.; Schwartz, S.B.; Windsor, E.A.; He, S.; Chang, B.; et al. Centrosomal-ciliary gene CEP290/NPHP6 mutations result in blindness with unexpected sparing of photoreceptors and visual brain: Implications for therapy of Leber congenital amaurosis. *Hum. Mutat.* **2007**, *28*, 1074–1083. [CrossRef] [PubMed]
7. Preising, M.N.; Schneider, U.; Friedburg, C.; Gruber, H.; Lindner, S. Lorenz, B. The Phenotypic spectrum of ophthalmic changes in CEP290 mutations. *Klin. Monbl. Augenheilkd* **2019**, *236*, 244–252.
8. Gerard, G.; Perrault, I.; Hanein, S.; Silva, E.; Bigot, K.; Defoort-Delhemmes, S.; Rio, M.; Munnich, A.; Scherman, D.; Kaplan, J.; et al. AON-mediated exon skipping restores ciliation in fibroblasts harboring the common leber congenital amaurosis CEP290 mutation. *Mol. Ther. Nucl. Acids* **2012**, *1*, e29. [CrossRef] [PubMed]
9. Collin, R.W.; den Hollander, A.I.; van der Velde-Visser, S.D.; Bennicelli, J.; Bennett, J.; Cremers, F.P. Antisense oligonucleotide (AON)-based therapy for leber congenital amaurosis caused by a frequent mutation in CEP290. *Mol. Ther. Nucl. Acids* **2012**, *1*, e14. [CrossRef]
10. Parfitt, D.A.; Lane, A.; Ramsden, C.M.; Carr, A.J.; Munro, P.M.; Jovanovic, K.; Schwarz, N.; Kanuga, N.; Muthiah, M.N.; Hull, S.; et al. Identification and correction of mechanisms underlying inherited blindness in human iPSC-derived optic cups. *Cell. Stem.* **2016**, *18*, 769–781. [CrossRef] [PubMed]

11. Dulla, K.; Aguila, M.; Lane, A.; Jovanovic, K.; Parfitt, D.A.; Schulkens, I.; Chan, H.L.; Schmidt, I.; Beumer, W.; Vorthoren, L.; et al. Splice-modulating oligonucleotide QR-110 restores CEP290 mRNA and function in human c.2991+1655A>G LCA10 models. *Mol. Ther. Nucl. Acids* **2018**, *12*, 730–740. [CrossRef] [PubMed]
12. Garanto, A.; Chung, D.C.; Duijkers, L.; Corral-Serrano, J.C.; Messchaert, M.; Xiao, R.; Bennett, J.; Vandenberghe, L.H.; Collin, R.W. In vitro and in vivo rescue of aberrant splicing in CEP290-associated LCA by antisense oligonucleotide delivery. *Hum. Mol. Genet.* **2016**, *25*, 2552–2563.
13. Cideciyan, A.V.; Jacobson, S.G.; Drack, A.V.; Ho, A.C.; Charng, J.; Garafalo, A.V.; Roman, A.J.; Sumaroka, A.; Han, I.C.; Hochstedler, M.D.; et al. Effect of an intravitreal antisense oligonucleotide on vision in Leber congenital amaurosis due to a photoreceptor cilium defect. *Nat. Med.* **2019**, *25*, 225. [CrossRef]
14. Bainbridge, J.W.; Smith, A.J.; Barker, S.S.; Robbie, S.; Henderson, R.; Balaggan, K.; Viswanathan, A.; Holder, G.E.; Stockman, A.; Tyler, N.; et al. Effect of gene therapy on visual function in Leber's congenital amaurosis. *N. Engl. J. Med.* **2008**, *358*, 2231–2239. [CrossRef] [PubMed]
15. Hauswirth, W.W.; Aleman, T.S.; Kaushal, S.; Cideciyan, A.V.; Schwartz, S.B.; Wang, L.; Conlon, T.J.; Boye, S.L.; Flotte, T.R.; Byrne, B.J.; et al. Treatment of leber congenital amaurosis due to rpe65 mutations by ocular subretinal injection of adeno-associated virus gene vector: short-term results of a phase I trial. *Hum. Gene Ther.* **2008**, *19*, 979–990. [CrossRef]
16. Maguire, A.M.; Simonelli, F.; Pierce, E.A.; Pugh, E.N., Jr.; Mingozzi, F.; Bennicelli, J.; Banfi, S.; Marshall, K.A.; Testa, F.; Surace, E.M.; et al. Safety and Efficacy of gene transfer for leber's congenital amaurosis. *N. Engl. J. Med.* **2008**, *358*, 2240–2248. [CrossRef] [PubMed]
17. Seo, S.; Mullins, R.F.; Dumitrescu, A.V.; Bhattarai, S.; Gratie, D.; Wang, K.; Stone, E.M.; Sheffield, V.; Drack, A.V. Subretinal gene therapy of mice with bardet-biedl syndrome type 1. *Investig. Ophthalmol. Vis. Sci.* **2013**, *54*, 6118–6132. [CrossRef] [PubMed]
18. Kloeckener-Gruissem, B.; Neidhart, J.; Magyar, I.; Plauchu, H.; Zech, J.C.; Morlé, L.; Palmer-Smith, S.M.; Macdonald, M.J.; Nas, V.; Fry, A.E.; et al. Novel VCAN mutations and evidence for unbalanced alternative splicing in the pathogenesis of Wagner syndrome. *Eur. J. Hum. Genet.* **2013**, *21*, 352–356. [CrossRef]
19. Papon, J.F.; Perrault, I.; Coste, A.; Louis, B.; Gérard, X.; Hanein, S.; Fares-Taie, L.; Gerber, S.; Defoort-Dhellemmes, S.; Vojtek, A.M.; et al. Abnormal respiratory cilia in non-syndromic Leber congenital amaurosis with CEP290 mutations. *J. Med. Genet.* **2010**, *47*, 829–834. [CrossRef]
20. Drivas, T.G.; Wojno, A.P.; Tucker, B.A.; Stone, E.M.; Bennett, J. Basal exon skipping and genetic pleiotropy: A predictive model of disease pathogenesis. *Sci. Trans. Med.* **2015**, *7*, 291ra97. [CrossRef]
21. Barny, I.; Perrault, I.; Michel, C.; Soussan, M.; Goudin, N.; Rio, M.; Thomas, S.; Attié-Bitach, T.; Hamel, C.; Dollfus, H.; et al. Basal exon skipping and nonsense-associated altered splicing allows bypassing complete CEP290 loss-of-function in individuals with unusually mild retinal disease. *Hum. Mol. Genet.* **2018**, *15*, 2689–2702. [CrossRef]
22. Littink, K.W.; Pott, J.W.; Collin, R.W.; Kroes, H.Y.; Verheij, J.B.; Blokland, E.A.; de Castro Miro, M.; Hoyng, C.B.; Klaver, C.C.; Joenekoop, R.K.; et al. A novel nonsense mutation in CEP290 induces exon skipping and leads to a relatively mild retinal phenotype. *Investig. Ophthalmol. Vis. Sci.* **2010**, *51*, 3646–3652. [CrossRef]
23. Roosing, S.; Cremers, F.P.M.; Riemslag, F.C.C.; Zonneveld-Vrieling, M.N.; Talsma, H.E.; Klessens-Godfroy, F.J.M.; den Hollander, A.I.; van den Born, L.I. A rare form of retinal dystrophy caused by hypomorphic nonsense mutations in CEP290. *Genes* **2017**, *8*, 208. [CrossRef]
24. Disterer, P.; Kryczka, A.; Liu, Y.; Badi, Y.E.; Wong, J.J.; Owen, J.S.; Khoo, B. Development of therapeutic splice-switching oligonucleotides. *Hum. Gene Ther.* **2014**, *25*, 587–598. [CrossRef]
25. Tsang, W.Y.; Bossard, C.; Khanna, H.; Peränen, J.; Swaroop, A.; Malhotra, V.; Dynlacht, B.D. CP110 Suppresses primary cilia formation through its interaction with cep290, a protein deficient in human ciliary disease. *Dev. Cell* **2008**, *15*, 187–197. [CrossRef]
26. Kim, J.; Krishnaswami, S.R.; Gleeson, J.G. CEP290 interacts with the centriolar satellite component PCM-1 and is required for Rab8 localization to the primary cilium. *Hum. Mol. Genet.* **2008**, *17*, 3796–3805. [CrossRef]
27. Stowe, T.R.; Wilkinson, C.J.; Iqbal, A.; Stearns, T. The centriolar satellite proteins Cep72 and Cep290 interact and are required for recruitment of BBS proteins to the cilium. *Mol. Biol. Cell* **2012**, *23*, 3322–3335. [CrossRef]
28. Ramsbottom, S.A.; Molinari, E.; Srivastava, S.; Silberman, F.; Henry, C.; Alkanderi, S.; Devlin, L.A.; White, K.; Steel, D.H.; Saunier, S.; et al. Targeted exon skipping of a CEP290 mutation rescues Joubert syndrome phenotypes in vitro and in a murine model. *Proc. Natl. Acad. Sci. USA* **2018**, *115*, 12489–12494. [CrossRef]

29. Drivas, T.G.; Holzbaur, E.L.F.; Bennett, J. Disruption of CEP290 microtubule/membrane-binding domains causes retinal degeneration. *J. Clin. Investig.* **2013**, *123*, 4525–4539. [CrossRef]
30. Rachel, R.A.; Yamamoto, E.A.; Dewanjee, M.K.; May-Simera, H.L.; Sergeev, Y.V.; Hackett, A.N.; Pohida, K.; Munasinghe, J.; Gotoh, N.; Wickstead, B.; et al. CEP290 alleles in mice disrupt tissue-specific cilia biogenesis and recapitulate features of syndromic ciliopathies. *Hum. Mol. Genet.* **2015**, *24*, 3775–3791. [CrossRef]
31. Chang, B.; Khanna, H.; Hawes, N.; Jimeno, D.; He, S.; Lillo, C.; Parapuram, S.K.; Cheng, H.; Scott, A.; Hurd, R.E.; et al. In-frame deletion in a novel centrosomal/ciliary protein CEP290/NPHP6 perturbs its interaction with RPGR and results in early-onset retinal degeneration in the rd16 mouse. *Hum. Mol. Genet.* **2006**, *15*, 1847–1857. [CrossRef]
32. Shimada, H.; Lu, Q.; Insinna-Kettenhofen, C.; Nagashima, K.; English, M.A.; Semler, E.M.; Mahgerefteh, J.; Cideciyan, A.V.; Li, T.; Brooks, B.P.; et al. In Vitro modeling using ciliopathy-patient-derived cells reveals distinct cilia dysfunctions caused by CEP290 mutations. *Cell Rep.* **2017**, *20*, 384–396. [CrossRef]
33. Barny, I.; Perrault, I.; Rio, M.; Dollfus, H.; Defoort-Dhellemmes, S.; Kaplan, J.; Rozet, J.-M.; Gerard, X. Description of two siblings with apparently severe CEP290 mutations and unusually mild retinal disease unrelated to basal exon skipping or nonsense-associated altered splicing. *Adv. Exp. Med. Biol.* (under review).
34. Valentine, C.R. The association of nonsense codons with exon skipping. *Mutat. Res./Rev. Mutat. Res.* **1998**, *411*, 87–117. [CrossRef]
35. Cartegni, L.; Chew, S.L.; Krainer, A.R. Listening to silence and understanding nonsense: exonic mutations that affect splicing. *Nat. Rev. Genet.* **2002**, *3*, 285. [CrossRef] [PubMed]
36. Shiga, N.; Takeshima, Y.; Sakamoto, H.; Inoue, K.; Yokota, Y.; Yokoyama, M.; Matsuo, M. Disruption of the splicing enhancer sequence within exon 27 of the dystrophin gene by a nonsense mutation induces partial skipping of the exon and is responsible for Becker muscular dystrophy. *J. Clin. Investig.* **1997**, *100*, 2204–2210. [CrossRef] [PubMed]
37. Coppieters, F.; Lefever, S.; Leroy, B.P.; Baere, E.D. CEP290, a gene with many faces: Mutation overview and presentation of CEP290base. *Hum. Mutat.* **2010**, *31*, 1097–1108. [CrossRef]
38. Mokrzan, E.M.; Lewis, J.S.; Mykytyn, K. Differences in renal tubule primary cilia length in a mouse model of bardet-biedl syndrome. *NEE* **2007**, *106*, e88–e96. [CrossRef] [PubMed]
39. Smith, L.A.; Bukanov, N.O.; Husson, H.; Russo, R.J.; Barry, T.C.; Taylor, A.L.; Beier, D.R.; Ibraghimov-Beskrovnaya, O. Development of Polycystic kidney disease in juvenile cystic kidney mice: insights into pathogenesis, ciliary abnormalities, and common features with human disease. *JASN* **2006**, *17*, 2821–2831. [CrossRef]
40. Sohara, E.; Luo, Y.; Zhang, J.; Manning, D.K.; Beier, D.R.; Zhou, J. Nek8 regulates the expression and localization of polycystin-1 and polycystin-2. *J. Am. Soc. Nephrol.* **2008**, *19*, 469–476. [CrossRef]
41. Tammachote, R.; Hommerding, C.J.; Sinders, R.M.; Miller, C.A.; Czarnecki, P.G.; Leightner, A.C.; Salisbury, J.L.; Ward, C.J.; Torres, V.E.; Gattone, V.H., 2nd; et al. Ciliary and centrosomal defects associated with mutation and depletion of the Meckel syndrome genes MKS1 and MKS3. *Hum. Mol. Genet.* **2009**, *18*, 3311–3323. [CrossRef]
42. He, M.; Subramanian, R.; Bangs, F.; Omelchenko, T.; Liem, K.F. Jr.; Kapoor, T.M.; Anderson, K.V. The kinesin-4 protein KIF7 regulates mammalian hedgehog signaling by organizing the cilia tip compartment. *Nat. Cell. Biol.* **2014**, *16*, 663–672. [CrossRef] [PubMed]
43. Sanders, A.A.; de Vrieze, E.; Alazami, A.M.; Alzahrani, F.; Malarkey, E.B.; Sorush, N.; Tebbe, L.; Kuhns, S.; van Dam, T.J.; Alhashem, A.; et al. KIAA0556 is a novel ciliary basal body component mutated in Joubert syndrome. *Genome Biol.* **2015**, *16*, 293. [CrossRef] [PubMed]
44. Stayner, C.; Poole, C.A.; McGlashan, S.R.; Pilanthananond, M.; Brauning, R.; Markie, D.; Lett, B.; Slobbe, L.; Chae, A.; Johnstone, A.C.; et al. An ovine hepatorenal fibrocystic model of a Meckel-like syndrome associated with dysmorphic primary cilia and TMEM67 mutations. *Sci. Rep.* **2017**, *7*, 1601. [CrossRef]
45. Nikopoulos, K.; Farinelli, P.; Giangreco, B.; Tsika, C.; Royer-Bertand, B.; Mbefo, M.K.; Bedoni, N.; Kjellström, U.; El Zaoui, I.; Di Gioia, S.A.; et al. Mutations in CEP78 cause cone-rod dystrophy and hearing loss associated with primary-cilia defects. *Am. J. Hum. Genet.* **2016**, *99*, 770–776. [CrossRef]
46. Srivastava, S.; Ramsbottom, S.A.; Molinari, E.; Alkanderi, S.; Filby, A.; White, K.; Henry, C.; Saunier, S.; Miles, C.G.; Sayer, J.A. A human patient-derived cellular model of Joubert syndrome reveals ciliary defects which can be rescued with targeted therapies. *Hum. Mol. Genet.* **2017**, *26*, 4657–4667. [CrossRef] [PubMed]

47. Garanto, A.; van Beersum, S.E.C.; Peters, T.A.; Roepman, R.; Cremers, F.P.M.; Collin, R.W.J. Unexpected CEP290 mRNA splicing in a humanized knock-in mouse model for leber congenital amaurosis. *PLoS ONE* **2013**, *8*, e79369. [CrossRef] [PubMed]
48. Marshall, W.F.; Qin, H.; Brenni, M.R.; Rosenbaum, J.L. Flagellar length control system: Testing a simple model based on intraflagellar transport and turnover. *Mol. Biol. Cell* **2005**, *16*, 270–278. [CrossRef]
49. Tanackovic, G.; Rivolta, C. PRPF31 alternative splicing and expression in human retina. *Ophthalmic Genet.* **2009**, *30*, 76–83. [CrossRef]

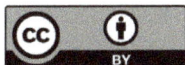

© 2019 by the authors. Licensee MDPI, Basel, Switzerland. This article is an open access article distributed under the terms and conditions of the Creative Commons Attribution (CC BY) license (http://creativecommons.org/licenses/by/4.0/).

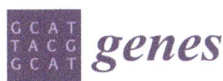

Article

Antisense Oligonucleotide Screening to Optimize the Rescue of the Splicing Defect Caused by the Recurrent Deep-Intronic *ABCA4* Variant c.4539+2001G>A in Stargardt Disease

Alejandro Garanto [1,*], Lonneke Duijkers [2], Tomasz Z. Tomkiewicz [1] and Rob W. J. Collin [1,*]

1. Department of Human Genetics and Donders Institute for Brain, Cognition and Behaviour, Radboud University Medical Center, 6525GA Nijmegen, The Netherlands; tomasz.tomkiewicz@radboudumc.nl
2. Department of Human Genetics, Radboud University Medical Center, 6525GA Nijmegen, The Netherlands; lonneke.duijkers@radboudumc.nl
* Correspondence: alex.garanto@radboudumc.nl (A.G.); rob.collin@radboudumc.nl (R.W.J.C.); Tel.: +31-24-36-14107 (A.G.); +31-24-36-13750 (R.W.J.C.)

Received: 16 May 2019; Accepted: 11 June 2019; Published: 14 June 2019

Abstract: Deep-sequencing of the *ABCA4* locus has revealed that ~10% of autosomal recessive Stargardt disease (STGD1) cases are caused by deep-intronic mutations. One of the most recurrent deep-intronic variants in the Belgian and Dutch STGD1 population is the c.4539+2001G>A mutation. This variant introduces a 345-nt pseudoexon to the *ABCA4* mRNA transcript in a retina-specific manner. Antisense oligonucleotides (AONs) are short sequences of RNA that can modulate splicing. In this work, we designed 26 different AONs to perform a thorough screening to identify the most effective AONs to correct splicing defects associated with c.4539+2001G>A. All AONs were tested in patient-derived induced pluripotent stem cells (iPSCs) that were differentiated to photoreceptor precursor cells (PPCs). AON efficacy was assessed through RNA analysis and was based on correction efficacy, and AONs were grouped and their properties assessed. We (a) identified nine AONs with significant correction efficacies (>50%), (b) confirmed that a single nucleotide mismatch was sufficient to significantly decrease AON efficacy, and (c) found potential correlations between efficacy and some of the parameters analyzed. Overall, our results show that AON-based splicing modulation holds great potential for treating Stargardt disease caused by splicing defects in *ABCA4*.

Keywords: antisense oligonucleotides; Stargardt disease; inherited retinal diseases; splicing modulation; RNA therapy; ABCA4; iPSC-derived photoreceptor precursor cells

1. Introduction

Stargardt disease (STGD1; MIM:248200) is an autosomal recessive condition affecting the retina, and was first described in 1909 by the German ophthalmologist Karl Stargardt [1]. The clinical hallmark of STGD1 is progressive bilateral impairment of central vision. Impairment in visual acuity and progressive bilateral atrophy of photoreceptors and the retinal pigment epithelium (RPE) are accompanied by the accumulation of toxic fluorescent deposits of lipofuscin in the macula [2,3]. The underlying genetic causes of the disease are mutations in the *ABCA4* gene that encodes the ATP-binding cassette transporter type 4 subfamily A (ABCA4). The *ABCA4* protein belongs to the superfamily of membrane-bound ATP-binding cassette transporters [4]. It translocates the visual cycle metabolites, all-*trans*-retinal and *N*-retinylidene-phosphatidyl ethanolamine (*N*-retinylidene-PE), from the lumen to the cytoplasmic side of photoreceptor disc membranes [5]. The decrease in *ABCA4* activity causes an accumulation of toxic retinal derivatives, which eventually results in RPE and photoreceptor cell death [6,7]. Over 900 disease-associated variants in *ABCA4* have been described [8,9], causing a wide range of phenotypes ranging from STGD1 to cone–rod dystrophy, depending on the severity of the mutation [10,11].

STGD1 cases can be explained by biallelic mutations in either the coding sequence or in the intronic regions of *ABCA4* [12]. Around 10% of cases carry intronic variants that result in the insertion of pseudoexons (PEs) into the final *ABCA4* mRNA transcript [4,9,13–20]. Such mutations are an ideal target for antisense oligonucleotide (AON) therapy. AONs are short synthetic RNA molecules that can interfere with the processing of pre-mRNA [21] and thereby modulate splicing. Modified AONs employed to correct splicing defects have been extensively studied in the field of inherited retinal diseases (IRDs) for genes such as *CEP290* [22–27], *USH2A* [28], *CHM* [29], *OPN1* [30], or *ABCA4* [18,20,31]. The first splicing modulation strategy described for a retinal disease was targeting a recurring deep-intronic variant (c.2991+1655A>G) in the *CEP290* gene, underlying recessive Leber congenital amaurosis (LCA; MIM:611755). This mutation results in the generation of a cryptic splice donor site leading to a 128-nt pseudoexon with a premature stop codon between exons 26 and 27. AONs used to block the pseudoexon showed successful restoration of the original mRNA both in vivo and in vitro [22,24–27] and have recently shown promising results in the first clinical trial with AONs for IRDs [32].

Another mutation that causes a pre-mRNA splicing defect and is amenable to AON therapy is the c.4539+2001G>A variant in *ABCA4* [13–15], which is recurrently found in the Belgian and Dutch STGD1 population. Recently, our group described the molecular mechanism by which c.4539+2001G>A and the adjacent c.4539+2028C>T mutations in *ABCA4* lead to insertion of a retina-specific 345-nt pseudoexon that is predicted to result in premature termination of protein synthesis (p.Arg1514Leufs*36). The c.4539+2001G>A variant enhances a predicted exonic splice enhancer and creates a new SRp55 motif. This was the first reported insertion of a pseudoexon into a retinal gene due to the creation of new exonic splicing enhancer (ESE) motifs rather than the generation of new cryptic splice sites, although other examples have been described previously [33,34]. By using AON technology, we were able to restore correct splicing with two of the four AONs (AON1–4) that were used (AON1 and AON4) [18].

In this study, we performed an in-depth screening of a large set of AONs targeting the entire pseudoexon region to identify the most effective AON(s) against the splicing defect caused by the c.4539+2001G>A mutation. In total, 26 AONs were screened in retinal precursor cells differentiated from patient-derived induced pluripotent stem cell (iPSC), and their efficacy in correcting splicing defects was assessed. Subsequently, properties of the most effective AONs were compared in order to identify potential parameters for a better design of AONs in the future.

2. Materials and Methods

2.1. Study Design

The objectives of this study were to (1) perform an in-depth screening of AONs targeting the pseudoexon introduced by the recurrent c.4539+2001G>A deep-intronic variant in *ABCA4*, (2) identify the best AON(s) to correct the pre-mRNA splicing defect caused by this mutation using patient-derived photoreceptor precursor cells (PPCs), and (3) identify potential correlations between AON characteristics and their efficacy that can provide new insights into a better AON design. Twenty-two new AONs targeting the pseudoexon were designed and tested together with four previously described AONs [18]. Fibroblast cells obtained from a skin biopsy of a Stargardt individual carrying the deep-intronic variant were cultured, reprogrammed into iPSCs, and subsequently differentiated to PPCs. All 26 AONs and two sense oligonucleotides (SONs) were designed along the pseudoexon. Upon AON delivery, subsequent RNA analysis by RT-PCR was performed to assess the efficacy of the splicing redirection for each AON. After semiquantification of the rescue, AONs were classified into different groups, and the properties of the AONs were compared to identify parameters that could improve the AON design. Two separate differentiation experiments were performed. RNA analysis was performed in triplicate to reduce technical variability.

2.2. AON Design

Previously, four AONs were designed targeting the top SC35 motifs and the mutation itself [18]. For the detailed screening that was the subject of this study, the entire pseudoexon plus the flanking regions were analyzed for their RNA structure to identify the open and closed regions. Subsequently, AONs were designed according to previously described guidelines independently of the potential motifs that they were targeting [35,36]. All AON sequences and properties are provided in Table 1. After AON design, targeted regions were analyzed to predict potential exonic splicing enhancer (ESE) motifs using either an ESE finder (http://krainer01.cshl.edu/cgi-bin/tools/ESE3/esefinder.cgi?process=home), which allows for the detection of SRSF1, SRSF2, SRSF5, and SRSF6, or using RBPmap (http://rbpmap.technion.ac.il/index.html), which allows for the identification of 94 potential binding sites for RNA binding proteins. All AONs were 2'OMe-PS (2'O-methyl phosphorothioate) and were purchased from Eurogentec (Liege, Belgium). Sequences and general parameters of the 26 AONs and 2 SONs are depicted in Table 1.

2.3. Subjects

A skin biopsy was collected from a Dutch individual with STGD1 carrying the *ABCA4* variants c.4539+2001G>A (p.Arg1514Leufs*36) and c.4892T>C (p.Leu1631Pro) to establish a fibroblast cell line, as described previously [18]. Our research was conducted according to the tenets of the Declaration of Helsinki and after gathering written informed consent from the STGD1 individual. The procedures for obtaining human skin biopsies to establish primary fibroblast cell lines were approved by the local ethical committee (2015-1543).

2.4. iPSC Differentiation into Photoreceptor Precursor Cells (PPCs)

Fibroblast cells were reprogrammed into iPSCs, as previously described [18]. PPCs were obtained after following a 2D differentiation protocol [37]. Briefly, iPSCs were dissociated with ReLeSR (Stemcell Technologies) and plated in 12-well plates coated with matrigel (Corning, Tewksbury, MA, USA) to form a monolayer. Essential-Flex E8 medium was changed to differentiation medium (CI) when reaching confluence. The CI medium consisted of DMEM/F12 supplemented with nonessential amino acids (NEAA, Sigma Aldrich, Saint Louis, CA, USA), B27 supplements (Thermo Fisher Scientific, Waltham, MA, USA), N2 supplements (Thermo Fisher Scientific), 100 ng/µL of insulin growth factor-1 (IGF-1, Sigma Aldrich), 10 ng/µL of recombinant fibroblast growth factor basic (bFGF, Sigma Aldrich), 10 µg/µL of Heparin (Sigma Aldrich), 200 µg/mL of recombinant human COCO (R&D Systems, Minneapolis, MN, USA), and 100 µg/mL of Primocin (Invivogen, Toulouse, France). Half of the medium was replaced every day for 30 days. On day 28, PPCs were treated with 1 µM of AON. AONs were first mixed with the medium without any transfection reagent and were subsequently added to the cells. Twenty-four hours later, cycloheximide (CHX) was added to the medium (final concentration 100 µg/mL), and on day 30 (48 h post-AON delivery and 24 h post-CHX treatment), cells were collected.

2.5. RNA Analysis

RNA was isolated from patient-derived PPCs using the Nucleospin RNA kit (Machery Nagel, Düren, Germany) following the manufacturer's instructions. One microgram of total RNA was used for cDNA synthesis using SuperScript VILO Master Mix (Thermo Fisher Scientific) and was subsequently diluted with H_2O to a final concentration of 20 ng/µL. Reverse transcription-PCR (RT-PCR) was performed with 10 µM of each primer, 2 µM of dNTPs, 2.5 mM of $MgCl_2$, 1 U of Taq polymerase (Roche, Basel, Switzerland), and 80 ng of cDNA in a total reaction of 25 µL using the following PCR conditions: 2 min at 94 °C, followed by 35 cycles of 30 s at 94 °C, 30 s at 58 °C, and 70 s at 72 °C, with a final extension of 2 min at 72 °C. Actin was amplified to serve as a loading control. All PCR products were resolved on 2% agarose gels and were confirmed by Sanger. Fiji software was used to perform a semiquantitative analysis of the bands in which the values were normalized against the housekeeping gene *ACTB* [38]. For that, the band representing the 345-nt pseudoexon, plus half of the value of the heteroduplexes, and the partial pseudoexon skipping band were counted as aberrant. The other half of the heteroduplexes together with the correct band were considered to be correct transcripts. We observed a nonspecific band that was not considered for the analysis. The list of primers is provided in the Supplementary Materials, Table S1.

2.6. qPCR

The cDNA samples were obtained as described above from iPSCs at day 0, and the nontreated PPCs at day 30 (both replicates) were used for quantitative real-time PCR (qPCR) to assess the differentiation process: qPCR was performed using GoTaq qPCR master mix (Promega, Madison, WI, USA). Three technical replicates were done for each of the two biological replicates. The list of primers is provided in the Supplementary Materials, Table S1.

2.7. AON Classification and Common Properties

Once the rescue was assessed, AONs were classified into 5 groups: Highly effective (>75% correction), effective (between 75% and 50%), moderately effective (between 50% and 25%), poorly effective (between 25% and 0%), and noneffective (no correction detected). For the study of the properties of each group, the groups poorly effective and noneffective were combined into one single group, as well as the highly effective and effective groups, generating three new groups: Effective, moderately effective, and poorly effective. Using this information, several potential correlations between AON properties, target motifs, and their efficacy were assessed, with the aim of establishing possible improvements in the AON design. Statistical analyses were performed using GraphPad Prism. Given the low numbers for some of the groups, normality could not be assessed, and therefore nonparametric tests were used.

Table 1. Antisense oligonucleotide (AON) sequences and general parameters.

AON#	Sequence (5' to 3')	L	Tm	GC	FE-A	FE-D	BE	Remarks
AON1	ACAGGAGUCCUCAGCAUUG	19	51.1	53	−0.1	−12.4	16.2	Specific for c.4539+2001G>A-pseudoexon
AON2	UUUUGUCCAGGGACCAAGG	19	51.1	53	−1.6	−15.6	23.1	Previously reported in Reference [18]
AON3	CUGUUACAUUUUGUCCAGG	19	46.8	42	−0.9	−7.3	20.7	Previously reported in Reference [18]
AON4	GGGGCACAGAGGACUGAGA	19	55.4	63	−0.8	−5.9	30.6	Previously reported in Reference [18]
AON5	GAGAGAAAAUAUUGCUUGAGAA	22	47.4	32	1.7	−5.0	27.5	Previously reported in Reference [18]
AON6	GCAGAUGAGCUGUGAUUCAA	20	49.7	45	−2.5	−8.8	24.0	
AON7	UAUGAUGCAGCAGAUGAGCUG	21	52.4	48	−3.9	−12.2	24.1	
AON8	UGGGAUCCCUAUGAUGCAGC	20	53.8	55	−1.1	−17.4	19.4	
AON9	AGAGGACUGAGACAAGUUCC	20	51.8	50	−4.2	−10.0	23.1	
AON10	GCUUCCUCUGGGCACAGA	20	55.9	60	−5.1	−12.0	28.4	
AON11	CCUCAGCAUGACAGCAA	18	48	50	−0.6	−3.2	16.1	
AON12	ACAGGAGCCUCAGCAUUG	19	53.2	58	−0.4	−9.3	11.1	One mismatch in c.4539+2001G>A-pseudoexon
AON13	UGGAGGCAGCCACAGAG	18	54.9	67	−1.3	−11.8	31.4	One mismatch in c.4539+2028C>T-pseudoexon
AON14	GAUGCUGGAGGGUUUUGAGUG	21	54.4	52	−1.7	−12.6	27.1	Perfect match in c.4539+2001G>A-pseudoexon Specific for c.4539+2028C>T-pseudoexon
AON15	GAUGCUGGAGAGUUUUGAGUG	21	52.4	48	−1.7	−14.2	20.2	One mismatch in c.4539+2001G>A-pseudoexon
AON16	GCCUUGACGUCCUGAUGCU	19	53.2	58	1.4	−10.3	20.4	
AON17	GCCAAGAGCUCAGGGUACAG	20	55.9	60	−0.9	−19.9	31.8	
AON18	CUUGGCCUCCCUCCCUC	18	57.2	72	1.4	−8.3	29.4	
AON19	AACACCAUGUAGGUAGGC	18	48	50	−1.6	−6.8	21.2	
AON20	GUUUAGGAAAUGAAACACCAUG	22	49.2	36	−0.7	−4.5	23.0	
AON21	GACCGCGUGGAAGUAAGG	18	52.6	61	−0.3	−14.9	22.1	
AON22	AUAAGUUUCUAAGCUGGACAG	21	48.5	38	−0.4	−8.1	27.2	
AON23	GGACCAAGGACCAACACUAC	20	53.8	55	−0.6	−9.7	27.9	
AON24	GGCUGUUACAUUUUGUCCAGG	21	52.4	48	−1.0	−7.5	28.5	
AON25	GGCAGGAACUGGCUUGCCUU	20	55.9	60	−8.6	−20.2	27.2	
AON26	AGAAGUGAAAGAAAAUGGCAGG	22	51.1	41	1.9	−3.0	23.3	
SON1	CAAUGCUGAGGACUCCUGU	19	51.1	53	−0.7	−11	6.0	Sense sequence of AON1 Previously reported in Reference [18]
SON2	UCUCAGUCCUCUGUGCCCC	19	55.4	63	−0.9	−5.6	3.4	Sense sequence of AON4

The nucleotides underlined represent the possible mismatch in relation to the mutation present in the pseudoexon (c.4539+2001G>A or c.4539+2028C>T). L: Length in nt; Tm: Melting temperature in °C; GC: GC content in %; FE-A: Free energy AON molecule; FE-D: Free energy AON dimer; BE: Binding energy to the target region. All energy values are in arbitrary units obtained using RNAstructure software (https://rna.urmc.rochester.edu/RNAstructureWeb/Servers/bifold/bifold.html).

3. Results

Previously, we showed that the variants c.4539+2001G>A and c.4539+2028C>T cause the insertion of a 345-nt pseudoexon in a retina-specific manner. Four AONs (AON1 to AON4) targeting this region were designed according to previously described guidelines [35,36,39] and were assessed in PPCs. Our results showed that two AONs (AON1 and AON4) were able to restore correct *ABCA4* splicing by skipping the pseudoexon in a mutation-dependent manner. AON1 was specific for the c.4539+2001G>A variant and was not able to correct the splicing defect caused by the c.4539+2028C>T mutation, suggesting that one nucleotide mismatch can already impair rescue efficacy. Here, we screened the entire pseudoexon region in order to identify potential new targets that can promote splicing redirection with a higher efficacy by designing 22 new AONs.

3.1. Screening and Selection of AONs

The entire pseudoexon (345 nt) together with its flanking regions were subjected to AON design. A total of 22 new AONs were designed throughout the entire region (Figure 1A). The AON design parameters, such as melting temperature (Tm), GC content, and free energy were assessed in order to have optimal sequences when possible (e.g., Tm > 48 °C, GC content between 40% and 60%). Subsequently, to further assess what AONs were targeting, we predicted the RNA structure of the region using mfold software [40]. We also checked the ESE motifs that were present in the region using an ESE finder (http://rulai.cshl.edu/) or the potential RNA binding protein sites using RBPmap (http://rbpmap.technion.ac.il/). Overall, all AONs were covering the pseudoexon or its splice sites and were targeting all types of regions (predicted to be more closed or open) and motifs.

Patient-derived iPSCs heterozygously carrying the c.4539+2001G>A mutation in conjunction with another *ABCA4* mutation on the other allele were differentiated into PPCs. Differentiation of the cells was assessed by qPCR. The results showed a differentiation toward retinal lineage with a clear increase in *ABCA4* expression (Supplementary Materials, Figure S1). As we already described, the 345-nt pseudoexon was only visible upon inhibition of nonsense-mediated decay (NMD) (Figure 1B). Therefore, PPCs were first treated with the corresponding AON and after 24 h were subjected to cycloheximide (CHX) treatment to inhibit NMD. RNA analysis was performed by RT-PCR (Figure 1B). We then semiquantified the amount of aberrant transcript (Figure 1C). Remarkably, three AONs were able to almost completely rescue the splicing defect (AON4, AON17, and AON18). Interestingly, we also observed that four AONs (AON7, AON13, AON14, and AON16) caused the appearance of additional bands. Some of them represented partial pseudoexon skipping, while others turned out to be potential artifacts due to mis-splicing, although we could not exactly determine the splicing sites. Sequencing results determined that the partial-exon skipping observed in AON14 and AON16-treated samples was a partial skipping of exon 30 (previously described in Reference [18]) together with partial skipping of the first 142 nt of the pseudoexon (splice acceptor site in c.4539+2035). In the case of AON13, we identified partial pseudoexon exclusion, but we could not determine the splice acceptor site. In the case of AON7, we could not determine both splice sites (acceptor and donor), and it was probably an aberrant mRNA caused by the AON treatment. Using the average of the cells not treated with AONs but subjected to CHX treatment and the ones treated with the sense oligonucleotide (SON), we established the basal levels (~29%) of the *ABCA4* aberrant transcript (Figure 1C). These values were used to establish the percentage of correction for each AON (Figure 2A). Five groups were determined: Highly effective (correction >75%, $n = 3$), effective (75%–50%, $n = 6$), moderately effective (50%–25%, $n = 8$), poorly effective (25%–0%, $n = 9$), and noneffective (0% or even increasing the amount of pseudoexon). These groups are depicted in Figure 2A according to different colors in the graph.

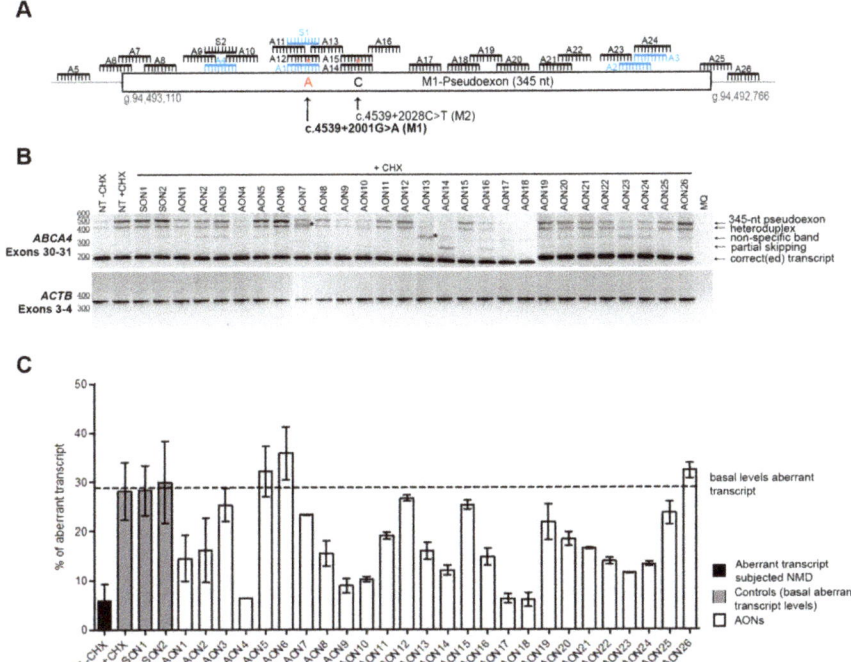

Figure 1. AON-based pseudoexon skipping efficacy. (**A**) Schematic representation of the 345-nt pseudoexon insertion caused by the c.4539+2001G>A mutation and the location of the 26 AONs and the 2 sense oligonucleotides (SONs). Blue oligonucleotides refer to previously studied molecules [18]. Red asterisks represent mismatches with the pseudoexon sequence created only by the c.4539+2001G>A mutation (namely an A at position c.4539+2001 and a C at position c.4539+2028). (**B**) Representative image of an RT-PCR performed on patient-derived photoreceptor precursor cells (PPCs) upon AON treatment. *ACTB* was used to normalize samples. An heteroduplex band was observed in all samples, containing the correct and the pseudoexon-included transcripts. AON-derived partial skipping was observed in samples AON14 and AON16. Double bands highlighted with an * (lanes AON7 and AON13) indicate artifacts derived from the AON treatment, and splice sites could not be identified upon Sanger sequencing. In most of the lanes, we identified a PCR artifact (nonspecific band). (**C**) Percentage of aberrant transcript after semiquantification. NT: Nontreated; CHX: Cycloheximide. Error bars indicate average ± SD.

3.2. Analysis of the Properties of the AONs

Once the efficacy of all AONs was estimated, we subdivided them into three larger groups: Effective ($n = 9$ comprising all AONs with an efficacy > 50%), moderately effective ($n = 8$ with efficacies between 25% and 50%), and poorly effective ($n = 7$, the rest). AONs containing a mismatch (AON12 and AON15) were not used in these analyses, as the decrease in the efficacy was due to the mismatch. This was shown by the fact that both AON1 and AON14 (perfectly matching the c.4539+2001G>A allele, but containing a mismatch for the PE induced by the c.4539+2028C>T mutation) correct the splice defect associated with c.4539+2001G>A.

We first analyzed the basic parameters: Melting temperature (Tm), GC content, and length (Figure 2B). We found a statistically significant correlation (two-tailed Spearman test) for the Tm and GC content parameters ($p = 0.0012$ and $p = 0.0041$, respectively). In both cases, the higher the value was, the more efficient the AON was (Supplementary Materials, Figure S2). The Tm average of the three groups ranged from 54.21 °C (effective) to 50.19 °C (poorly effective). The differences in Tm between groups was statistically different ($p = 0.0292$, nonparametric one-way ANOVA), while the GC content was nearly significant ($p = 0.0611$). When comparing all different groups separately, statistically significant differences were observed between the groups of effective AONs and poorly effective AONs for Tm ($p = 0.0256$, Mann–Whitney test) and GC content ($p = 0.0127$). No differences were observed for the length of the AONs.

Other important parameters when designing AONs are the free energy of the AON molecule itself, the dimer, and the binding energy to the target. The free energy of the AON molecule and its dimer did not show any correlation nor difference between groups. Interestingly, the binding energy showed a significant correlation ($p = 0.0391$) with efficacy. We analyzed the groups separately, and although no statistically significant differences were found, the effective group showed a trend toward significance when compared to the moderately effective ($p = 0.0673$, Mann–Whitney test) and the poorly effective ($p = 0.0712$, Mann–Whitney test) groups. Consistently, the highest binding energies corresponded to the three most effective AONs (AON4, AON17, and AON18). Interestingly, when these three values were separated, the tendency of the effective group disappeared. In contrast, these three AONs only showed a statistically significant higher binding energy compared to the other three groups (Figure 2C).

Next, we checked the common serine and arginine-rich splicing factors (SRSFs): SF2 (SRSF1), SC35 (SRSF2), SRp40 (SRSF4), and SRp55 (SRSF5)) using an ESE finder (Supplementary Materials, Figure S3). All motifs that were partially or completely covered by an AON were counted and assigned to the particular AON. We did not find any correlation between the percentage of correction and the presence of these motifs. However, we noticed that the strength of some of the motifs was different between groups. For that, we categorized all the motifs found by assigning them a number according to the strength of the predicted score (lowest = 1, second lowest = 2, etc.). After that, the average for each AON was calculated. Interestingly, a statistically significant correlation ($p = 0.0066$, two-tailed Spearman test) was observed for the categorized SRp40 motifs. In this case, the strongest motifs were correlating with the poorly or moderately effective AONs, and the lowest with the effective ones (Figure 2D). However, when pooling all groups together, differences were not statistically significant. No other differences were detected for any of the other three SRSF motifs, except for SC35, where significant differences were observed when comparing effective versus moderately effective AONs ($p = 0.0316$, Mann–Whitney test; Supplementary Materials, Figure S3).

Finally, we used RBPmap to predict potential RNA protein-binding motifs. Again, each motif detected in the region was assigned to each AON when partial or complete overlap occurred. First, manual filtering of the motifs was done by checking which motifs were common to all AONs in each group. Unfortunately, none of the motifs were shared between all effective AONs. AON18 was the one behaving differently than the rest, almost not sharing any motif with the others. When AON18 was left out of the filtering, SRSF3 appeared as a common motif not only in the effective group, but also in the poorly and moderately effective groups. When assessed in more detail (Figure 2D), a statistically significant negative correlation was observed ($p = 0.0188$, two-tailed Spearman test). The analysis per group revealed a significant difference between the effective and poorly effective groups ($p = 0.0431$) and close to significance between the moderately and poorly effective groups ($p = 0.0622$). Categorized SRSF3 did not show significant differences. The second most recurrent motif in the poorly effective group was MBNL1. Given the fact that all but one poorly acting AON contained this predicted motif, we performed statistical analyses to determine whether the presence of MBNL1 motifs correlated with the lower performance of some AONs. Indeed, a significant correlation was observed ($p = 0.0025$), implying an association between the presence of these motifs and a low AON performance (Figure 2D). When differences between groups were assessed, only the effective group showed a statistically significant lower number of MBNL1 when compared to the poorly effective group ($p = 0.0309$). The total amount of motifs detected by RBPmap showed a nearly significant negative correlation with efficiency ($p = 0.0522$). However, when groups were analyzed separately, this trend completely disappeared (Supplementary Materials, Figure S4).

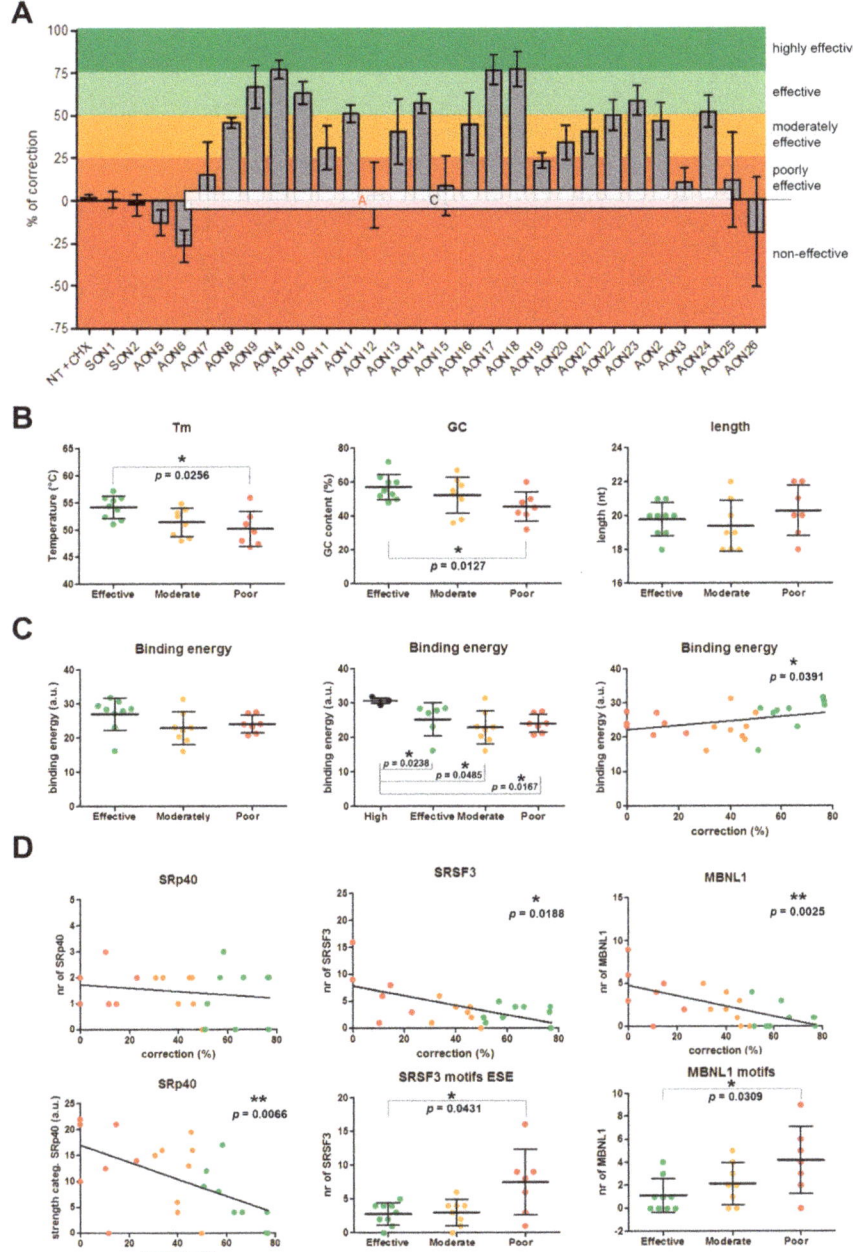

Figure 2. Assessment of AON efficacy and correlations. (**A**) Percentage of correction for each AON. AONs are located according to their position in the c.4539+2001G>A-specific pseudoexon. Colors indicate the efficacy classification that was established. (**B–C**) Representation of the statistical analyses for general parameters taken into account for AON design. (**D**) Analysis of the influence of certain motifs in AON efficacy. Error bars in all graphs indicate average ± SD.

4. Discussion

The fact that the eye is an isolated, immunoprivileged, and easily accessible organ makes it a very attractive model for molecular therapies. In addition, IRDs are progressive diseases that offer a window of opportunity for treatment. However, the high genetic heterogeneity in IRDs hampers the development of new therapies. AONs have been shown to be an auspicious approach to treat splicing defects causing IRDs. They have been shown to be safe and easy to deliver to the retina without the necessity of any vector. Furthermore, recent results from a phase 1/2 clinical trial to correct the splicing defect introduced by a deep-intronic mutation in *CEP290* showed the great potential that these molecules hold. In this study, we screened 26 AONs targeting a pseudoexon product of a recurrent deep-intronic mutation (c.4539+2001G>A) in the *ABCA4* gene with the intention of identifying the most promising AON molecules to eventually treat STGD1.

We designed and tested 26 different AONs located across the 345-nt pseudoexon. In total, three highly effective AONs were identified: AON4, AON17, and AON18. All of them showed similar efficacies (76.42%–76.97%). Another six AONs (AON1, AON9, AON10, AON14, AON23, and AON24) corrected the pre-mRNA splicing defect with an efficacy of more than 50%. Previously, we showed that AON1 was only effective when the change c.4539+2001G>A was present, as the pseudoexon containing the change c.4539+2028C>T was not removed. This highlighted the fact that for 2'OMe/PS chemically modified AONs, one mismatch could dramatically affect the splicing redirection efficacy. Here, we demonstrated again that one mismatch was enough to prevent AON-based splicing modulation. For that, we generated the same AON1 but with a wild-type nucleotide (AON12). Furthermore, we also designed an AON specific for the c.4539+2028C>T variant (AON15) and a corresponding AON with a wild-type change (AON14). As expected, the mutation-specific AON (AON15) did not redirect splicing in this cell line, while the one perfectly matching the target did (AON14). Interestingly, AON14, although its correction efficacy was around 50%, is not considered a very promising AON for future studies since it was one of the four AONs (together with AON7, AON13, and AON16) that showed novel aberrant bands in RT-PCR. In this particular case, both AON14 and AON16 caused an unexpected (AONs binding on top of the novel splice acceptor site at position c.4539+2035) partial pseudoexon exclusion together with an already described partial exon 30 skipping [18]. However, this was clearly induced by these two AONs, which bind in the same region. However, for AON7 and AON13, we were not able to determine how the aberrant band was generated due to the lack of predicted splicing sites, and therefore we considered them artifacts. We previously observed a similar effect for another variant, and we concluded that this was either a PCR artifact or, due to the fact that AONs can interfere with RNA structure and the splicing machinery, some aberrant mis-spliced transcripts that may have appeared [20].

After classifying the AONs into three groups, we tried to identify common properties that could eventually lead to a better AON design. When analyzing the groups, we found correlations with the Tm and the GC content. Previously published guidelines [35,36,39] have indicated that Tm should be above 48 °C and the GC content between 40% and 60%. Based on our analyses, it seems that if the temperature is higher than 51 °C and the GC content close to 60%, the chances of designing an AON with a good efficacy are higher. According to previous guidelines, the binding energy should stay between 21 and 28. However, our best AON molecules had binding energies to the target of more than 30. Moreover, based on correlations that we were able to identify, AONs targeting predicted SRSF3 or MBNL1, as well as strong predicted SRp40 motifs, might show poorer efficacies. Although some of these parameters have been shown before to be relevant to AON design, it is important to mention that the efficacy of an AON molecule also can depend on the type of cell, tissue, or organ. In that sense, the parameters established above might be valid only for AONs delivered to retinal cells, and further confirmation in cells of other origins needs to be addressed. Unfortunately, this comparison was not possible in our case due to the fact that although *ABCA4* is lowly expressed in fibroblast cells, the splicing defects observed for some mutations, including c.4539+2001G>A, are not recapitulated in those cells. Most probably this is because the splicing retinal machinery may have different efficacies or recognition sites [41,42].

In our previous studies, AON1 showed an efficacy of ~75% [18]. However, in this study, only ~51% correction was detected, although the PPCs were derived from the same patient iPSC line. One explanation could be that in our previous study, we only detected around 25% of pseudoexon insertion, while in this study we were able to detect more pseudoexon-including transcripts (~30%). This could therefore have modified the correction ratio. In addition, the inhibition of NMD by CHX is not always complete, and therefore variability in the detection of the pseudoexon transcript (subjected to NMD) might have been variable between experiments and samples. Another possible explanation could be differences between the AON batches. All of these factors, either alone or in combination, could have influenced the differences observed between the two studies.

Finally, as discussed above, AON4, AON17, and AON18 showed the highest efficacies. However, AON18 did not show that much similarity to the other two AONs other than a high binding energy. AON18 did not share obvious targeted predicted motifs with either of the two highly effective AONs (Supplementary Materials, Figure S5). We also checked the secondary structure of the RNA and all three AON target partially closed regions. Therefore, the slightly higher efficacy might have been related to the binding to the target itself and the disruption of the secondary structure rather than the motifs that were blocked by the molecule. In addition, when comparing the sequences to see which one could be a potential candidate for further development, we observed that all three AONs contained stretches of Gs and Cs (which are recommended to be avoided). AON4 and AON17 contained a G stretch of four and three Gs, respectively, while AON18 contained two stretches of three and four Cs. Nevertheless, given their efficacy, all three molecules might be potential good candidates for further therapeutic studies.

5. Conclusions

In conclusion, we designed 26 AONs targeting a 345-nt pseudoexon caused by the recurrent c.4539+2001G>A deep-intronic mutation in *ABCA4*. In total, nine AONs showed promising efficacies (correction above 50%). We identified three AONs promoting a correction superior to 75%. For AON design, we suggest increasing the minimum Tm to 50 or 51 °C, the GC content close to 60%, and the binding energy to around 30 to target retinal pseudoexons, although this needs to be tested and confirmed using other targets. Overall, we demonstrated that AON-based splicing modulation holds great potential for treating Stargardt disease caused by splicing defects in *ABCA4*.

6. Patents

A.G. and R.W.J.C. are inventors on a filed patent (PCT/EP2017/1082627) that is related to the contents of this manuscript.

Supplementary Materials: The following are available online at http://www.mdpi.com/2073-4425/10/6/452/s1, Table S1: List of primers; Figure S1: Analysis by qPCR of iPSCs and photoreceptor precursor cells; Figure S2: Representation of the correlation on general parameters; Figure S3: Representation of the analyses performed on regular exonic splicing enhancers; Figur S4: Analysis of all predicted RNA binding sites using RBPmap; Figure S5: Schematic representation of the percentage of correction with exonic splicing enhancers and silencers.

Author Contributions: Conceptualization: A.G. and R.W.J.C.; methodology and experimental work: A.G. and L.D.; results analysis: A.G., L.D., and R.W.J.C.; writing and reviewing the manuscript: all authors; funding acquisition: A.G. and R.W.J.C.

Funding: This work was supported by the Algemene Nederlandse Vereniging ter Voorkoming van Blindheid, Stichting Blinden-Penning, Landelijke Stichting voor Blinden en Slechtzienden, Stichting Oogfonds Nederland, Stichting Macula Degeneratie Fonds, and Stichting Retina Nederland Fonds (who contributed through UitZicht 2015-31 and 2018-21), together with the Rotterdamse Stichting Blindenbelangen, Stichting Blindenhulp, Stichting tot Verbetering van het Lot der Blinden, Stichting voor Ooglijders, and Stichting Dowilvo (to A.G. and R.W.J.C.). This work was also supported by the Foundation Fighting Blindness USA, grant no. PPA-0517-0717-RAD (to A.G. and R.W.J.C.). The funding organizations had no role in the design or conduct of this research. They provided unrestricted grants.

Acknowledgments: The authors would like to thank the Stem Cell Technology Center of the Radboudumc for providing iPSCs.

Conflicts of Interest: A.G. and R.W.J.C. declare that they are inventors on a filed patent (PCT/EP2017/1082627) that is related to the contents of this manuscript. The rest of the authors declare no conflicts of interest.

References

1. Stargardt, K. Über familiäre, progressive Degeneration in der Maculagegend des Auges. *Albrecht von Graefes Archiv für Ophthalmologie* **1909**, *71*, 534–550. [CrossRef]
2. Birnbach, C.D.; Jarvelainen, M.; Possin, D.E.; Milam, A.H. Histopathology and immunocytochemistry of the neurosensory retina in fundus flavimaculatus. *Ophthalmology* **1994**, *101*, 1211–1219. [CrossRef]
3. Sahel, J.A.; Marazova, K.; Audo, I. Clinical characteristics and current therapies for inherited retinal degenerations. *Cold Spring Harb. Perspect. Med.* **2014**, *5*, a017111. [CrossRef] [PubMed]
4. Zernant, J.; Xie, Y.A.; Ayuso, C.; Riveiro-Alvarez, R.; Lopez-Martinez, M.A.; Simonelli, F.; Testa, F.; Gorin, M.B.; Strom, S.P.; Bertelsen, M.; et al. Analysis of the *ABCA4* genomic locus in Stargardt disease. *Hum. Mol. Genet.* **2014**, *23*, 6797–6806. [CrossRef] [PubMed]
5. Vasiliou, V.; Vasiliou, K.; Nebert, D.W. Human ATP-binding cassette (ABC) transporter family. *Hum. Genom.* **2009**, *3*, 281–290. [CrossRef]
6. Molday, R.S. Insights into the Molecular Properties of *ABCA4* and Its Role in the Visual Cycle and Stargardt Disease. *Prog. Mol. Biol. Transl. Sci.* **2015**, *134*, 415–431. [PubMed]
7. Molday, R.S.; Zhong, M.; Quazi, F. The role of the photoreceptor ABC transporter *ABCA4* in lipid transport and Stargardt macular degeneration. *Biochim. Biophys. Acta* **2009**, *1791*, 573–583. [CrossRef]
8. Quazi, F.; Lenevich, S.; Molday, R.S. ABCA4 is an N-retinylidene-phosphatidylethanolamine and phosphatidylethanolamine importer. *Nat. Commun.* **2012**, *3*, 925. [CrossRef]
9. Cornelis, S.S.; Bax, N.M.; Zernant, J.; Allikmets, R.; Fritsche, L.G.; den Dunnen, J.T.; Ajmal, M.; Hoyng, C.B.; Cremers, F.P. In Silico Functional Meta-Analysis of 5,962 *ABCA4* Variants in 3,928 Retinal Dystrophy Cases. *Hum. Mutat.* **2017**, *38*, 400–408. [CrossRef]
10. Maugeri, A.; van Driel, M.A.; van de Pol, D.J.; Klevering, B.J.; van Haren, F.J.; Tijmes, N.; Bergen, A.A.; Rohrschneider, K.; Blankenagel, A.; Pinckers, A.J.; et al. The 2588G→C mutation in the ABCR gene is a mild frequent founder mutation in the Western European population and allows the classification of ABCR mutations in patients with Stargardt disease. *Am. J. Hum. Genet.* **1999**, *64*, 1024–1035. [CrossRef]
11. Sheffield, V.C.; Stone, E.M. Genomics and the eye. *N. Engl. J. Med.* **2011**, *364*, 1932–1942. [CrossRef] [PubMed]
12. Zernant, J.; Collison, F.T.; Lee, W.; Fishman, G.A.; Noupuu, K.; Yuan, B.; Cai, C.; Lupski, J.R.; Yannuzzi, L.A.; Tsang, S.H.; et al. Genetic and clinical analysis of *ABCA4*-associated disease in African American patients. *Hum. Mutat.* **2014**, *35*, 1187–1194. [CrossRef] [PubMed]
13. Braun, T.A.; Mullins, R.F.; Wagner, A.H.; Andorf, J.L.; Johnston, R.M.; Bakall, B.B.; Deluca, A.P.; Fishman, G.A.; Lam, B.L.; Weleber, R.G.; et al. Non-exomic and synonymous variants in *ABCA4* are an important cause of Stargardt disease. *Hum. Mol. Genet.* **2013**, *22*, 5136–5145. [CrossRef] [PubMed]
14. Bauwens, M.; De Zaeytijd, J.; Weisschuh, N.; Kohl, S.; Meire, F.; Dahan, K.; Depasse, F.; De Jaegere, S.; De Ravel, T.; De Rademaeker, M.; et al. An augmented *ABCA4* screen targeting noncoding regions reveals a deep intronic founder variant in Belgian Stargardt patients. *Hum. Mutat.* **2015**, *36*, 39–42. [CrossRef] [PubMed]
15. Bax, N.M.; Sangermano, R.; Roosing, S.; Thiadens, A.A.; Hoefsloot, L.H.; van den Born, L.I.; Phan, M.; Klevering, B.J.; Westeneng-van Haaften, C.; Braun, T.A.; et al. Heterozygous deep-intronic variants and deletions in *ABCA4* in persons with retinal dystrophies and one exonic *ABCA4* variant. *Hum. Mutat.* **2015**, *36*, 43–47. [CrossRef] [PubMed]
16. Sangermano, R.; Bax, N.M.; Bauwens, M.; van den Born, L.I.; De Baere, E.; Garanto, A.; Collin, R.W.; Goercharn-Ramlal, A.S.; den Engelsman-van Dijk, A.H.; Rohrschneider, K.; et al. Photoreceptor Progenitor mRNA Analysis Reveals Exon Skipping Resulting from the *ABCA4* c.5461-10T→C Mutation in Stargardt Disease. *Ophthalmology* **2016**, *123*, 1375–1385. [CrossRef] [PubMed]
17. Zernant, J.; Lee, W.; Nagasaki, T.; Collison, F.T.; Fishman, G.A.; Bertelsen, M.; Rosenberg, T.; Gouras, P.; Tsang, S.H.; Allikmets, R. Extremely hypomorphic and severe deep intronic variants in the *ABCA4* locus result in varying Stargardt disease phenotypes. *Mol. Case Stud.* **2018**, *4*, a002733. [CrossRef]

18. Albert, S.; Garanto, A.; Sangermano, R.; Khan, M.; Bax, N.M.; Hoyng, C.B.; Zernant, J.; Lee, W.; Allikmets, R.; Collin, R.W.J.; et al. Identification and Rescue of Splice Defects Caused by Two Neighboring Deep-Intronic *ABCA4* Mutations Underlying Stargardt Disease. *Am. J. Hum. Genet.* **2018**, *102*, 517–527. [CrossRef]
19. Sangermano, R.; Khan, M.; Cornelis, S.S.; Richelle, V.; Albert, S.; Garanto, A.; Elmelik, D.; Qamar, R.; Lugtenberg, D.; van den Born, L.I.; et al. *ABCA4* midigenes reveal the full splice spectrum of all reported noncanonical splice site variants in Stargardt disease. *Genome Res.* **2018**, *28*, 100–110. [CrossRef]
20. Sangermano, R.; Garanto, A.; Khan, M.; Runhart, E.H.; Bauwens, M.; Bax, N.M.; van den Born, L.I.; Khan, M.I.; Cornelis, S.S.; Verheij, J.B.G.M.; et al. Deep-intronic *ABCA4* variants explain missing heritability in Stargardt disease and allow correction of splice defects by antisense oligonucleotides. *Genet. Med.* **2019**. [CrossRef]
21. Shen, X.; Corey, D.R. Chemistry, mechanism and clinical status of antisense oligonucleotides and duplex RNAs. *Nucleic Acids Res.* **2018**, *46*, 1584–1600. [CrossRef] [PubMed]
22. Collin, R.W.; den Hollander, A.I.; van der Velde-Visser, S.D.; Bennicelli, J.; Bennett, J.; Cremers, F.P. Antisense Oligonucleotide (AON)-based Therapy for Leber Congenital Amaurosis Caused by a Frequent Mutation in CEP290. *Mol. Ther. Nucleic Acids* **2012**, *1*, e14. [CrossRef] [PubMed]
23. Gerard, X.; Perrault, I.; Hanein, S.; Silva, E.; Bigot, K.; Defoort-Delhemmes, S.; Rio, M.; Munnich, A.; Scherman, D.; Kaplan, J.; et al. AON-mediated Exon Skipping Restores Ciliation in Fibroblasts Harboring the Common Leber Congenital Amaurosis CEP290 Mutation. *Mol. Ther. Nucleic Acids* **2012**, *1*, e29. [CrossRef] [PubMed]
24. Garanto, A.; Chung, D.C.; Duijkers, L.; Corral-Serrano, J.C.; Messchaert, M.; Xiao, R.; Bennett, J.; Vandenberghe, L.H.; Collin, R.W. In vitro and in vivo rescue of aberrant splicing in CEP290-associated LCA by antisense oligonucleotide delivery. *Hum. Mol. Genet.* **2016**, *25*, 2552–2563. [PubMed]
25. Parfitt, D.A.; Lane, A.; Ramsden, C.M.; Carr, A.J.; Munro, P.M.; Jovanovic, K.; Schwarz, N.; Kanuga, N.; Muthiah, M.N.; Hull, S.; et al. Identification and Correction of Mechanisms Underlying Inherited Blindness in Human iPSC-Derived Optic Cups. *Cell Stem Cell* **2016**, *18*, 769–781. [CrossRef] [PubMed]
26. Duijkers, L.; van den Born, L.I.; Neidhardt, J.; Bax, N.M.; Pierrache, L.H.M.; Klevering, B.J.; Collin, R.W.J.; Garanto, A. Antisense Oligonucleotide-Based Splicing Correction in Individuals with Leber Congenital Amaurosis due to Compound Heterozygosity for the c.2991+1655A>G Mutation in CEP290. *Int. J. Mol. Sci.* **2018**, *19*, 753. [CrossRef] [PubMed]
27. Dulla, K.; Aguila, M.; Lane, A.; Jovanovic, K.; Parfitt, D.A.; Schulkens, I.; Chan, H.L.; Schmidt, I.; Beumer, W.; Vorthoren, L.; et al. Splice-Modulating Oligonucleotide QR-110 Restores CEP290 mRNA and Function in Human c.2991+1655A>G LCA10 Models. *Mol. Ther. Nucleic Acids* **2018**, *12*, 730–740. [CrossRef] [PubMed]
28. Slijkerman, R.W.; Vache, C.; Dona, M.; Garcia-Garcia, G.; Claustres, M.; Hetterschijt, L.; Peters, T.A.; Hartel, B.P.; Pennings, R.J.; Millan, J.M.; et al. Antisense Oligonucleotide-based Splice Correction for USH2A-associated Retinal Degeneration Caused by a Frequent Deep-intronic Mutation. *Mol. Ther. Nucleic Acids* **2016**, *5*, e381. [CrossRef]
29. Garanto, A.; van der Velde-Visser, S.D.; Cremers, F.P.M.; Collin, R.W.J. Antisense Oligonucleotide-Based Splice Correction of a Deep-Intronic Mutation in CHM Underlying Choroideremia. *Adv. Exp. Med. Biol.* **2018**, *1074*, 83–89.
30. Bonifert, T.; Gonzalez Menendez, I.; Battke, F.; Theurer, Y.; Synofzik, M.; Schols, L.; Wissinger, B. Antisense Oligonucleotide Mediated Splice Correction of a Deep Intronic Mutation in OPA1. *Mol. Ther. Nucleic Acids* **2016**, *5*, e390. [CrossRef]
31. Bauwens, M.; Garanto, A.; Sangermano, R.; Naessens, S.; Weisschuh, N.; De Zaeytijd, J.; Khan, M.; Sadler, F.; Balikova, I.; Van Cauwenbergh, C.; et al. *ABCA4*-associated disease as a model for missing heritability in autosomal recessive disorders: Novel noncoding splice, cis-regulatory, structural, and recurrent hypomorphic variants. *Genet. Med. Off. J. Am. Coll. Med. Genet.* **2019**. [CrossRef] [PubMed]
32. Cideciyan, A.V.; Jacobson, S.G.; Drack, A.V.; Ho, A.C.; Charng, J.; Garafalo, A.V.; Roman, A.J.; Sumaroka, A.; Han, I.C.; Hochstedler, M.D.; et al. Effect of an intravitreal antisense oligonucleotide on vision in Leber congenital amaurosis due to a photoreceptor cilium defect. *Nat. Med.* **2019**, *25*, 225–228. [CrossRef] [PubMed]
33. Homolova, K.; Zavadakova, P.; Doktor, T.K.; Schroeder, L.D.; Kozich, V.; Andresen, B.S. The deep intronic c.903+469T>C mutation in the MTRR gene creates an SF2/ASF binding exonic splicing enhancer, which leads to pseudoexon activation and causes the cblE type of homocystinuria. *Hum. Mutat.* **2010**, *31*, 437–444. [CrossRef] [PubMed]

34. Rincon, A.; Aguado, C.; Desviat, L.R.; Sanchez-Alcudia, R.; Ugarte, M.; Perez, B. Propionic and methylmalonic acidemia: Antisense therapeutics for intronic variations causing aberrantly spliced messenger RNA. *Am. J. Hum. Genet.* **2007**, *81*, 1262–1270. [CrossRef] [PubMed]
35. Aartsma-Rus, A. Overview on AON design. *Methods Mol. Biol.* **2012**, *867*, 117–129. [PubMed]
36. Collin, R.W.; Garanto, A. Applications of antisense oligonucleotides for the treatment of inherited retinal diseases. *Curr. Opin. Ophthalmol.* **2017**, *28*, 260–266. [CrossRef] [PubMed]
37. Flamier, A.; Barabino, A.; Gilbert, B. Differentiation of Human Embryonic Stem Cells into Cone Photoreceptors. *Bio-Protoc.* **2016**, *6*, e1870. [CrossRef]
38. Schindelin, J.; Arganda-Carreras, I.; Frise, E.; Kaynig, V.; Longair, M.; Pietzsch, T.; Preibisch, S.; Rueden, C.; Saalfeld, S.; Schmid, B.; et al. Fiji: An open-source platform for biological-image analysis. *Nat. Methods* **2012**, *9*, 676–682. [CrossRef] [PubMed]
39. Slijkerman, R.; Kremer, H.; van Wijk, E. Antisense Oligonucleotide Design and Evaluation of Splice-Modulating Properties Using Cell-Based Assays. *Methods Mol. Biol.* **2018**, *1828*, 519–530.
40. Zuker, M. Mfold web server for nucleic acid folding and hybridization prediction. *Nucleic Acid Res.* **2013**, *31*, 3406–3415. [CrossRef]
41. Garanto, A.; Riera, M.; Pomares, E.; Permanyer, J.; de Castro-Miro, M.; Sava, F.; Abril, J.F.; Marfany, G.; Gonzalez-Duarte, R. High transcriptional complexity of the retinitis pigmentosa CERKL gene in human and mouse. *Investig. Ophthalmol. Vis. Sci.* **2011**, *52*, 5202–5214. [CrossRef] [PubMed]
42. Murphy, D.; Cieply, B.; Carstens, R.; Ramamurthy, V.; Stoilov, P. The Musashi 1 Controls the Splicing of Photoreceptor-Specific Exons in the Vertebrate Retina. *PLoS Genet.* **2016**, *12*, e1006256. [CrossRef] [PubMed]

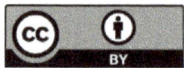

© 2019 by the authors. Licensee MDPI, Basel, Switzerland. This article is an open access article distributed under the terms and conditions of the Creative Commons Attribution (CC BY) license (http://creativecommons.org/licenses/by/4.0/).

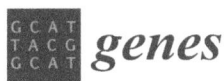

Review

Balancing the Photoreceptor Proteome: Proteostasis Network Therapeutics for Inherited Retinal Disease

Siebren Faber and Ronald Roepman *

Department of Human Genetics and Radboud Institute for Molecular Life Sciences,
Radboud University Medical Center, Geert Grooteplein Zuid 10, 6525 GA Nijmegen, The Netherlands
* Correspondence: ronald.roepman@radboudumc.nl

Received: 10 June 2019; Accepted: 16 July 2019; Published: 24 July 2019

Abstract: The light sensing outer segments of photoreceptors (PRs) are renewed every ten days due to their high photoactivity, especially of the cones during daytime vision. This demands a tremendous amount of energy, as well as a high turnover of their main biosynthetic compounds, membranes, and proteins. Therefore, a refined proteostasis network (PN), regulating the protein balance, is crucial for PR viability. In many inherited retinal diseases (IRDs) this balance is disrupted leading to protein accumulation in the inner segment and eventually the death of PRs. Various studies have been focusing on therapeutically targeting the different branches of the PR PN to restore the protein balance and ultimately to treat inherited blindness. This review first describes the different branches of the PN in detail. Subsequently, insights are provided on how therapeutic compounds directed against the different PN branches might slow down or even arrest the appalling, progressive blinding conditions. These insights are supported by findings of PN modulators in other research disciplines.

Keywords: protein trafficking; protein folding; protein degradation; chaperones; chaperonins; heat shock response; unfolded protein response; autophagy; therapy

1. Introduction

The rod and cone photoreceptor (PR) cells are the most abundant cell types in the human retina, with ~6.4 million cones and up to 125 million rods per adult retina [1]. PRs are highly specialized, polarized neurons of neuroepithelial origin, consisting of morphologically and functionally distinct cellular compartments, including a synaptic terminal, an inner segment (IS), an outer segment (OS), and a connecting cilium bridging the IS and OS. The classical division into rods and cones is based on their different OS morphology and differential expression of subtypes of opsin. The rod outer segments are long, thin, rod-shaped organelles containing rhodopsin in large stacks of membranous discs, allowing to process variations in dim-light conditions, but they lose this ability in bright light conditions. The OSs of cones represent a shorter conical organelle containing either S-opsin, M-opsin, or L-opsin, which are less sensitive compared to rhodopsin, but are perfectly suited to process bright light of different wavelengths, allowing color vision [2].

Despite the difference in photosensitivity, the process of converting light stimuli into biochemical signals, the phototransduction cascade, is almost indistinguishable between rods and cones [3,4]. In rods, upon capture of a photon, the chromophore 11-*cis* retinal, which is conjugated to a rhodopsin molecule, undergoes a conformational change that isomerizes it to all-*trans* retinal leading to the activation of rod opsin. The activated opsin molecule is now able to bind and subsequently activate the G-protein, transducin. Transducin consists of three subunits: G_α, G_β, and G_γ. In its inactive state, G_α is bound to a GDP. When transducin gets activated by rhodopsin, this GDP is replaced by a GTP and subsequently G_α dissociates from the $G_{\beta\gamma}$ subunit. The GTP bound G_α is now able to displace one of the two inhibitory γ-subunits of cGMP-specific 3′,5′-cyclic phosphodiesterase (PDE6) causing the exposure of one of the two catalytic sites of the PDE6$_{\alpha\beta}$ heterodimer (PDE6$_{\alpha'}$ for cones). The exposed catalytic sites are now able to hydrolyze multiple cGMP molecules to 5′-GMP. In the dark state, cGMP binds to its specific cation channel allowing a steady movement of cations into the OS, which is compensated by the efflux of cations from the OS by Na$^+$/Ca^{2+}, K$^+$ exchangers (NCKXs) [5]. Due to the hydrolysis of cGMP, its levels decrease causing the closure of cation channels in the OS. The resulting hyperpolarization of the OS membrane spreads throughout the cell, eventually reaching the synaptic terminal. Here, the hyperpolarization causes closure of calcium channels and subsequently a decrease in calcium-dependent synaptic glutamate release [3,4], which activates the glutamate receptors of the bipolar cells postsynaptically, transducing the brain-bound electrical signal [6].

The phototransduction cascade, carried out in only a few milliseconds, is based on capture of one single photon in dim light. However, in bright daylight conditions, immense amounts of photons are caught by the human PRs, mainly cones, every second, which causes toxic photo-oxidative damage to the OS components. These components, which include most proteins involved in the phototransduction cascade, are therefore continuously renewed (~10% every day for human PRs), by incorporating newly synthesized PR discs at the OS base, and shedding the oldest membrane discs at the cell's tip [7,8]. The shed OS tips are subsequently phagocytosed by the retinal pigment epithelium (RPE) cells, which is the highest active phagocytic process in our body [9,10]. Because of this highly active protein turnover, a mutation in a gene encoding a protein involved in this machinery most often leads to PR cell death, a classical hallmark of many inherited retinal diseases (IRDs).

IRDs are a genetically heterogeneous group of rare eye disorders with a progressive manifestation causing vision loss or even complete blindness [11]. Mutations in many genes that are required for PR function were found to be causative for IRDs. These include genes encoding proteins involved in protein trafficking, splicing, energy metabolism, and photoreceptor structure [12]. The compartments of PRs most prominently implicated in IRDs are the OS and the connecting cilium. The connecting cilium correlates with the transition zone of a primary cilium and functions as a gatekeeper to regulate the molecular composition of the OS. Thus, the OS, connecting cilium, and the immediately adjacent basal body, form the photoreceptor sensory cilium, one of the most highly specialized primary cilia, fully optimized for photoreception and transduction [13,14]. Hence, IRDs with defects in these compartments are referred to as retinal ciliopathies [11].

Defects in the conserved ciliary processes mostly manifest as syndromic ciliopathy conditions, affecting multiple organs. The most prominent ciliopathies in which the retina is affected are Bardet–Biedl syndrome (BBS), Joubert syndrome (JS), Meckel–Gruber syndrome (MKS), and Senior–Løken syndrome (SLS) [4,11]. Because PRs are highly specialized, polarized neurons, retinal ciliopathies often also occur in a nonsyndromic fashion, affecting ciliary proteins specific to rods and/or cones. Based on the PR cell type affected, different IRDs can be categorized, including retinitis pigmentosa (RP), Leber congenital amaurosis (LCA), cone-rod dystrophy (CRD), and achromatopsia (ACHM) [4,11].

RP is the most common form of inherited blindness worldwide, with a prevalence of about 1:4000 people. The cells that are affected initially in RP are the rods leading to night blindness and loss of peripheral vision. Secondary, cones are most often also affected as the disease progresses [15].

LCA is the most severe form of inherited retinal degeneration, causing patients to suffer from severe visual impairment to complete blindness before the first year of life. With LCA, both rods and cones are affected at early stages often leading to complete blindness [16].

Another early onset form of hereditary retinal dystrophy is CRD, which manifest in the opposite order compared to RP, since in CRD cones are initially affected, followed by the loss of rods [17].

A disease in which specifically the cones deteriorate is ACHM, most often leading to complete color blindness [18].

Apart from some specific exceptions, most of the above described blinding conditions are still considered incurable. However, significant and promising progress has been made with therapeutic studies targeting specific genes and/or mutations, most prominently by employing gene augmentation and antisense-oligo nucleotide (AON)-based techniques [19,20]. Yet, a major disadvantage of these treatments is that they are complex and invasive for the patient. On top of that, for nearly every mutation, a personalized approach needs to be developed. Therefore, there is a high interest in pharmacological agents with a broad range of disease targets. To discover such agents, a growing number of studies have focused on a common phenomenon seen in many IRDs before the actual death of rods and cones: the accumulation and/or misfolding of proteins in the inner segment of the photoreceptors [21].

This phenomenon can be explained by the malfunction of several processes, all involved in protein homeostasis or proteostasis. A first process is the disruption of protein transport from the IS to the OS (Figure 1A). As the OS lacks the biosynthesis machinery for proteins and lipids, all of the components required for OS morphogenesis, maintenance, and sensory functions must be transported from the endoplasmic reticulum (ER), located in the IS, to the OS [2], across the connective connecting cilium stalk. Therefore, defects in this transport most often lead to the accumulation of proteins in the IS. Another process involved in the accumulation of proteins in the IS is the dysregulation of pathways involved in protein degradation, including ER-associated degradation (ERAD) and autophagy (Figure 1C). Finally, also incorrect folding of specific proteins due to loss-of-function mutations can results in protein accumulation in the IS (Figure 1B). An accumulation of misfolded proteins in the ER membrane or in the cytoplasm of the PRs can induce the heat shock response (HSR) and/or the unfolded protein response (UPR). Continuous activation of these responses will ultimately lead to death of PRs [21].

In this review the above mentioned branches of the proteostasis network will be described in detail. Subsequently, we will explain how potential therapeutic agents directed against these branches might slow down or even arrest the dramatic blinding conditions, supported by findings of PN modulators in other research disciplines.

2. The Different Branches of the Proteostasis Network

2.1. Pathways Involved in Protein Trafficking

2.1.1. Chaperones Involved in Lipid-Dependent Trafficking

Many PR-specific proteins depend on post-translational lipid modifications, including prenylation and myristoylation, for correct localization to the OS and their anchoring at one of the OS membranes [22]. Protein prenylation involves the transfer of either a farnesyl or a geranylgeranyl moiety to the C-terminal cysteine(s) of the target protein by farnesyltransferase (FTase) and geranylgeranyltransferase (GGTase-I), respectively [23]. Several chaperones are involved in this prenylation process, including AIPL1, PDE6D, and UNC119.

Aryl hydrocarbon receptor (AhR)-interacting protein-like 1 (AIPL1) was first discovered in association with Leber congenital amaurosis (LCA) [24]. Mutations in the *AIPL1* gene encoding for AIPL1 results in LCA4, one of the most severe forms of LCA leading to blindness in early childhood [25]. Since then, studies were set up to unravel the function of the AIPL1 protein. Studies in AIPL1 knockdown and knockout mouse models revealed that AIPL1 functions as a chaperone for PDE6 [26,27]. In these mouse models protein levels and activity of PDE6 were severely reduced, whereas other photoreceptor proteins were unaffected. Other studies suggest that AIPL1 is also necessary for the maintenance of PRs by enhancing the essential farnesylation reaction [28,29]. Several retinal proteins, including PDE, transducin, and rhodopsin kinase (GRK1) are known to be farnesylated [30]. These findings are in line with the observed rapid degeneration of rods and cones in the animal models, as well as in LCA4 patients.

Another chaperone, mainly involved in the trafficking of prenylated proteins, is PDE6D [8,31]. In mice, knockout of PDE6D results in mislocalization of prenylated PR proteins, including PDE6, GRK1, and Gγ [32]. In human, mutations in PDE6D are associated with Joubert syndrome (JS) [33,34]. This syndromic condition can be explained by mislocalization of other critical cargos of PDE6D important for the development and stability of the primary cilium. These cargos include inositol polyphosphate

5-phosphatase E (INPP5E) and retinitis pigmentosa GTPase regulator (RPGR) [33,35]. The trafficking of these cargos comprises of several steps [36,37]. First, PDE6D solubilizes the prenylated protein from the ER by sequestering the hydrophobic farnesyl or geranylgeranyl tail. Subsequently, PDE6D targets the cargo to the destination membrane by association with a peripherally membrane bound docking protein. Finally, binding of the displacement factor ARL3 to PDE6D causes a reduction in size of the hydrophobic cavity resulting in the release of the cargo [38]. PDE6D can now travel back to repeat its cycle.

UNC119 shares significant sequence and structural homology with the prenyl-binding protein PDE6D [37]. Similar to PDE6D, UNC119 is also a subject of ARL3-dependent cargo release, and therefore the transport mechanism of PDE6D and UNC119 are highly identical. However, a remarkable difference between PDE6D and UNC119 is the ARL3-dependent release of their cargo. In contrast to PDE6D, the hydrophobic pocket of UNC119 is expanded upon binding of ARL3, thereby weakening the interaction with the cargo instead of squeezing the lipid out of the hydrophobic pocket [39]. This might be partly explained by the binding of different lipid moieties of both chaperones. Whereas PDE6D sequesters prenylated proteins, UNC119 is known to bind myristoylated cargo [31,40]. UNC119 has been shown to be important in the trafficking of transducin, which is myristoylated on its α-subunit [41]. In UNC119 knockout mice, the trafficking of transducin to the OS during dark adaptation was significantly impaired, contributing to the observed slow retinal degeneration [42]. The observed mislocalization of transducin in these mice is not complete, supporting the fact that transducin is trafficked by other proteins, including PDE6D. Interestingly, a study performed in *Pde6d;Unc119* double-knockout mice showed partially improved rhodopsin kinase (GRK1) expression and trafficking in cones compared to *Pde6d* single-knockout mice [43]. Based on these findings, the authors suggest that the transport by PDE6D and UNC119 in cones might be interdependent. The improvement found in only cones is in line with the relatively mild phenotype seen in patients with a truncating mutation in UNC119, which is associated with late onset CRD [44].

2.2. Pathways Involved in Protein Folding

2.2.1. Chaperonins, Phosducins and Ric8A

In addition to the classic and ubiquitous molecular chaperones from the heat shock protein superfamily (discussed below), various studies have focused on chaperones and co-chaperones involved in folding and assembly of PR-specific proteins.

One of the PR-specific proteins that needs targeted guidance for its correct folding and assembly is transducin. The folding and assembly of the full transducin protein complex is performed in two distinct steps. In the first step, the so-called chaperonins or CCTs (chaperonins containing TCP-1) are involved. CCTs are protein-folding ATPase complexes consisting of two stacked rings, which form a central cavity [45]. The β-subunit of transducin (G_β) is able to enter this cavity. Once transducin enters, ATP binding occurs, resulting in the closure of the cavity by hydrolysis of the just bound ATP molecule [46]. In addition to ATP, the folding of G_β requires a co-chaperone, phosducin-like protein 1 (PhLP1). Binding of PhLP1 induces conformational changes of CCT that lock the β-propeller structure of G_β. Subsequently, G_β rotates inside the cavity followed by its release in complex with PhLP1. PhLP1 is required for the formation of the $G_{\beta\gamma}$ dimer [47].

The second step involves the trafficking of the $G_{\beta\gamma}$ dimer to the OS by phosducin, another member of the phosducin family of proteins. Phosducin forms a complex with $G_{\beta\gamma}$ by sequestering the hydrophobic farnesyl residue of G_γ [48]. The farnesyl residue serves as a membrane anchor, which targets $G_{\beta\gamma}$ to the OS [49]. Another speculated function of phosducin is the protection of $G_{\beta\gamma}$ against ubiquitination and degradation by the proteasome [50].

CCTs are also involved in the folding and assembly of the BBSome [51], a protein complex that regulates the ciliary import, export, and intraciliary trafficking of molecules [52]. Mutations in genes coding for BBSome proteins most often result in the development of Bardet–Biedl syndrome, one of the syndromic ciliopathy conditions in which the retina is affected [53], as indicated in the introduction. For some of the BBSome proteins it was shown that these proteins contain a β-propeller fold, similar to G_β [54]. Whether or not the folding and assembly of the BBSome proteins is comparable to the situation of G_β remains to be elucidated.

It remains largely unknown if the α-subunit of transducin also needs assistance in correct folding and trafficking to the OS before it forms a heterotrimeric complex with $G_{\beta\gamma}$. However, evidence is emerging that resistance to inhibitors of cholinesterase 8 (RIC8) proteins function as ubiquitous chaperones for G_α [55]. The two known isoforms—RIC8A and RIC8B—each regulate specific classes of G_α [56]. Although the specific PR class of Gα and its relation to RIC8 has not been investigated, it has been shown that a closely related form interacts with RIC8A [57]. The proposed mode of action of RIC8A is to positively regulate G_α by acting as a guanine nucleotide exchange factor (GEF). RIC8A preferentially binds GDP-bound G_α and causes GDP release. Subsequently, RIC8A assists in organizing a de novo nucleotide-binding pocket for binding of GTP. The RIC8A-G_α complex breaks apart when a GTP molecule binds. Subsequent hydrolysis of GTP results in the binding of G_α to the $G_{\beta\gamma}$ yielding the fully assembled heterotrimeric complex [58]. Taken together, CCT together with PhLP1 regulate the folding of the transducin β-subunit. Subsequently, G_β forms a dimer with G_γ by guidance of PhLP1. Finally, the $G_{\beta\gamma}$ dimer is trafficked to the OS by phosducin, where it can bind to G_α. RIC8A has been proposed as the chaperone of G_α and its assembly to the $G_{\beta\gamma}$ dimer.

2.2.2. Heat Shock Response (HSR)

The HSR is known to be present in every living organism, and functions as an essential survival mechanism against extracellular challenges, such as increased temperatures, and intracellular stressors such as oxidative stress, that lead to protein misfolding [21,59]. The HSR is featured by an extremely rapid activation of gene expression, leading to a remarkable increase in molecular chaperones, including heat shock proteins (HSPs) [60]. In vertebrates, the HSR is regulated by a family of transcription factors, which includes six members (HSF1-4, HSFX, and HSFY) [59]. HSF1 is believed to be the master regulator of molecular chaperone synthesis upon protein misfolding [61]. Under normal physiological conditions, monomeric HSF1 is repressed and localized in the cytosol by interacting with molecular chaperones, including HSP90, HSP70, and the chaperonin CCT. When a threshold of misfolded proteins is reached, the chaperones dissociate from HSF1 leading to trimerization and nuclear accumulation of HSF1 followed by transcriptional activation of HSPs. The major HSPs involved in the HSR include HSP90, HSP70, and HSP60 [61].

HSP90 and HSP70 are able to associate with the hydrophobic regions of the protein, and thereby preventing binding to other hydrophobic moieties [61]. Subsequently, they assist in the folding of these hydrophobic regions in such a way that the hydrophobic groups are not exposed. Furthermore, they aid in overcoming the energy thresholds of the intermediate folding states of the protein [62]. Similar to HSP90 and HSP70, the chaperonin HSP60 is also able to bind hydrophobic residues of proteins. In contrast, the barrel-shaped HSP60 is more passively involved in the folding of proteins by creating a favorable microenvironment for the hydrophobic regions in its central cavity [63].

2.2.3. Unfolded Protein Response (UPR)

A more specific cellular stress response related to the ER is the UPR. The UPR is activated in response to an accumulation of unfolded and/or misfolded proteins in the lumen of the ER [64]. The activation of the UPR aims to reduce ER stress and restore proteostasis in three distinct ways: an initial response to reduce protein synthesis, a second wave of increased production of molecular chaperones involved in protein folding to increase folding capacity, and finally the degradation of misfolded proteins when the folding capacity is insufficient to restore functional protein balance. It is generally accepted that a member of the HSP70 family, BiP/GRP78, is the key regulator in the activation of the UPR [65]. BiP has been shown to associate with all three transmembrane sensors of the UPR, including inositol requiring enzyme-1 (IRE1) α and β, protein kinase RNA (PKR)-like ER kinase

(PERK), and activating transcription factor 6 (ATF6) α and β. Under normal physiological conditions, BiP associates with the ER luminal domain of IRE1 and PERK via its ATPase domain, maintaining them in an inactive monomeric state.

The interaction of BiP with ATF6 masks a binding site to coat protein-II (COP-II) vesicles, thereby preventing ATF6 translocation to the Golgi. Upon ER stress, BiP dissociates from the sensors and binds to misfolded proteins. Subsequently, IRE1 and PERK are able to oligomerize followed by their trans-autophosphorylation and ATF6 traffics to the Golgi for further processing and activation.

Dissociation of BiP from IRE1 results in the activation of its RNase domain. This activation is sustained by binding of HSP47 to the luminal domain of IRE1, thereby hindering the binding of BiP [66]. Subsequently, a single mRNA encoding for X-box binding protein 1 (XBP1) is targeted for non-conventional splicing [67].

These spliced XBP1s trigger the expression of molecular chaperones and components of ERAD in order to relieve the load on the ER and eventually restore protein balance [68]. One of the upregulated chaperones is the ER resident co-chaperone ERdj4, which eases and stabilizes the binding of BiP [69]. Furthermore, it has been shown that protein disulfide isomerase A6 (PDIA6) plays an important role in the conversion of IRE1 to its monomeric state [70]. Based on these findings, it is speculated that ERdj4 and PDIA6 are important regulators of the IRE1 negative feedback loop. Activation of PERK leads to phosphorylation of the α-subunit of eukaryotic translation initiation factor 2 (eIF2α), thereby hindering the conversion of eIF2-GDP to eIF2-GTP by the GEF eIF2B [71]. The inactivation of eIF2α leads to overall decrease in mRNA translation and thus protein synthesis. Although, global mRNA translation is reduced, some specific mRNAs are favored to be translated, including activation transcription factor 4 (ATF4) [72]. ATF4 is able to activate the transcription of various genes involved in protein folding, autophagy, and apoptosis, including CCAAT/enhancer-binding protein (C/EBP) homologous protein (*CHOP*), ER oxidoreductin 1 (*ERO1*), and growth arrest and DNA damage-inducible protein (*GADD34*). GADD34 plays a role in the negative feedback loop for PERK by acting as a cofactor in the dephosphorylation of eIF2α [73]. CHOP and ERO1 mainly play a role in prolonged PERK activation [74], which will be discussed below.

Under ER stress, ATF6 binds to COP-II vesicles and traffics to the Golgi [75]. Here, it is cleaved by proteases S1P and S2P resulting in a cytosolic fragment [76]. This fragment travels into the nucleus to regulate transcription of specific UPR genes, including *CHOP* and *XBP1*. Interestingly, XBP1s and ATF6 are able to heterodimerize, and subsequently induce the expression of genes involved in ERAD [77].

2.3. Pathways Involved in Protein Degradation

2.3.1. ER-associated Degradation (ERAD)

Folding and maturation of proteins is a complicated process that is highly susceptible to errors. Up to 30% of all newly synthesized proteins are affected by such errors and are therefore degraded by the proteasome before they reach their defective mature state [78]. An important player in proteasomal-dependent protein degradation is ERAD. The process of ERAD can be divided into three consecutive steps: recognition of misfolded proteins in the ER, retrotranslocation of these proteins into the cytosol, and ubiquitin-dependent degradation by the ubiquitin–proteasome system (UPS) [79].

The recognition of misfolded proteins depends on the detection of substructures within proteins, including exposed hydrophobic regions, unpaired cysteine residues, and immature glycans [80]. The latter involves the lectin-type chaperones calnexin and calreticulin, which can bind to glycans possessing the $Glc_3Man_9GlcNAc_2$ structure produced by deglucosylation [81]. Incompletely or misfolded proteins undergo multiple rounds of reglucosylation by uridine diphosphate (UDP)-glucose:glycoprotein glucosyltransferase (UGGT) and subsequent folding by reassociation with calnexin or calreticulin, eventually resulting in the mature protein conformation [82].

On the other hand, terminally misfolded proteins must be extracted from this calnexin/calreticulin cycle. This extraction is regulated by the removal of terminal mannose residues from core glycans by mannosidases, including ER mannosidase I (ERMANI), ER degradation-enhancing α-mannosidase-like protein 1 (EDEM1), EDEM3, or Golgi-resident mannosidase α class 1C member 1 (MAN1C1) [83–85]. In this way, ERAD can discriminate between terminally misfolded proteins and their fully functional counterparts.

Since the ubiquitin-dependent degradation by the UPS is performed in the cytosol, terminally misfolded proteins subjected to ERAD have to be transported through the ER membrane via a transmembrane channel, called the retrotranslocon [86]. The exact composition of this channel is yet unknown. However, it has been shown that the membrane protein Derlin-1 and various E3 ubiquitin ligases are part of the retrotranslocon complex [87]. Once a small part of the substrate for ERAD is exposed to the surface of the ER, the substrate becomes a subject for poly-ubiquitination. Subsequently, the p97/valosin-containing protein (VCP), which is a member of the type II AAA+ protein family of ATPases, together with its cofactors, possessing ubiquitin-binding domains (UBDs), cooperatively produce a driving force for the retrotranslocation [88].

Retrotranslocated substrates for ERAD often possess exposed hydrophobic domains. Therefore, it is important that these substrates should be rapidly transported to the UPS for degradation to prevent aggregation. A chaperone complex consisting of BCL-2-associated athanogene 6 (BAG6), ubiquitin-like protein 4A (UBL4A), transmembrane domain recognition complex 35 (TRC35), and co-chaperone small glutamine-rich TPR-containing protein α (SGTA) has been shown to play an important role in the trafficking of ERAD substrates to the UPS by binding to the hydrophobic domains [89].

2.3.2. Autophagy

Another very important process involved in protein degradation is autophagy. Multiple forms of autophagy are known, including macroautophagy, chaperone-mediated autophagy (CMA), and microautophagy [90].

Macroautophagy is the most common form of autophagy and therefore often referred to simply as autophagy. Autophagy consists of multiple consecutive phases, including initiation, nucleation, elongation, closure, and fusion to the lysosome. The initiation phase is tightly regulated by AMP-activated protein kinase (AMPK) and mammalian target of rapamycin complex I (mTORC1) [91]. In addition, factors expressed resulting from ER stress are also able to trigger the initiation phase.

It all starts with the formation of the Unc-51-like kinase 1 (ULK1) complex followed by the phosphorylation of the class III phosphoinositide 3-kinase (PI3KC3) complex I leading to the nucleation of the phagophore [91,92]. Subsequently, autophagosome elongation and closure requires two ubiquitin-like conjugation systems, including an ATG7 dependent system and an ATG5-ATG12 dependent system. Together they are responsible for the lipidation, by phosphatidyethanolamine (PE), from cleavage of microtubule-associated protein 1 light chain 3 (LC3). Membrane sources in form of lipids needed for the elongation of the autophagosomal membrane are provided by ATG9-dependent vesicle trafficking. After closure of the autophagosomal membrane, the autophagosome has to fuse with the lysosome to form an autolysosome in order to degrade its enclosed cargo [93].

A selective form of autophagy is CMA, which to date is only identified in mammals [94]. This form of autophagy is specific for proteins containing a KFERQ motif in their amino acid sequence [95]. Heat shock cognate of the HSP70 family, HSC70, is able to recognize this motif and subsequently targets these proteins to the lysosome [96]. Here, it binds to the lysosomal receptor LAMP-2A and facilitates, together with its co-chaperones, in the unfolding process of the substrate in order to translocate it into the lysosome [97].

Microautophagy is a process in which cytoplasmic cargo is directly engulfed into the lysosome [98]. This process is triggered by the same stimuli compared to common autophagy, but in contrast it mainly facilitates the degradation of smaller substrates, including misfolded proteins. Similar to CMA, Hsc70 is involved in the protein cargo selection for degradation [99].

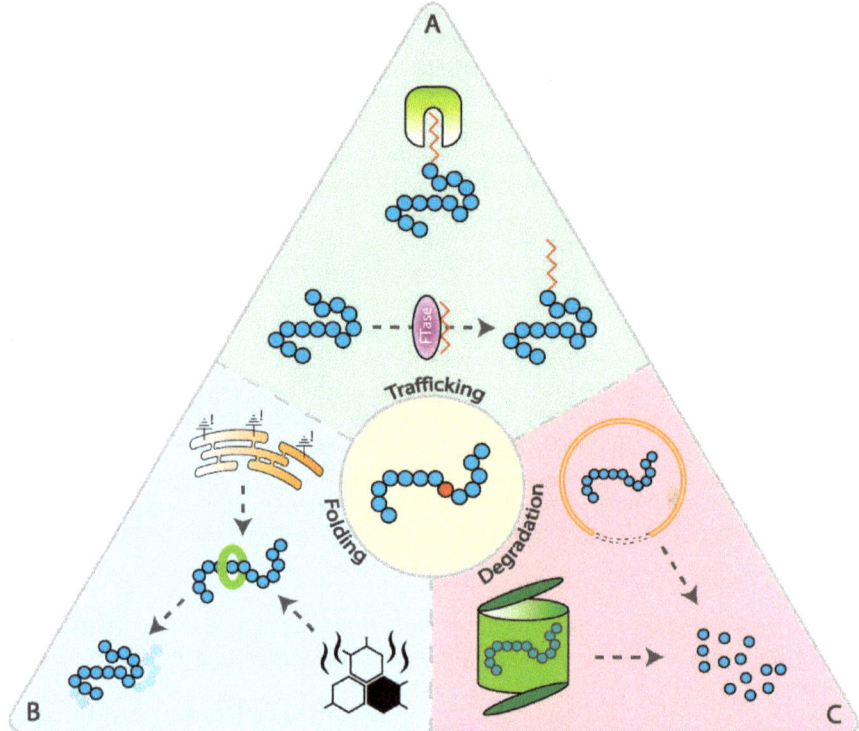

Figure 1. Schematic representation of the different branches of the proteostasis network, divided into trafficking, folding and degradation. (A) Trafficking: Protein prenylation involves the transfer of either a farnesyl or a geranylgeranyl moiety to the C-terminal cysteine(s) of the target protein by farnesyltransferase (FTase) and geranylgeranyltransferase (GGTase-I), respectively. Chaperones involved in regulation of this prenylation process and trafficking of prenylated proteins, include AIPL1, PDE6D, and UNC119 (depicted in green). (B) Folding: Two responses that are activated upon protein misfolding are the unfolded protein response (UPR) and the heat shock response (HSR). Both responses result in enhanced expression of chaperones (depicted in green) in order to restore the correct folding of proteins. (C) Degradation: ER-associated degradation (ERAD) results in the degradation of proteins by the ubiquitin–proteasome system (UPS). Another pathway of protein degradation is autophagy. Background colors in figure (green, blue, and red) correspond with background colors of Table 1.

Table 1. Therapeutic compounds directed against the different branches of the proteostasis network (PN). Therapeutic compounds are divided based on which branch of the PN they target, including trafficking (green), folding (blue), and degradation (red). Subgroups include compounds directed against protein lipid-modifications, (co-)chaperonins, HSR, UPR, ERAD, and autophagy. * Compounds that are not yet available.

Target	Compounds *	Function	Effect on PRs	References
Protein lipid-modifications	FTase inhibitors	Inhibits the farnesylation of proteins	(Proposed) underprenylation and mislocalization of many PR proteins	[100,101]
	GGTase-I inhibitors	Inhibits the geranylgeranylation of proteins	(Proposed) underprenylation and mislocalization of many PR proteins	[102]
(Co-)chaperonins	CCT inducers *	Improves folding of transducin and possibly other PR proteins	Undetermined	[103]
	PhLP1 inducers *	Improves function of CCTs and possibly CCT-independent functions	Malformation of OS by transgenic expression of a PhLP1 dominant-negative mutant	[47,103,104]
	CCT-BBSome stabilizers *	Stabilizes BBSome formation and thereby the export of molecules from the OS	Undetermined	[105]
	Small molecule Ric8 inhibitors *	Prevents folding of disease-causing Gα	Undetermined	[106,107]
Heat shock response (HSR)	geldanamycin, tanespimycin, alvespimycin	1st generation HSP90 inhibitors	Geldanamycin not suitable for future experiments because of poor applicability and toxicity; Tanespimycin reduced mutant protein accumulation in rat RP model (R135L); prolonged treatment with alvespimycin leads to PR cell death	[108–112]
	luminespib, onalespib, ganetespib, HSP990	Newer generation HSP90 inhibitors	HSP90 treatment in a RP rat model (P23H) enhances visual function and delayed PR degeneration, but prolonged treatment led to visual impairment by GRK1 and PDE6 reduction; prolonged treatment with ganetespib led to PR cell death	[109,111,112]
	AAV-HSF-1	Overexpressing HSF-1 and thereby transcriptional activation of HSPs	Subretinal injection of AAV-Hsf-1 in a RP rat model (P23H) improved visual reponse	[113]
	Arimoclomol	Induces HSR and UPR, only in stressed cells	Prolonged PR survival and improved visual responses in P23H transgenic rats	[114]
Unfolded protein response (UPR)	AAV-BiP	Relieves ER stress by reducing cleaved ATF6, phosphorylated eIF2α and CHOP	Subretinal delivery of AAV5-BiP reduced PR cell death and improved visual responses in P23H transgenic rats	[115,116]
	CHOP inhibitors *	Inhibits proapoptotic transcription activity of CHOP	CHOP knockout in a transgenic mouse model of RP (T17M) led to PR cell death and strong impairment in visual function; CHOP knockout in P23H RHO mice had no effect on PR survival in young mice, but partly protected PR degeneration in older mice	[117–119]
	ATF4 inhibitors *	Inhibits downstream transcription activation of Chop, Ero1, and Gadd34	ATF4 knockdown in T17M RHO mice decreased retinal degeneration and improved PR survival	[120]
	GSK2606414A	Specific PERK inhibitor	Treatment with GSK2606414A in P23H RHO rats accelerated PR cell death and further impaired visual function	[121]
	Salubrinal	Inhibitor of eIF2α dephosphorylation	Treatment with salubrinal in P23H RHO rats improved PR survival	[121]

Table 1. *Cont.*

Target	Compounds *	Function	Effect on PRs	References
	KIRA6	Allosterically inhibits IRE1α RNase activity	Intravitreal injection of KIRA6 in P23H RHO rats increased PR survival	[122]
	Reactive electrophilic species (RES) modulators *	Modulate the effects of RES on IRE1	Undetermined	[123–128]
	Ceapins	Selective inhibitors of ATF6α	Undetermined	[129,130]
ER-associated degradation (ERAD)	Kyoto University Substances (KUSs)	Inhibits VCP's ATPase activity, without affecting the cellular functions of VCP	Individual treatment with KUS121 and KUS187 in a *rd10* mouse model preserved ONL thickness and improved visual function	[131]
	AAA+ protein derivatives *	Unfolding of misfolded proteins	Transgenic expression of PAN in Gy-/- mice increased PR survival and preserved visual function	[132]
	DUB/USP modulators	Modulating the ubiquitin cleavage from proteins, thereby modulating proteasomal degradation	Undetermined	[133–135]
Autophagy	Rapamycin, everolimus, temsirolimus, ridaforolimus	Inhibiting mTOR pathway by directly binding to mTORC1	Improved rod survival in P23H-3 rats	[136]
	Metformin	Activation of AMP-activated protein kinase (AMPK)	Metformin treatment protected against retinal cell death in diabetic mice, whereas it accelerated PR degeneration in P23H RHO mice	[137,138]
	Valproic acid (VPA)	Upregulates autophagy by inhibiting inositol synthesis	VPA treatment in BBS12-/- mice, P23H RHO *Xenopus laevis*, and a *rd1* mouse model resulted in PR protection, whereas treatment in T17M RHO X. *laevis*, a P23H-1 rat model, and a *rd10* mouse model exacerbated PR degeneration	[139–141]

3. Therapeutic Approaches to Restore Protein Balance

The light sensing OS of PRs requires renewal every ten days due to its high photoactivity, especially of the cones during daytime vision. This demands a high turnover of biosynthetic compounds, including membranes and proteins). Therefore, a well-balanced proteostasis network is of particular importance for the PRs. For many IRDs it has been shown that this balance in the PRs is disrupted, leading to protein accumulation in the IS and eventually the death of photoreceptors. For this reason, several studies have focused on therapeutically targeting the three main branches of the PR proteostasis network to restore the protein balance. The different therapeutic approaches and their effects on PRs are discussed below and summarized in Table 1.

3.1. Therapeutic Strategies Involved in Protein Trafficking

3.1.1. Targeting Protein Lipid Modifications

Agents targeting prenylation have been extensively studied in cancer research. The first agents tested were FTase inhibitors used to target the farnesylation of K-Ras, which was shown to induce several forms of cancer, including colorectal cancer and lung cancer [142]. Although some clinical improvements were seen for different forms of cancer, these improvements could not be related to inhibition of K-Ras. Subsequent experiments revealed that K-Ras was geranylgeranylated when farnesylation was blocked by FTase inhibitors [143]. Therefore, inhibitors of GGTase-I emerged as potential target for cancer therapy. However, a phase I clinical trial investigating a dual FTase and GGTase-I inhibitor showed dose-limiting side effects in patients with locally advanced pancreatic cancer, indicating that inhibition of prenylation has a broad detrimental effect on human health [102]. FTase inhibitors are also of particular interest in the Hutchinson–Gilford progeria syndrome (HGPS) research field. HGPS is a rare premature-aging disease caused by a dominant de novo point mutation in the *LMNA* gene, resulting in the expression of a mutant form of lamin A, also known as progerin [144]. Progerin remains persistently farnesylated, which makes it a suitable candidate for FTase inhibitors [100]. Although, promising improvements in bone structure, vascular stiffness, and hearing have been obtained using FTase inhibitors in HGPS patients, nothing is reported about possible dose-limiting side effects [101].

Despite the promising results of using FTase and GGTase-I inhibitors for targeting several forms of cancer and HGPS, the side effects are of major concern; especially in the highly compartmentalized PRs, where many proteins depend on prenylation for subcellular trafficking and anchoring. General inhibition of prenylation would probably lead to underprenylation of many PR proteins leading to mislocalization and accumulation of these proteins in the IS. Therefore, inhibition of prenylation in PRs will rather accelerate protein accumulation than decreasing it.

3.2. Therapeutic Strategies Involved in Protein Folding

3.2.1. Targeting Chaperonins and Their Co-chaperones

The type II chaperonin CCT is proposed to be involved in the folding of approximately 10% of newly translated cytosolic proteins [145]. Besides ATP, CCT also needs the co-chaperone PhLP1 for the correct folding of these proteins [47]. It has been shown that inhibition of CCT by the transgenic expression of a dominant-negative mutant of PhLP1 results in the malformation of the OS in mouse photoreceptors [103]. Proteomic analysis revealed that the expression of several important PR proteins was affected, including PDE6, rhodopsin, transducin, peripherin 2, ROM1, musashi-1, and UNC-119. It could be possible that CCT is responsible for the folding of these proteins. Yet, only transducin has been shown to be a direct substrate of CCT. Therefore, a more plausible explanation would be that PhLP1 regulates the expression of these proteins in a CCT-independent manner.

Besides transducin, the BBSome is also a substrate for CCT for its correct folding and assembly. It has been shown that some of the BBSome proteins, including BBS6, BBS10, and BBS12, can form a

CCT-like complex together with CCT subunits. Interestingly, 50% of clinically diagnosed BBS cases are caused by a mutation in one of these three genes. Furthermore, mutations in these genes result in a more severe phenotype compared to other BBS proteins [105].

These findings highlight the importance of chaperone defects as pathogenic factors and therefore as potential therapeutic targets. Surprisingly, chaperonins and their co-chaperones, such as PhLP1, have not been investigated in relation to therapy. Especially PhLP1 would be an interesting therapeutic target, because of its proposed CCT-dependent and CCT-independent regulation of important PR proteins [104].

In cancer research, RIC8, functioning as GEF and chaperone for G_α, has been proposed as a potential therapeutic target, since it has been shown that constitutive activation of G_α by somatic mutations leads to development of various cancers [106]. Therefore, inhibition of RIC8 by small molecules might reduce tumorigenesis. A constitutive active mutant of rod G_α has also been associated to a form of congenital stationary night blindness [107]. RIC8 inhibition might therefore also alleviate or delay this phenotype. However, as described earlier, the function of RIC8 in the PR has not been investigated and inhibition of RIC8 would only be applicable to this specific mutation.

3.2.2. Targeting the Heat Shock Response (HSR)

HSP90, a component involved in the HSR, is commonly overexpressed in multiple forms of cancer [146]. It has been proposed that cancer cells increase their HSP90 expression and thereby change their proteostasis network in order to adapt to dysregulated and misfolded protein synthesis as a consequence of rapid cell division [147]. For this reason, many studies have focused on investigating HSP90 inhibitors. The first HSP90 inhibitor identified was geldanamycin, but this never reached the clinical testing phase because of its poor applicability and toxicity [108]. Nevertheless, geldanamycin paved the way for production of geldanamycin analogs, including 17-AAG/tanespimycin and 17-DMAG/alvespimycin [109]. Although clinical testing was halted for these agents, it did provide proof-of-principle that HSP90 is a target for cancer therapy. Now, a new generation of HSP90 inhibitors, including luminespib, onalespib, and ganetespib, show greater potency in clinical testing [109].

HSP90 inhibitors have also been tested in models for retinal degeneration. Systemic administration of 17-AAG accompanied by inner-blood retina barrier modulation in a mouse model of RP (RP10) protects against photoreceptor degeneration induced by aggregating RP10-associated mutant IMPDH1 protein [110]. Furthermore, HSP90 inhibition by 17-AAG in a transgenic rat model of RP (R135L) reduced the intracellular accumulation of the mutant protein and restored the localization of this protein comparable to wild type controls [111]. Administration of another HSP90 inhibitor, HSP990, in a different transgenic rat model of RP (P23H) resulted in enhanced visual function and delayed photoreceptor degeneration. However, prolonged treatment with HSP990 leads to a reduction in GRK1 and PDE6 protein levels followed by visual impairment [111]. The visual impairment caused by prolonged HSP90 inhibition is in line with findings from a study in which four HSP90 inhibitors were tested, including 17-AAG, 17-DMAG, luminespib, and ganetespib, in a rat retinal damage model. Here, it was shown that prolonged inhibition with 17-DMAG and ganetespib results in PR cell death, whereas there was no PR injury detected upon treatment with the other two agents [112].

These contradictory findings might be explained by the different modes of action of the HSP90 inhibitors, since the effect of 17-AAG was dependent on HSF1 in the P23H rat model, whereas its effect was HSF1-independent in the R135L model. This is further supported by the notion that HSP90 is known to facilitate the folding and assembly of more than 300 proteins [146]. Alternatively, agents that induce the HSR in other ways might be more suitable as potential treatments for IRDs. A direct way to target the HSR is by overexpressing the *HSF-1* gene. A study in the p23H RHO RD rat model showed a significant increase of scotopic electroretinogram (ERG) amplitudes compared to untreated controls upon ectopic overexpression of *HSF-1* by subretinal injection of AAV-*HSF-1* [113].

The hydroxylamine derivative arimoclomol might be a more indirect alternative agent to induce the HSR. Treatment of transgenic rats, carrying a P23H rhodopsin mutation, with arimoclomol resulted in improved PR OS structure and reduced rhodopsin accumulation in the IS, accompanied by prolonged PR survival and improved visual responses [114]. It was shown that these improvements were mediated by both the HSR and the UPR, thereby indicating that these responses are intertwined. Another great advantage of arimoclomol is that it only acts on stressed cells. In this way, potential side effects, as a consequence of inducing an HSR response in healthy cells present in the retina, are avoided.

3.2.3. Targeting the Unfolded Protein Response (UPR)

As described earlier, the UPR senses ER stress by using three transmembrane sensors, including IRE1, PERK, and ATF6. In IRDs, mutations causing defective proteins can result in prolonged ER stress. It has been shown that upon prolonged ER stress, downstream effectors of the PERK pathway, ATF4 and CHOP heterodimerize. This results in increased protein synthesis, protein misfolding, and oxidative stress, eventually leading to cell death [148]. Another branch of the UPR that gets hyperactivated upon prolonged ER stress is IRE1. Hyperactive IRE1 cleaves microRNAs that normally inhibit proapoptotic targets, thereby inducing apoptosis [149]. Because apoptosis as a consequence of ER stress is often seen in PRs of IRD patients, therapeutically targeting UPR regulators or pathways involved in one of the three branches of the UPR might promote PR survival and thereby visual function.

As discussed earlier, it is commonly accepted that BiP/GRP78 is the key regulator in the activation of the UPR. Therefore, BiP might be a potential therapeutic target for relieving ER stress. Indeed, studies have shown that subretinal delivery of AAV5-BiP to a transgenic rat model of RP (P23H) results in reduction of PR cell death and improved ERG amplitudes [115]. Furthermore, a study in primary human retinal pigmented epithelium cells (hRPE) showed that AAV2-BiP promotes the survival of these cells under ER stress [116]. Both studies suggest that these improvements are due to a suppression of apoptosis by downregulation of CHOP protein levels. For this reason, reducing CHOP levels might be a promising strategy to alleviate ER stress. This notion is supported by a large body of evidence in the field of Alzheimer's Disease, cardiac hypertrophy, and diabetes, wherein they link CHOP to these disease conditions [150].

Recently, several studies investigated the effect of CHOP reduction in the context of photoreceptor degeneration. A first study was performed in a transgenic mouse model of RP (T17M) [117]. Subsequently, these mice were crossed with CHOP knockout mice in order to get T17M RHO CHOPP$^{-/-}$ mice. Complete knockdown of CHOP in these mice resulted in photoreceptor cell death, indicated by significant thinning of the outer nuclear layer, accompanied by a strong impairment in visual function. In a similar experimental setup comparing P23H RHO CHOPP$^{-/-}$ mice with P23H RHO mice, they found no effect on PR survival in young animals. In older mice, however, the central retina of the CHOPP$^{-/-}$ mice was partly protected against degeneration [118]. Another study in transgenic mice expressing human P23H rhodopsin also showed that knockout of CHOP had no effect on the rescue of retinal degeneration [119]. These studies indicated that complete ablation of CHOP has no positive effect in early developmental stages. As already described earlier, CHOP is mainly involved in prolonged PERK activation. Therefore, reducing CHOP levels to physiological levels during prolonged ER stress might be a better solution. This notion is supported by above described findings in older mice.

Interestingly, knocking down the proapoptotic partner of CHOP, ATF4 in a T17M rhodopsin mutant mouse model resulted in decreased retinal degeneration and improved PR survival [120].

Further support that the PERK branch of the UPR might be a promising therapeutic target comes from studies investigating ER stress related diseases, including Alzheimer's Disease (AD), amyotrophic lateral disease (ALS), Parkinson's Disease, and prion diseases [151,152].

In an Alzheimer's disease mouse model it was shown that deletion of PERK resulted in decreased phosphorylation of eIF2α and prevented deficits in protein synthesis leading to an improvement of the AD phenotype in these mice [153]. Comparable results were obtained in prion-diseased mice by overexpressing GADD34, which plays a role in the negative feedback loop for PERK by acting as a cofactor in the dephosphorylation of eIF2α [154]. Treatment of the prion-diseased mice with salubrinal, an inhibitor of eIF2α dephosphorylation, had the opposite effect compared to GADD34 overexpression, thereby supporting the positive effects of eIF2α dephosphorylation. The positive effect of the inhibition of the PERK pathway is further supported by a study investigating the effect of the specific PERK inhibitor, GSK2606414A, in prion-diseased mice [155]. Treatment with this inhibitor showed reduced neuronal cell death leading to increased survival of these mice.

Surprisingly, opposing results were found for GSK2606414A and salubrinal treatment when administered in P23H RHO transgenic rats. GSK2606414A treatment resulted in accelerated photoreceptor cell death and further impaired visual function, whereas salubrinal treatment was found to improve photoreceptor survival [121]. It could be possible that in some disease conditions or models the PERK pathway is protective, whereas in other conditions it is rather a secondary effect of the disease process. Therefore, targeting other branches of the UPR might overcome this issue.

Targeting the IRE1 branch of the UPR has been shown to be beneficial in multiple rodent models, including a P23H RHO rat model [122]. In this model, intravitreal injection of KIRA6, which allosterically inhibits the RNase domain of IRE1, showed increased photoreceptor survival.

Recently, an emerging role of reactive electrophilic species (RES) as key regulators for the UPR, more specifically the IRE1 pathway, have been described [123]. Furthermore, RES have been reported to be involved in ER-stress related diseases, including neurodegenerative diseases, amyotrophic lateral sclerosis (ALS), and cancer [124–126]. The RES nitric oxide (NO) has been shown to modulate PDI and IRE1 through S-nitrosylation and thereby inhibiting the IRE1 branch of the UPR [127,128]. Therefore, modulation by RES might be a new potential therapeutic strategy for ER stress-associated diseases, including IRDs.

Maybe the most interesting sensor of the UPR, in context of IRDs, is ATF6, because mutations in ATF6 have been shown to cause autosomal recessive achromatopsia and early onset photoreceptor degeneration, also affecting the macula [156,157].

Until recently, no compounds were available that specifically target the ATF6 branch of the UPR. However, by cell-based screens a new class of pyrazole amides, named Ceapins, were identified as selective inhibitors of ATF6α [129,130]. Ceapins selectively prevent transport of AFT6α to the Golgi apparatus during ER stress. Interestingly, Ceapins have no toxic impact on unstressed cells, whereas they increase ER stress sensitivity upon ER stress induction.

3.3. Therapeutic Strategies Involved in Protein Degradation

3.3.1. Targeting the ER-associated Degradation (ERAD)

One of the essential players in ERAD is p97/VCP, belonging to the type II AAA+ protein family of ATPases. Because of its essential role in ERAD, VCP is proposed as a novel therapeutic target for the treatment of various diseases, including cystic fibrosis, cancer, and neurodegenerative disorders [131]. Besides its function in retrotranslocation and protein degradation, VCP is also involved in many other cellular processes, including mitosis, nuclear reformation, DNA/RNA repair, aggresome formation and inflammatory signaling [158]. Therefore, for therapeutic applicability, selective intervention of VCP is required to minimize the side effects. Small compounds, named Kyoto University Substances (KUSs), might fulfill these criteria. KUSs have been shown to specifically inhibit VCP's ATPase activity, without affecting the cellular functions of VCP [131]. Administering KUSs, more specifically KUS121 or KUS187, by intraperitoneal injection in a *rd10* mouse model resulted in preserved outer nuclear layer (ONL) thickness and improved visual function measured by ERG.

Because of the unfolding properties of VCP also other AAA+ proteins have been proposed as potent therapeutic agents, especially in solving protein misfolding and aggregation in neurodegenerative diseases. Although not functionally related to ERAD, the repurposing of two AAA+ proteins, including Hsp104 and proteasome-activating nucleotidase (PAN) were shown to protect from protein misfolding in several neurodegenerative animal models [159]. Furthermore, transgenic expression of PAN in rods of mice lacking the γ-subunit of transducin ($G_\gamma^{-/-}$) resulted in increased photoreceptor survival accompanied by preserved visual function [132].

Another possible therapeutic target of ERAD could be the enhancement of proteosomal degradation. Important players in this process are the deubiquitination enzymes (DUBs), also known as ubiquitin-specific proteases (USPs). USPs are known to cleave ubiquitin moieties from proteins and thereby preventing these proteins from proteosomal degradation [133]. Therefore, inhibiting USPs might work as a therapeutic approach to stimulate the degradation of misfolded proteins by the proteasome. In cancer research inhibition of specific USPs, including USP7 and USP10, has already been shown to have beneficial effects, by acting on the tumor suppressor p53 [134].

Depending on the type of mutation, p53 can either gain oncogenic properties or lose its tumor suppressor ability [160]. Therefore, based on the mutant form of p53, either increasing or lowering the levels of p53 could be beneficial. Inhibiting USP7, a negative regulator of p53, leads to increased p53 levels, whereas inhibiting USP10, a positive regulator of p53, leads to reduction of p53 levels [134]. With this in mind, the causative mutation for the disease has to be known, as well as the specificity of the USP inhibitor before administering it to the patient. From discrepancies in findings of different studies it cannot be concluded whether p53 is involved in the pathogenesis of PR cell death [161,162]. However, a recent study found a biallelic mutation in *USP45* associated with LCA. This indicates that USPs can play important roles in the pathogenesis of PR degeneration [163].

Another important issue to address is that DUBs associated with VCP have been suggested to promote protein turnover by assisting in retrotranslocation instead of their traditional function in preventing proteasomal degradation. Therefore, inducing these specific VCP associated DUBs might have therapeutic potential [135].

3.3.2. Targeting Autophagy

One of the best known inducers of autophagy is rapamycin, which directly binds to mTORC1, thereby inhibiting the mTOR pathway [164]. Because of its limited absorption, studies have been focusing on investigating rapamycin analogs or rapalogs, including everolimus, temsirolimus, and ridaforolimus. These mTORC1 inhibitors were highlighted as promising therapeutic agents in various protein misfolding associated diseases, including neurodegenerative diseases and multiple forms of cancer [165,166]. Also, a study in an RP rat model has shown the therapeutic potential of rapamycin in treating blindness [136]. In this study, rod cell degeneration was slowed down, without affecting cones, in a P23H rat model upon systemic administration of rapamycin. In contrast, other studies showed that activation of the mTOR pathway promotes cone survival [167–169]. Taken together, these results indicate that activation of autophagy is particularly protective for rods, but can have opposing effects on cones.

Studies investigating other mTOR inhibitors, including ATP-competitive mTOR inhibitors, are emerging [170]. Furthermore, indirect modulators of the mTOR pathway, including metformin and nilotinib have also been shown to play a protective role in diabetes, cancer, and neurodegenerative diseases via indirect activation of AMPK [171–173]. Contradictory results are found in mouse models of retinal degeneration when treated with metformin. In diabetic mice, metformin treatment protected against retinal cell death, whereas in a P23H RHO mouse model it accelerated the photoreceptor degeneration, indicating different modes of action by metformin [137,138].

In addition to autophagy upregulators acting on the mTOR pathway, also mTOR-independent autophagy upregulators have been widely studied, mainly in Huntington's disease [174]. One such agent is valproic acid (VPA), which upregulates autophagy by inhibiting inositol synthesis. In line with findings in neurodegeneration models, VPA treatment in models for photoreceptor degeneration can be detrimental or protective [139,175]. In a mouse model for Bardet–Biedl syndrome ($BBS12^{-/-}$), as well as in a *Xenopus laevis* model for RP (P23H) treatment with VPA resulted in photoreceptor protection [139,140]. In contrast, a T17M *X. laevis* model of RP and the P23H-1 rat model showed exacerbated photoreceptor degeneration upon VPA treatment [15,139]. Even in mouse models with a different mutation in the same gene (PDE6) this discrepancy in outcome was observed: VPA treatment reduced photoreceptor loss in the *rd1* model, whereas VPA treatment slightly accelerated photoreceptor loss in the *rd10* model [141]. Taken together, these studies indicate that the outcome of VPA treatment depends on the genotype and even on the type of mutation. The conflicting results might be partly explained by the different modes of action by VPA, since VPA is also acting as a histone deacetylase (HDAC) inhibitor, thereby altering expression of different genes [176].

4. Discussion and Outlook

The OS of the PR can be considered as a highly specialized cilium responsible for the conversion of light stimuli into electrical signals, also known as the phototransduction cascade. This cascade requires a tremendous amount of energy as well as a continuous OS protein turnover to maintain cellular homeostasis. Therefore, a perfectly balanced proteostasis network is of particular importance for the PRs. In many IRDs this balance is disrupted leading to protein accumulation in the IS and ultimately to PR cell death. Several attempts were made to restore this balance by therapeutically targeting different branches of the proteostasis network, including protein trafficking, folding, and degradation. For therapeutic intervention, it has to be taken into account that these different branches consist of tightly intertwined processes, which depend on each other and influence each other's function and activation. For example, administration of the AMPK activator metformin to P23H RHO mice resulted in enhanced trafficking of rhodopsin to the rod OSs. However, it still led to reduced PR function and survival. Apparently, metformin did not succeed in full restoration of the correct folding of rhodopsin, leading to increased destabilization of the OSs [137]. Taken together, enhancing protein trafficking without improving protein folding will accelerate the disease progression rather than diminishing it. Recently, also an intimate cross-talk between the UPR, more specifically IRE1, and ERAD has been described [177]. On one hand, splicing of XBP1s by activated IRE1 promotes the expression of ERAD components, while on the other hand ERAD serves as a feedback loop for IRE1 by targeting it for degradation. This cross-talk is probably further extended to other branches of the UPR, since it has been shown that the turnover of ATF6 is also regulated by ERAD [178].

Another issue that has to be taken into account for therapeutic intervention is that in some disease conditions certain branches of the proteostasis network are protective, whereas in other disease conditions it is a consequence of the disease process. Therefore, it is often not clear which branch of the proteostasis network would be the most effective target to treat a certain disease type. Even different mutations in the same gene causing similar disease conditions can have an effect on the treatment outcome, indicated by contradictory findings in VPA treatment in the *rd1* and *rd10* mouse models [141]. This discrepancy might be partly explained by the severity of the gene mutations leading to different rates of disease progression, since *rd1* mice show rapid degeneration of PRs, whereas the *rd10* mouse model represents a more slowly progressive form of RP. With this in mind, therapeutic compounds that have an positive effect on slow progressing forms of RP might not be suitable for fast progressing forms of RP and early onset forms of blindness, such as LCA.

The animal model used for therapeutic testing, especially animals carrying a transgene, can also influence therapeutic outcome. One such animal model carrying a transgene is the P23H RHO rat model. Numerous different lines with various transgene expression exist [179–181]. It has been shown that the amount of expression of the transgene can have an effect on the disease phenotype. Even overexpression of wild type human rod opsin has been shown to induce PR degeneration [182]. In contrast, it has been shown that overexpression of wild type RHO partially rescues visual responses in a P23H RHO rat model [113]. Nevertheless, studies using the P23H RHO rat model presented in this review should be interpreted with caution, especially when translating therapeutic outcome to the patient situation.

Instead of directly targeting the different branches of the proteostasis network, mimicking the actions of these branches might also be a valuable therapeutic approach. The main action of the PERK pathway of the UPR is reducing the protein synthesis and thereby reducing the ER-stress load. This action can also be regulated by targeting the epigenome, including histone acetylation. Enzymes that play an important role in this acetylation process are the histone deacetylases (HDACs). Inhibiting these HDACs was shown to be protective for PR cell death. Administration of the HDAC6 inhibitor tubastatin A in an inherited blindness zebrafish model resulted in the rescue of retinal morphology and visual function [183]. However, further investigation of the underlying molecular mechanisms is necessary, since poor efficacy and safety have been reported for other HDAC inhibitors, including VPA [176,184].

Another way to influence protein synthesis is by the regulation of splicing. The importance of splicing in the retina is indicated by mutations found in the ubiquitously expressed pre-mRNA processing factors (PRPFs), which only cause retinal-specific degeneration [185]. In situ gene editing of a pathogenic, dominant mutation in PRPF31 resulted in the rescue of protein expression as well as the phenotype [186]. The proof-of-principle for targeting splicing as potential therapeutic strategy is further supported by the application of antisense oligonucleotides for the treatment of inherited retinal diseases, including CEP290 associated LCA [20,187].

In addition to influencing protein synthesis, degeneration of PRs, which is the ultimate consequence of sustained ER-stress and a key hallmark of IRDs, can also been seen as a therapeutic target. A broad range of therapeutic agents is available that can be protective for PR cell death, including cell death inhibitors, caspase modulators, and neurotrophic factors. Individual treatment of P23H-1 rats with the known cell death inhibitors calpeptin, N-acetylcysteine, and necrostatin-1s all resulted in improved photoreceptor function [188]. Furthermore, the chemical chaperone tauroursodeoxycholic acid (TUDCA), which inhibits apoptosis by preventing BAX from being transported to the mitochondria to initiate caspase release, has been shown to preserve cones in a LCA mouse model upon systemic injection [189]. On top of that, direct inhibition of caspases by subretinal AAV delivered X-linked inhibitor of apoptosis (XIAP) in two RP rat models protected PR structure and function [190]. Finally, neurotrophic factors, including CNTF, BDNF, GDNF, LEDGF, PEDF, and RdCVF were also found to have positive effects on PR survival [191]. However, the therapeutic potential of neurotrophic factors as a general treatment may not outweigh the plausible risk of side effects. These side effects can be reduced by carefully selecting the proper administration route, which accounts for every therapeutic agent described in this review. In general, there are three possible delivery methods to reach the eye: systemic, topical, and local. Each of these methods have their advantages and disadvantages [192]. Systemic delivery is often accompanied by systemic side effects and drugs need to pass the blood–retinal barrier first to perform their function, but it is less invasive compared to intraocular injections. Topical delivery in form of eye drops or ointments is not invasive, but the chance that the therapeutic compound reaches its destination is often an issue. Intraocular injection is the most invasive delivery method, but most often also the most effective one. Furthermore, with this method the involvement of the immune system is largely circumvented, as the eye is a largely immune-privileged organ, thereby further reducing the risk of potential side effects. Intraocular delivery can be performed by injecting the therapeutic compound by itself, but the cell penetrance and thus delivery efficiency is much higher when the compound is packed into nanoparticles, for example [192].

Immense progress has been made in optimizing the delivery methods in combination with the drug formulation, especially for gene augmentation and antisense-oligo nucleotide (AON)-based treatments. Now, an increasing number of studies are aimed at developing broader applicable treatments, and therefore are focused on therapies targetting the proteostatis network. Many of these studies show hopeful results in delaying blinding conditions [111,114,121,122,131]. However, much effort has still to be made to first efficiently halt the progression of IRD, let alone fully restore vision.

Funding: This work was funded by Gelderse Blindenstichting, Janivo Stichting, Landelijke Stichting voor Blinden en Slechtzienden, Retina Nederland, Rotterdamse Stichting Blindenbelangen, Stichting Beheer Het Schild, Stichting Blinden-Penning, Stichting Steunfonds Uitzicht, Stichting tot Verbetering van het Lot der Blinden 'Het Lot', Stichting voor gehandicapte kinderen Dowilvo, the Netherlands Organisation for Health Research and Development (ZonMW, #91216051) and the Foundation Fighting Blindness, USA (PPA-0717-0719-RAD).

Acknowledgments: The authors would like to acknowledge Marius Ueffing for valuable advice on P23H RHO models.

Conflicts of Interest: The authors declare no conflict of interest.

References

1. Osterberg, G. Topography of the layer of rods and cones in the human retina. *Acta Ophthalmol. Suppl.* **1935**, *6*, 1–103.
2. May-Simera, H.; Nagel-Wolfrum, K.; Wolfrum, U. Cilia-The sensory antennae in the eye. *Prog. Retin. Eye Res.* **2017**, *60*, 144–180. [CrossRef] [PubMed]
3. Arshavsky, V.Y.; Lamb, T.D.; Pugh, E.N., Jr. G proteins and phototransduction. *Annu. Rev. Physiol.* **2002**, *64*, 153–187. [CrossRef] [PubMed]
4. Sokolov, M.; Yadav, R.P.; Brooks, C.; Artemyev, N.O. Chaperones and retinal disorders. *Adv. Protein Chem. Struct. Biol.* **2019**, *114*, 85–117. [CrossRef] [PubMed]
5. Krizaj, D. Calcium regulation in photoreceptors. *Front. Biosci. A J. Virtual Libr.* **2002**, *7*, 2023–2044. [CrossRef]
6. Martemyanov, A.K. The Transduction Cascade in Retinal ON-Bipolar Cells: Signal Processing and Disease. *Annu. Rev. Vis. Sci.* **2017**, *3*, 25–51. [CrossRef] [PubMed]
7. Young, R.W.R. The renewal of photoreceptor cell outer segments. *J. Cell Biol.* **1967**, *33*, 61–72. [CrossRef] [PubMed]
8. Baehr, W. Membrane protein transport in photoreceptors: The function of PDEdelta: The Proctor lecture. *Investig. Ophthalmol. Vis. Sci.* **2014**, *55*, 8653–8666. [CrossRef]
9. Leveillard, T.; Sahel, J.A. Metabolic and redox signaling in the retina. *Cell Mol. Life Sci.* **2017**, *74*, 3649–3665. [CrossRef]
10. Narayan, D.S.; Chidlow, G.; Wood, J.P.; Casson, R.J. Glucose metabolism in mammalian photoreceptor inner and outer segments. *Clin. Exp. Ophthalmol.* **2017**, *45*, 730–741. [CrossRef]
11. Bujakowska, K.M.; Liu, Q.; Pierce, E.A. Photoreceptor Cilia and Retinal Ciliopathies. *Cold Spring Harb. Perspect. Biol.* **2017**, *9*. [CrossRef] [PubMed]
12. Daiger, S.P.; Sullivan, L.S.; Rossiter, B.J.F. Cloned and/or Mapped Human Genes Causing Retinal Degeneration or Related Diseases. Available online: https://sph.uth.edu/retnet/ (accessed on 23 July 2019).
13. Roepman, R. Protein networks and complexes in photoreceptor cilia. *Sub-Cell. Biochem.* **2007**, *43*, 209–235.
14. Liu, Q. The proteome of the mouse photoreceptor sensory cilium complex. *Mol. Cell. Proteom.* **2007**, *6*, 1299–1317. [CrossRef] [PubMed]
15. Athanasiou, D.; Aguila, M.; Bellingham, J.; Li, W.; McCulley, C.; Reeves, P.J.; Cheetham, M.E. The molecular and cellular basis of rhodopsin retinitis pigmentosa reveals potential strategies for therapy. *Prog. Retin. Eye Res.* **2018**, *62*, 1–23. [CrossRef] [PubMed]
16. den Hollander, A.I.; Koenekoop, R.K.; Mohamed, M.D.; Arts, H.H.; Boldt, K.; Towns, K.V.; Sedmak, T.; Beer, M.; Nagel-Wolfrum, K.; McKibbin, M.; et al. Mutations in LCA5, encoding the ciliary protein lebercilin, cause Leber congenital amaurosis. *Nat. Genet.* **2007**, *39*, 889–895. [CrossRef] [PubMed]
17. Hamel, C.P. Cone rod dystrophies. *Orphanet J. Rare Dis.* **2007**, *2*, 7. [CrossRef] [PubMed]
18. Hirji, N.; Aboshiha, J.; Georgiou, M.; Bainbridge, J.; Michaelides, M. Achromatopsia: Clinical features, molecular genetics, animal models and therapeutic options. *Ophthalmic Genet.* **2018**, *39*, 149–157. [CrossRef] [PubMed]
19. Song, J.Y.; Aravand, P.; Nikonov, S.; Leo, L.; Lyubarsky, A.; Bennicelli, J.L.; Pan, J.; Wei, Z.; Shpylchak, I.; Herrera, P.; et al. Amelioration of neurosensory structure and function in animal and cellular models of a congenital blindness. *Mol. Ther.* **2018**. [CrossRef]
20. Garanto, A.; Chung, D.C.; Duijkers, L.; Corral-Serrano, J.C.; Messchaert, M.; Xiao, R.; Bennett, J.; Vandenberghe, L.H.; Collin, R.W. In vitro and in vivo rescue of aberrant splicing in CEP290-associated LCA by antisense oligonucleotide delivery. *Hum. Mol. Genet.* **2016**, *25*, 2552–2563. [CrossRef]
21. Athanasiou, D.; Aguila, M.; Bevilacqua, D.; Novoselov, S.S.; Parfitt, D.A.; Cheetham, M.E. The cell stress machinery and retinal degeneration. *FEBS Lett.* **2013**, *587*, 2008–2017. [CrossRef]
22. Maurer-Stroh, S.; Koranda, M.; Benetka, W.; Schneider, G.; Sirota, F.L.; Eisenhaber, F. Towards complete sets of farnesylated and geranylgeranylated proteins. *PLoS Comput. Biol.* **2007**, *3*, e66. [CrossRef] [PubMed]
23. Casey, P.J.P. Protein prenyltransferases. *J. Biol. Chem.* **1996**, *271*, 5289–5292. [CrossRef] [PubMed]

24. Sohocki, M.M.M. Mutations in a new photoreceptor-pineal gene on 17p cause Leber congenital amaurosis. *Nat. Genet.* **2000**, *24*, 79–83. [CrossRef] [PubMed]
25. den Hollander, A.I. Leber congenital amaurosis: Genes, proteins and disease mechanisms. *Prog. Retin. Eye Res.* **2008**, *27*, 391–419. [CrossRef] [PubMed]
26. Liu, X. AIPL1, the protein that is defective in Leber congenital amaurosis, is essential for the biosynthesis of retinal rod cGMP phosphodiesterase. *Proc. Natl. Acad. Sci. USA* **2004**, *101*, 13903–13908. [CrossRef] [PubMed]
27. Ramamurthy, V. Leber congenital amaurosis linked to AIPL1: A mouse model reveals destabilization of cGMP phosphodiesterase. *Proc. Natl. Acad. Sci. USA* **2004**, *101*, 13897–13902. [CrossRef] [PubMed]
28. Ramamurthy, V. AIPL1, a protein implicated in Leber's congenital amaurosis, interacts with and aids in processing of farnesylated proteins. *Proc. Natl. Acad. Sci. USA* **2003**, *100*, 12630–12635. [CrossRef] [PubMed]
29. Yadav, R.P.; Artemyev, N.O. AIPL1: A specialized chaperone for the phototransduction effector. *Cell Signal.* **2017**, *40*, 183–189. [CrossRef] [PubMed]
30. Roosing, S.; Collin, R.W.; den Hollander, A.I.; Cremers, F.P.; Siemiatkowska, A.M. Prenylation defects in inherited retinal diseases. *J. Med. Genet.* **2014**, *51*, 143–151. [CrossRef] [PubMed]
31. Zhang, H.; Constantine, R.; Frederick, J.M.; Baehr, W. The prenyl-binding protein PrBP/delta: A chaperone participating in intracellular trafficking. *Vis. Res.* **2012**, *75*, 19–25. [CrossRef]
32. Zhang, H.H. Deletion of PrBP/delta impedes transport of GRK1 and PDE6 catalytic subunits to photoreceptor outer segments. *Proc. Natl. Acad. Sci. USA* **2007**, *104*, 8857–8862. [CrossRef] [PubMed]
33. Thomas, S. A homozygous PDE6D mutation in Joubert syndrome impairs targeting of farnesylated INPP5E protein to the primary cilium. *Hum. Mutat.* **2014**, *35*, 137–146. [CrossRef] [PubMed]
34. Megarbane, A.; Hmaimess, G.; Bizzari, S.; El-Bazzal, L.; Al-Ali, M.T.; Stora, S.; Delague, V.; El-Hayek, S. A novel PDE6D mutation in a patient with Joubert syndrome type 22 (JBTS22). *Eur. J. Med. Genet.* **2018**. [CrossRef]
35. Rao, K.N.; Zhang, W.; Li, L.; Anand, M.; Khanna, H. Prenylated retinal ciliopathy protein RPGR interacts with PDE6delta and regulates ciliary localization of Joubert syndrome-associated protein INPP5E. *Hum. Mol. Genet.* **2016**, *25*, 4533–4545. [CrossRef] [PubMed]
36. Qureshi, B.M.; Schmidt, A.; Behrmann, E.; Burger, J.; Mielke, T.; Spahn, C.M.T.; Heck, M.; Scheerer, P. Mechanistic insights into the role of prenyl-binding protein PrBP/delta in membrane dissociation of phosphodiesterase 6. *Nat. Commun.* **2018**, *9*, 90. [CrossRef] [PubMed]
37. Hanke-Gogokhia, C.; Frederick, J.M.; Zhang, H.; Baehr, W. Binary Function of ARL3-GTP Revealed by Gene Knockouts. *Adv. Exp. Med. Biol.* **2018**, *1074*, 317–325. [CrossRef] [PubMed]
38. Ismail, A.S. Arl2-GTP and Arl3-GTP regulate a GDI-like transport system for farnesylated cargo. *Nat. Chem. Biol.* **2011**, *7*, 942–949. [CrossRef]
39. Fansa, K.E. Sorting of lipidated cargo by the Arl2/Arl3 system. *Small GTPases* **2016**, *7*, 222–230. [CrossRef] [PubMed]
40. Constantine, R. Uncoordinated (UNC)119: Coordinating the trafficking of myristoylated proteins. *Vis. Res.* **2012**, *75*, 26–32. [CrossRef] [PubMed]
41. Zhang, H. UNC119 is required for G protein trafficking in sensory neurons. *Nat. Neurosci.* **2011**, *14*, 874–880. [CrossRef] [PubMed]
42. Ishiba, Y. Targeted inactivation of synaptic HRG4 (UNC119) causes dysfunction in the distal photoreceptor and slow retinal degeneration, revealing a new function. *Exp. Eye Res.* **2007**, *84*, 473–485. [CrossRef] [PubMed]
43. Zhang, H.; Frederick, J.M.; Baehr, W. Unc119 gene deletion partially rescues the GRK1 transport defect of Pde6d (-/-) cones. *Adv. Exp. Med. Biol.* **2014**, *801*, 487–493. [CrossRef]
44. Kobayashi, A.A. HRG4 (UNC119) mutation found in cone-rod dystrophy causes retinal degeneration in a transgenic model. *Investig. Ophthalmol. Vis. Sci.* **2000**, *41*, 3268–3277.
45. Zhang, J. Mechanism of folding chamber closure in a group II chaperonin. *Sci. Am.* **2010**, *463*, 379–383. [CrossRef] [PubMed]
46. Wells, A.C. Role of the chaperonin CCT/TRiC complex in G protein betagamma-dimer assembly. *J. Biol. Chem.* **2006**, *281*, 20221–20232. [CrossRef] [PubMed]
47. Lukov, L.G. Phosducin-like protein acts as a molecular chaperone for G protein betagamma dimer assembly. *EMBO J.* **2005**, *24*, 1965–1975. [CrossRef] [PubMed]

48. Loew, A.A. Phosducin induces a structural change in transducin β γ. *Structure* **1998**, *6*, 1007–1019. [CrossRef]
49. Brooks, C. Farnesylation of the Transducin G Protein γ Subunit Is a Prerequisite for Its Ciliary Targeting in Rod Photoreceptors. *Front. Mol. Neurosci.* **2018**, *11*, 16. [CrossRef]
50. Obin, M. Ubiquitylation of the transducin betagamma subunit complex. Regulation by phosducin. *J. Biol. Chem.* **2002**, *277*, 44566–44575. [CrossRef]
51. Zhang, Q. Intrinsic protein-protein interaction-mediated and chaperonin-assisted sequential assembly of stable bardet-biedl syndrome protein complex, the BBSome. *J. Biol. Chem.* **2012**, *287*, 20625–20635. [CrossRef]
52. Klink, B.U. A recombinant BBSome core complex and how it interacts with ciliary cargo. *eLife* **2017**, *6*, e27434. [CrossRef] [PubMed]
53. Forsythe, E. Bardet-Biedl syndrome. *Eur. J. Hum. Genet.* **2013**, *21*, 8–13. [CrossRef] [PubMed]
54. Jin, H. The conserved Bardet-Biedl syndrome proteins assemble a coat that traffics membrane proteins to cilia. *Cell* **2010**, *141*, 1208–1219. [CrossRef] [PubMed]
55. Chan, P. Molecular chaperoning function of Ric-8 is to fold nascent heterotrimeric G protein a subunits. *Proc. Natl. Acad. Sci. USA* **2013**, *110*, 3794–3799. [CrossRef] [PubMed]
56. Tall, G.G. Ric-8 regulation of heterotrimeric G proteins. *J. Recept. Signal Transduct.* **2013**, *33*, 139–143. [CrossRef]
57. Fenech, C. Ric-8A, a Gα protein guanine nucleotide exchange factor potentiates taste receptor signaling. *Front. Cell. Neurosci.* **2009**, *3*, 11. [CrossRef] [PubMed]
58. Sprang, R.S. Structural basis of effector regulation and signal termination in heterotrimeric Gα proteins. *Adv. Protein Chem.* **2007**, *74*, 1–65.
59. Joutsen, J.; Sistonen, L. Tailoring of Proteostasis Networks with Heat Shock Factors. *Cold Spring Harb. Perspect. Biol.* **2019**, *11*. [CrossRef]
60. Morimoto, R.I.R. The heat-shock response: Regulation and function of heat-shock proteins and molecular chaperones. *Essays Biochem.* **1997**, *32*, 17–29.
61. Vabulas, R.M.R.M. Protein folding in the cytoplasm and the heat shock response. *Cold Spring Harbor Perspect. Biol.* **2010**, *2*, a004390. [CrossRef]
62. Hartl, F.U.; Bracher, A.; Hayer-Hartl, M. Molecular chaperones in protein folding and proteostasis. *Nature* **2011**, *475*, 324–332. [CrossRef] [PubMed]
63. Apetri, C.A. Chaperonin chamber accelerates protein folding through passive action of preventing aggregation. *Proc. Natl. Acad. Sci. USA* **2008**, *105*, 17351–17355. [CrossRef] [PubMed]
64. Walter, P. The unfolded protein response: From stress pathway to homeostatic regulation. *Science* **2011**, *334*, 1081–1086. [CrossRef] [PubMed]
65. Bertolotti, A.A. Dynamic interaction of BiP and ER stress transducers in the unfolded-protein response. *Nat. Cell Biol.* **2000**, *2*, 326–332. [CrossRef] [PubMed]
66. Lamriben, L. Activating and Repressing IRE1a: The Hsp47 and BiP Tug of War. *Mol. Cell* **2018**, *69*, 159–160. [CrossRef] [PubMed]
67. Calfon, M. IRE1 couples endoplasmic reticulum load to secretory capacity by processing the XBP-1 mRNA. *Sci. Am.* **2002**, *415*, 92–96. [CrossRef] [PubMed]
68. Lee, A.H. XBP-1 regulates a subset of endoplasmic reticulum resident chaperone genes in the unfolded protein response. *Mol. Cell. Biol.* **2003**, *23*, 7448–7459. [CrossRef] [PubMed]
69. Fritz, M.J. Deficiency of the BiP cochaperone ERdj4 causes constitutive endoplasmic reticulum stress and metabolic defects. *Mol. Biol. Cell* **2014**, *25*, 431–440. [CrossRef]
70. Eletto, D. Protein disulfide isomerase A6 controls the decay of IRE1a signaling via disulfide-dependent association. *Mol. Cell* **2014**, *53*, 562–576. [CrossRef] [PubMed]
71. Harding, H.P.H. Protein translation and folding are coupled by an endoplasmic-reticulum-resident kinase. *Sci. Am.* **1999**, *397*, 271–274.
72. Vattem, M.K. Reinitiation involving upstream ORFs regulates ATF4 mRNA translation in mammalian cells. *Proc. Natl. Acad. Sci. USA* **2004**, *101*, 11269–11274. [CrossRef] [PubMed]
73. Novoa, I.I. Feedback inhibition of the unfolded protein response by GADD34-mediated dephosphorylation of eIF2α. *J. Cell Biol.* **2001**, *153*, 1011–1022. [CrossRef] [PubMed]
74. Marciniak, J.S. CHOP induces death by promoting protein synthesis and oxidation in the stressed endoplasmic reticulum. *Gen. Dev.* **2004**, *18*, 3066–3077. [CrossRef] [PubMed]

75. Shen, J. ER stress regulation of ATF6 localization by dissociation of BiP/GRP78 binding and unmasking of Golgi localization signals. *Dev. Cell* **2002**, *3*, 99–111. [CrossRef]
76. Haze, K.K. Mammalian transcription factor ATF6 is synthesized as a transmembrane protein and activated by proteolysis in response to endoplasmic reticulum stress. *Mol. Biol. Cell* **1999**, *10*, 3787–3799. [CrossRef] [PubMed]
77. Yamamoto, K. Transcriptional induction of mammalian ER quality control proteins is mediated by single or combined action of ATF6α and XBP1. *Dev. Cell* **2007**, *13*, 365–376. [CrossRef] [PubMed]
78. Schubert, U.U. Rapid degradation of a large fraction of newly synthesized proteins by proteasomes. *Sci. Am.* **2000**, *404*, 770–774. [CrossRef] [PubMed]
79. Olzmann, A.J. The mammalian endoplasmic reticulum-associated degradation system. *Cold Spring Harbor Perspect. Biol.* **2013**, *5*. [CrossRef] [PubMed]
80. Helenius, A. Roles of N-linked glycans in the endoplasmic reticulum. *Ann. Rev. Biochem.* **2004**, *73*, 1019–1049. [CrossRef]
81. Aebi, M. N-glycan structures: Recognition and processing in the ER. *Trends Biochem. Sci.* **2010**, *35*, 74–82. [CrossRef] [PubMed]
82. Hebert, N.D. ERAD substrates: Which way out? *Semin. Cell Dev. Biol.* **2010**, *21*, 526–532. [CrossRef] [PubMed]
83. Gonzalez, D.S.D. Identification, expression, and characterization of a cDNA encoding human endoplasmic reticulum mannosidase I, the enzyme that catalyzes the first mannose trimming step in mammalian Asn-linked oligosaccharide biosynthesis. *J. Biol. Chem.* **1999**, *274*, 21375–21386. [CrossRef] [PubMed]
84. Olivari, S. EDEM1 regulates ER-associated degradation by accelerating de-mannosylation of folding-defective polypeptides and by inhibiting their covalent aggregation. *Biochem. Biophys. Res. Commun.* **2006**, *349*, 1278–1284. [CrossRef] [PubMed]
85. Hirao, K. EDEM3, a soluble EDEM homolog, enhances glycoprotein endoplasmic reticulum-associated degradation and mannose trimming. *J. Biol. Chem.* **2006**, *281*, 9650–9658. [CrossRef] [PubMed]
86. Hampton, Y.R. Finding the will and the way of ERAD substrate retrotranslocation. *Curr. Opin. Cell Biol.* **2012**, *24*, 460–466. [CrossRef] [PubMed]
87. Ye, Y. A membrane protein complex mediates retro-translocation from the ER lumen into the cytosol. *Sci. Am.* **2004**, *429*, 841–847. [CrossRef] [PubMed]
88. Meyer, H. Emerging functions of the VCP/p97 AAA-ATPase in the ubiquitin system. *Nat. Cell Biol.* **2012**, *14*, 117–123. [CrossRef] [PubMed]
89. Xu, Y. SGTA recognizes a noncanonical ubiquitin-like domain in the Bag6-Ubl4A-Trc35 complex to promote endoplasmic reticulum-associated degradation. *Cell Rep.* **2012**, *2*, 1633–1644. [CrossRef] [PubMed]
90. Boya, P.; Esteban-Martinez, L.; Serrano-Puebla, A.; Gomez-Sintes, R.; Villarejo-Zori, B. Autophagy in the eye: Development, degeneration, and aging. *Prog. Retin. Eye Res.* **2016**, *55*, 206–245. [CrossRef] [PubMed]
91. Wong, P.M. The ULK1 complex: Sensing nutrient signals for autophagy activation. *Autophagy* **2013**, *9*, 124–137. [CrossRef] [PubMed]
92. Walker, S. Making autophagosomes: Localized synthesis of phosphatidylinositol 3-phosphate holds the clue. *Autophagy* **2008**, *4*, 1093–1096. [CrossRef] [PubMed]
93. Frost, L.S.; Mitchell, C.H.; Boesze-Battaglia, K. Autophagy in the eye: Implications for ocular cell health. *Exp. Eye Res.* **2014**, *124*, 56–66. [CrossRef] [PubMed]
94. Arias, E. Chaperone-mediated autophagy in protein quality control. *Curr. Opin. Cell Biol.* **2011**, *23*, 184–189. [CrossRef] [PubMed]
95. Dice, J.F.J. Peptide sequences that target cytosolic proteins for lysosomal proteolysis. *Trends Biochem. Sci.* **1990**, *15*, 305–309. [CrossRef]
96. Chiang, H.L.H. A role for a 70-kilodalton heat shock protein in lysosomal degradation of intracellular proteins. *Science* **1989**, *246*, 382–385. [CrossRef] [PubMed]
97. Cuervo, A.M.A. A receptor for the selective uptake and degradation of proteins by lysosomes. *Science* **1996**, *273*, 501–503. [CrossRef] [PubMed]
98. Sahu, R. Microautophagy of cytosolic proteins by late endosomes. *Dev. Cell* **2011**, *20*, 131–139. [CrossRef] [PubMed]
99. Morozova, K. Structural and Biological Interaction of hsc-70 Protein with Phosphatidylserine in Endosomal Microautophagy. *J. Biol. Chem.* **2016**, *291*, 18096–18106. [CrossRef]

100. Capell, C.B. Inhibiting farnesylation of progerin prevents the characteristic nuclear blebbing of Hutchinson-Gilford progeria syndrome. *Proc. Natl. Acad. Sci. USA* **2005**, *102*, 12879–12884. [CrossRef]
101. Gordon, B.L. Clinical Trial of the Protein Farnesylation Inhibitors Lonafarnib, Pravastatin, and Zoledronic Acid in Children With Hutchinson-Gilford Progeria Syndrome. *Circ. J. Am. Heart Assoc.* **2016**, *134*, 114–125. [CrossRef]
102. Martin, E.N. A phase I trial of the dual farnesyltransferase and geranylgeranyltransferase inhibitor L-778,123 and radiotherapy for locally advanced pancreatic cancer. *Clin. Cancer Res.* **2004**, *10*, 5447–5454. [CrossRef] [PubMed]
103. Posokhova, E. Disruption of the chaperonin containing TCP-1 function affects protein networks essential for rod outer segment morphogenesis and survival. *Mol. Cell. Proteom.* **2011**, *10*. [CrossRef] [PubMed]
104. Willardson, M.B. Function of phosducin-like proteins in G protein signaling and chaperone-assisted protein folding. *Cell Signal.* **2007**, *19*, 2417–2427. [CrossRef] [PubMed]
105. Álvarez-Satta, M. Bardet-Biedl Syndrome as a Chaperonopathy: Dissecting the Major Role of Chaperonin-Like BBS Proteins (BBS6-BBS10-BBS12). *Front. Mol. Biosci.* **2017**, *4*, 55. [CrossRef] [PubMed]
106. Papasergi, M.M. The G protein a chaperone Ric-8 as a potential therapeutic target. *Mol. Pharmacol.* **2015**, *87*, 52–63. [CrossRef] [PubMed]
107. Szabo, V. p.Gln200Glu, a putative constitutively active mutant of rod α-transducin (*GNAT1*) in autosomal dominant congenital stationary night blindness. *Hum. Mutat.* **2007**, *28*, 741–742. [CrossRef] [PubMed]
108. Supko, J.G.J. Preclinical pharmacologic evaluation of geldanamycin as an antitumor agent. *Cancer Chemother. Pharmacol.* **1995**, *36*, 305–315. [CrossRef]
109. Jhaveri, K. Advances in the clinical development of heat shock protein 90 (Hsp90) inhibitors in cancers. *Biochim. Biophys. Acta* **2012**, *1823*, 742–755. [CrossRef]
110. Tam, C.S.L. Prevention of autosomal dominant retinitis pigmentosa by systemic drug therapy targeting heat shock protein 90 (Hsp90). *Hum. Mol. Genet.* **2010**, *19*, 4421–4436. [CrossRef]
111. Aguilà, M. Hsp90 inhibition protects against inherited retinal degeneration. *Hum. Mol. Genet.* **2014**, *23*, 2164–2175. [CrossRef]
112. Zhou, D. A rat retinal damage model predicts for potential clinical visual disturbances induced by Hsp90 inhibitors. *Toxicol. Appl. Pharmacol.* **2013**, *273*, 401–409. [CrossRef] [PubMed]
113. Gorbatyuk, S.M. Functional rescue of P23H rhodopsin photoreceptors by gene delivery. *Adv. Exp. Med. Biol.* **2012**, *723*, 191–197. [PubMed]
114. Parfitt, D.A.; Aguila, M.; McCulley, C.H.; Bevilacqua, D.; Mendes, H.F.; Athanasiou, D.; Novoselov, S.S.; Kanuga, N.; Munro, P.M.; Coffey, P.J.; et al. The heat-shock response co-inducer arimoclomol protects against retinal degeneration in rhodopsin retinitis pigmentosa. *Cell Death Dis.* **2014**, *5*, e1236. [CrossRef] [PubMed]
115. Gorbatyuk, S.M. Restoration of visual function in P23H rhodopsin transgenic rats by gene delivery of BiP/Grp78. *Proc. Natl. Acad. Sci. USA* **2010**, *107*, 5961–5966. [CrossRef] [PubMed]
116. Ghaderi, S.; Ahmadian, S.; Soheili, Z.S.; Ahmadieh, H.; Samiei, S.; Kheitan, S.; Pirmardan, E.R. AAV delivery of GRP78/BiP promotes adaptation of human RPE cell to ER stress. *J. Cell Biochem.* **2018**, *119*, 1355–1367. [CrossRef] [PubMed]
117. Nashine, S. Ablation of C/EBP homologous protein does not protect T17M RHO mice from retinal degeneration. *PLoS ONE* **2013**, *8*. [CrossRef] [PubMed]
118. Adekeye, A. Ablation of the proapoptotic genes CHOP or Ask1 does not prevent or delay loss of visual function in a P23H transgenic mouse model of retinitis pigmentosa. *PLoS ONE* **2014**, *9*. [CrossRef] [PubMed]
119. Chiang, W.C. Ablation of Chop Transiently Enhances Photoreceptor Survival but Does Not Prevent Retinal Degeneration in Transgenic Mice Expressing Human P23H Rhodopsin. *Adv. Exp. Med. Biol.* **2016**, *854*, 185–191.
120. Bhootada, Y.; Kotla, P.; Zolotukhin, S.; Gorbatyuk, O.; Bebok, Z.; Athar, M.; Gorbatyuk, M. Limited ATF4 Expression in Degenerating Retinas with Ongoing ER Stress Promotes Photoreceptor Survival in a Mouse Model of Autosomal Dominant Retinitis Pigmentosa. *PLoS ONE* **2016**, *11*, e0154779. [CrossRef]
121. Athanasiou, D.; Aguila, M.; Bellingham, J.; Kanuga, N.; Adamson, P.; Cheetham, M.E. The role of the ER stress-response protein PERK in rhodopsin retinitis pigmentosa. *Hum. Mol. Genet.* **2017**, *26*, 4896–4905. [CrossRef]
122. Ghosh, R. Allosteric inhibition of the IRE1a RNase preserves cell viability and function during endoplasmic reticulum stress. *Cell* **2014**, *158*, 534–548. [CrossRef]

123. Takasugi, N. The Emerging Role of Electrophiles as a Key Regulator for Endoplasmic Reticulum (ER) Stress. *Int. J. Mol. Sci.* **2019**, *20*, 1783. [CrossRef] [PubMed]
124. Nakamura, T. Aberrant protein S-nitrosylation contributes to the pathophysiology of neurodegenerative diseases. *Neurobiol. Dis.* **2015**, *84*, 99–108. [CrossRef] [PubMed]
125. Groeger, L.A. Signaling actions of electrophiles: Anti-inflammatory therapeutic candidates. *Mol. Interv.* **2010**, *10*, 39–50. [CrossRef] [PubMed]
126. Sakanyan, V. Reactive Chemicals and Electrophilic Stress in Cancer: A Minireview. *High-Throughput* **2018**, *7*, 12. [CrossRef]
127. Uehara, T. S-nitrosylated protein-disulphide isomerase links protein misfolding to neurodegeneration. *Sci. Am.* **2006**, *441*, 513–517. [CrossRef] [PubMed]
128. Nakato, R. Regulation of the unfolded protein response via S-nitrosylation of sensors of endoplasmic reticulum stress. *Sci. Rep.* **2015**, *5*, 14812. [CrossRef]
129. Gallagher, M.C. Ceapins are a new class of unfolded protein response inhibitors, selectively targeting the ATF6a branch. *eLife* **2016**, *5*, e11878. [CrossRef]
130. Gallagher, M.C. Ceapins inhibit ATF6a signaling by selectively preventing transport of ATF6a to the Golgi apparatus during ER stress. *eLife* **2016**, *5*, e11880. [CrossRef]
131. Kakizuka, A. VCP, a Major ATPase in the Cells, as a Novel Drug Target for Currently Incurable Disorders. In *Innovative Medicine: Basic Research and Development*; Nakao, K., Minato, N., Uemoto, S., Eds.; Springer: Tokyo, Japan, 2015.
132. Brooks, C. Archaeal Unfoldase Counteracts Protein Misfolding Retinopathy in Mice. *J. Neurosci.* **2018**, *38*, 7248–7254. [CrossRef]
133. Wilkinson, K.D.K. Regulation of ubiquitin-dependent processes by deubiquitinating enzymes. *FASEB J.* **1997**, *11*, 1245–1256. [CrossRef] [PubMed]
134. Zhang, W. Generation and Validation of Intracellular Ubiquitin Variant Inhibitors for USP7 and USP10. *J. Mol. Biol.* **2017**, *429*, 3546–3560. [CrossRef] [PubMed]
135. Liu, Y. Roles of p97-associated deubiquitinases in protein quality control at the endoplasmic reticulum. *Curr. Protein Pept. Sci.* **2012**, *13*, 436–446. [CrossRef] [PubMed]
136. Sizova, S.O. Modulation of cellular signaling pathways in P23H rhodopsin photoreceptors. *Cell. Signal.* **2014**, *26*, 665–672. [CrossRef] [PubMed]
137. Athanasiou, D.; Aguila, M.; Opefi, C.A.; South, K.; Bellingham, J.; Bevilacqua, D.; Munro, P.M.; Kanuga, N.; Mackenzie, F.E.; Dubis, A.M.; et al. Rescue of mutant rhodopsin traffic by metformin-induced AMPK activation accelerates photoreceptor degeneration. *Hum. Mol. Genet.* **2017**, *26*, 305–319. [CrossRef] [PubMed]
138. Kim, Y.S. Metformin protects against retinal cell death in diabetic mice. *Biochem. Biophys. Res. Commun.* **2017**, *492*, 397–403. [CrossRef] [PubMed]
139. Vent-Schmidt, R.Y.J.; Wen, R.H.; Zong, Z.; Chiu, C.N.; Tam, B.M.; May, C.G.; Moritz, O.L. Opposing Effects of Valproic Acid Treatment Mediated by Histone Deacetylase Inhibitor Activity in Four Transgenic, X. laevis Models of Retinitis Pigmentosa. *J. Neurosci.* **2017**, *37*, 1039–1054. [CrossRef] [PubMed]
140. Mockel, A.; Obringer, C.; Hakvoort, T.B.; Seeliger, M.; Lamers, W.H.; Stoetzel, C.; Dollfus, H.; Marion, V. Pharmacological modulation of the retinal unfolded protein response in Bardet-Biedl syndrome reduces apoptosis and preserves light detection ability. *J. Biol. Chem.* **2012**, *287*, 37483–37494. [CrossRef] [PubMed]
141. Mitton, P.K. Different effects of valproic acid on photoreceptor loss in Rd1 and Rd10 retinal degeneration mice. *Mol. Vis.* **2014**, *20*, 1527–1544.
142. Reuter, C.W.C. Targeting the Ras signaling pathway: A rational, mechanism-based treatment for hematologic malignancies? *Blood* **2000**, *96*, 1655–1669.
143. Whyte, D.B.D. K- and N-Ras are geranylgeranylated in cells treated with farnesyl protein transferase inhibitors. *J. Biol. Chem.* **1997**, *272*, 14459–14464. [CrossRef] [PubMed]
144. Eriksson, M. Recurrent de novo point mutations in lamin A cause Hutchinson-Gilford progeria syndrome. *Sci. Am.* **2003**, *423*, 293–298. [CrossRef] [PubMed]
145. Thulasiraman, V.V. In vivo newly translated polypeptides are sequestered in a protected folding environment. *EMBO J.* **1999**, *18*, 85–95. [CrossRef] [PubMed]
146. Butler Lisa, M.L. Maximizing the Therapeutic Potential of HSP90 Inhibitors. *Mol. Cancer Res.* **2015**, *13*, 1445–1451. [CrossRef] [PubMed]

147. Workman, P. Drugging the cancer chaperone HSP90: Combinatorial therapeutic exploitation of oncogene addiction and tumor stress. *Ann. N. Y. Acad. Sci.* **2007**, *1113*, 202–216. [CrossRef] [PubMed]
148. Han, J. ER-stress-induced transcriptional regulation increases protein synthesis leading to cell death. *Nat. Cell Biol.* **2013**, *15*, 481–490. [CrossRef] [PubMed]
149. Upton, J.P. IRE1a cleaves select microRNAs during ER stress to derepress translation of proapoptotic Caspase-2. *Science* **2012**, *338*, 818–822. [CrossRef] [PubMed]
150. Yang, Y. Transcription Factor C/EBP Homologous Protein in Health and Diseases. *Front. Immunol.* **2017**, *8*, 1612. [CrossRef] [PubMed]
151. Milisav, I. Unfolded Protein Response and Macroautophagy in Alzheimer's, Parkinson's and Prion Diseases. *Molecules* **2015**, *20*, 22718–22756. [CrossRef] [PubMed]
152. Wang, L. The unfolded protein response in familial amyotrophic lateral sclerosis. *Hum. Mol. Genet.* **2011**, *20*, 1008–1015. [CrossRef] [PubMed]
153. Ma, T. Suppression of eIF2a kinases alleviates Alzheimer's disease-related plasticity and memory deficits. *Nat. Neurosci.* **2013**, *16*, 1299–1305. [CrossRef] [PubMed]
154. Moreno, A.J. Sustained translational repression by eIF2a-P mediates prion neurodegeneration. *Sci. Am.* **2012**, *485*, 507–511.
155. Moreno, A.J. Oral treatment targeting the unfolded protein response prevents neurodegeneration and clinical disease in prion-infected mice. *Sci. Transl. Med.* **2013**, *5*, 206ra138. [CrossRef] [PubMed]
156. Xu, M. ATF6 Is Mutated in Early Onset Photoreceptor Degeneration With Macular Involvement. *Investig. Ophthalmol. Vis. Sci.* **2015**, *56*, 3889–3895. [CrossRef] [PubMed]
157. Ansar, M. Mutation of ATF6 causes autosomal recessive achromatopsia. *Hum. Genet.* **2015**, *134*, 941–950. [CrossRef] [PubMed]
158. Bug, M. Expanding into new markets–VCP/p97 in endocytosis and autophagy. *J. Struct. Biol.* **2012**, *179*, 78–82. [CrossRef] [PubMed]
159. March, Z.M.; Mack, K.L.; Shorter, J. AAA+ Protein-Based Technologies to Counter Neurodegenerative Disease. *Biophys. J.* **2019**. [CrossRef] [PubMed]
160. Rivlin, N. Mutations in the p53 Tumor Suppressor Gene: Important Milestones at the Various Steps of Tumorigenesis. *Genes Cancer* **2011**, *2*, 466–474. [CrossRef] [PubMed]
161. Vuong, L. p53 selectively regulates developmental apoptosis of rod photoreceptors. *PLoS ONE* **2013**, *8*, e67381. [CrossRef]
162. Yoshizawa, K. N-methyl-N-nitrosourea-induced retinal degeneration in mice is independent of the p53 gene. *Mol. Vis.* **2009**, *15*, 2919–2925. [PubMed]
163. Yi, Z. Biallelic mutations in USP45, encoding a deubiquitinating enzyme, are associated with Leber congenital amaurosis. *J. Med. Genet.* **2019**, *56*, 325–331. [CrossRef] [PubMed]
164. Ballou, M.L. Rapamycin and mTOR kinase inhibitors. *J. Chem. Biol.* **2008**, *1*, 27–36. [CrossRef] [PubMed]
165. Walters, E.H. mTORC Inhibitors as Broad-Spectrum Therapeutics for Age-Related Diseases. *Int. J. Mol. Sci.* **2018**, *19*, 2325. [CrossRef] [PubMed]
166. Meng, L.H. Toward rapamycin analog (rapalog)-based precision cancer therapy. *Acta Pharmacol. Sin.* **2015**, *36*, 1163–1169. [CrossRef] [PubMed]
167. Venkatesh, A. Activated mTORC1 promotes long-term cone survival in retinitis pigmentosa mice. *J. Clin. Investig.* **2015**, *125*, 1446–1458. [CrossRef] [PubMed]
168. Rajala, A. Constitutive Activation Mutant mTOR Promote Cone Survival in Retinitis Pigmentosa Mice. *Adv. Exp. Med. Biol.* **2018**, *1074*, 491–497. [PubMed]
169. Punzo, C.; Kornacker, K.; Cepko, C.L. Stimulation of the insulin/mTOR pathway delays cone death in a mouse model of retinitis pigmentosa. *Nat. Neurosci.* **2009**, *12*, 44–52. [CrossRef] [PubMed]
170. Benjamin, D. Rapamycin passes the torch: A new generation of mTOR inhibitors. *Nat. Rev. Drug Discov.* **2011**, *10*, 868–880. [CrossRef] [PubMed]
171. Rotermund, C. The Therapeutic Potential of Metformin in Neurodegenerative Diseases. *Front. Endocrinol.* **2018**, *9*, 400. [CrossRef] [PubMed]
172. Buzzai, M. Systemic treatment with the antidiabetic drug metformin selectively impairs p53-deficient tumor cell growth. *Cancer Res.* **2007**, *67*, 6745–6752. [CrossRef]
173. Kurelac, I. The multifaceted effects of metformin on tumor microenvironment. *Semin. Cell Dev. Biol.* **2019**. [CrossRef] [PubMed]

174. Williams, A. Novel targets for Huntington's disease in an mTOR-independent autophagy pathway. *Nat. Chem. Biol.* **2008**, *4*, 295–305. [CrossRef] [PubMed]
175. Campello, L.; Esteve-Rudd, J.; Cuenca, N.; Martin-Nieto, J. The ubiquitin-proteasome system in retinal health and disease. *Mol. Neurobiol.* **2013**, *47*, 790–810. [CrossRef] [PubMed]
176. Chuang, D.M. Multiple roles of HDAC inhibition in neurodegenerative conditions. *Trends Neurosci.* **2009**, *32*, 591–601. [CrossRef] [PubMed]
177. Hwang, J.; Qi, L. Quality Control in the Endoplasmic Reticulum: Crosstalk between ERAD and UPR pathways. *Trends Biochem. Sci.* **2018**, *43*, 593–605. [CrossRef] [PubMed]
178. Horimoto, S. The unfolded protein response transducer ATF6 represents a novel transmembrane-type endoplasmic reticulum-associated degradation substrate requiring both mannose trimming and SEL1L protein. *J. Biol. Chem.* **2013**, *288*, 31517–31527. [CrossRef] [PubMed]
179. Orhan, E. Genotypic and phenotypic characterization of P23H line 1 rat model. *PLoS ONE* **2015**, *10*, e0127319. [CrossRef] [PubMed]
180. Monai, N. Characterization of photoreceptor degeneration in the rhodopsin P23H transgenic rat line 2 using optical coherence tomography. *PLoS ONE* **2018**, *13*, e0193778. [CrossRef]
181. Machida, S.S. P23H rhodopsin transgenic rat: Correlation of retinal function with histopathology. *Investig. Ophthalmol. Vis. Sci.* **2000**, *41*, 3200–3209.
182. Olsson, J.E.J. Transgenic mice with a rhodopsin mutation (Pro23His): A mouse model of autosomal dominant retinitis pigmentosa. *Neuron* **1992**, *9*, 815–830. [CrossRef]
183. Leyk, J.; Daly, C.; Janssen-Bienhold, U.; Kennedy, B.N.; Richter-Landsberg, C. HDAC6 inhibition by tubastatin A is protective against oxidative stress in a photoreceptor cell line and restores visual function in a zebrafish model of inherited blindness. *Cell Death Dis.* **2017**, *8*, e3028. [CrossRef] [PubMed]
184. Daly, C. Histone Deacetylase: Therapeutic Targets in Retinal Degeneration. *Adv. Exp. Med. Biol.* **2016**, *854*, 455–461. [PubMed]
185. Tanackovic, G. PRPF mutations are associated with generalized defects in spliceosome formation and pre-mRNA splicing in patients with retinitis pigmentosa. *Hum. Mol. Genet.* **2011**, *20*, 2116–2130. [CrossRef] [PubMed]
186. Buskin, A. Disrupted alternative splicing for genes implicated in splicing and ciliogenesis causes PRPF31 retinitis pigmentosa. *Nat. Commun.* **2018**, *9*, 4234. [CrossRef] [PubMed]
187. Collin, W.J.R. Applications of antisense oligonucleotides for the treatment of inherited retinal diseases. *Curr. Opin. Ophthalmol.* **2017**, *28*, 260–266. [CrossRef] [PubMed]
188. Viringipurampeer, I.A.; Metcalfe, A.L.; Bashar, A.E.; Sivak, O.; Yanai, A.; Mohammadi, Z.; Moritz, O.L.; Gregory-Evans, C.Y.; Gregory-Evans, K. NLRP3 inflammasome activation drives bystander cone photoreceptor cell death in a P23H rhodopsin model of retinal degeneration. *Hum. Mol. Genet.* **2016**, *25*, 1501–1516. [CrossRef] [PubMed]
189. Zhang, T.; Baehr, W.; Fu, Y. Chemical chaperone TUDCA preserves cone photoreceptors in a mouse model of Leber congenital amaurosis. *Investig. Ophthalmol. Vis. Sci.* **2012**, *53*, 3349–3356. [CrossRef] [PubMed]
190. Leonard, C.K. XIAP protection of photoreceptors in animal models of retinitis pigmentosa. *PLoS ONE* **2007**, *2*, e314. [CrossRef]
191. Thanos, C. Delivery of neurotrophic factors and therapeutic proteins for retinal diseases. *Exp. Opin. Biol. Ther.* **2005**, *5*, 1443–1452. [CrossRef]
192. Himawan, E.; Ekstrom, P.; Buzgo, M.; Gaillard, P.; Stefansson, E.; Marigo, V.; Loftsson, T.; Paquet-Durand, F. Drug delivery to retinal photoreceptors. *Drug Discov. Today* **2019**. [CrossRef]

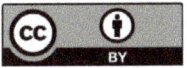

© 2019 by the authors. Licensee MDPI, Basel, Switzerland. This article is an open access article distributed under the terms and conditions of the Creative Commons Attribution (CC BY) license (http://creativecommons.org/licenses/by/4.0/).

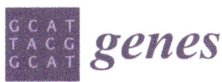

Review

The cGMP Pathway and Inherited Photoreceptor Degeneration: Targets, Compounds, and Biomarkers

Arianna Tolone [1,†], Soumaya Belhadj [1,†], Andreas Rentsch [2], Frank Schwede [2] and François Paquet-Durand [1,*]

1. Institute for Ophthalmic Research, University of Tübingen, Elfriede-Aulhorn-Strasse 5-7, 72076 Tübingen, Germany; arianna.tolone@uni-tuebingen.de (A.T.); soumaya.belhadj@uni-tuebingen.de (S.B.)
2. Biolog Life Science Institute, 28199 Bremen, Germany; ar@biolog.de (A.R.); fs@biolog.de (F.S.)
* Correspondence: francois.paquet-durand@klinikum.uni-tuebingen.de; Tel.: +49-7071-29-87430
† These authors contributed equally to this work.

Received: 15 April 2019; Accepted: 11 June 2019; Published: 14 June 2019

Abstract: Photoreceptor physiology and pathophysiology is intricately linked to guanosine-3′,5′-cyclic monophosphate (cGMP)-signaling. Here, we discuss the importance of cGMP-signaling for the pathogenesis of hereditary retinal degeneration. Excessive accumulation of cGMP in photoreceptors is a common denominator in cell death caused by a variety of different gene mutations. The cGMP-dependent cell death pathway may be targeted for the treatment of inherited photoreceptor degeneration, using specifically designed and formulated inhibitory cGMP analogues. Moreover, cGMP-signaling and its down-stream targets may be exploited for the development of novel biomarkers that could facilitate monitoring of disease progression and reveal the response to treatment in future clinical trials. We then briefly present the importance of appropriate formulations for delivery to the retina, both for drug and biomarker applications. Finally, the review touches on important aspects of future clinical translation, highlighting the need for interdisciplinary cooperation of researchers from a diverse range of fields.

Keywords: retina; cyclic GMP; apoptosis; necrosis; drug delivery systems; translational medicine

---

1. The Retina and Inherited Photoreceptor Degeneration

The retina transforms photons of light in electro-chemical signals, processes these signals, and transmits light-dependent information to different areas of the central nervous system [1]. The human retina is affected by a large number of hereditary, typically monogenic diseases, causing severe vision impairment or blindness [2,3]. Genetic diseases causing the degeneration and loss of the light-sensitive photoreceptors in the retina are grouped under the term inherited retinal degeneration (IRD) [4,5]. Photoreceptor loss in IRD-type diseases in most cases remains untreatable, making it a major unresolved medical problem [2,6]. This review focuses on the guanosine-3′,5′-cyclic monophosphate (cGMP)-signaling pathway and its role in IRD and how the components of this pathway may be exploited both for the development of new therapies as well as for new biomarkers for the evaluation of treatment efficacy.

In IRD-type diseases, the causative genetic defect typically causes a primary degeneration of rod photoreceptors (rods), with subsequent, secondary loss of cone photoreceptors (cones), eventually leading to complete blindness [4]. The result is an almost complete loss of the outer nuclear layer (ONL) and outer plexiform layer of the retina, while the inner retina remains intact initially (Figure 1). However, eventually in the inner retina the dendrites of bipolar and horizontal cells retract and an extensive gliotic scar may form [7]. The secondary degeneration of cones can be a surprisingly slow process, with some cones surviving for many years beyond the main degeneration phase [8].

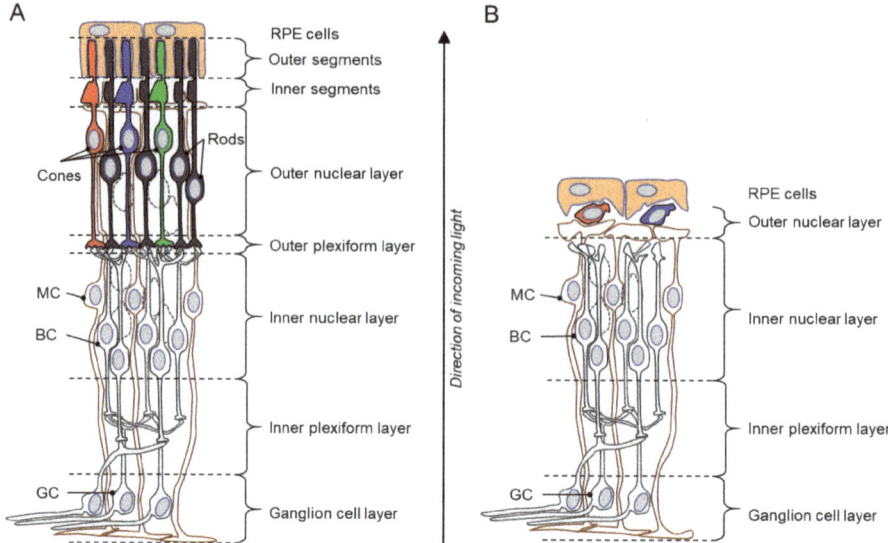

Figure 1. Schematic drawings of a healthy retina and a inherited retinal degeneration (IRD) retina. (**A**) Illustration of the various layers of an intact, healthy retina, from the retinal pigment epithelium (RPE) to the ganglion cell layer. Rod photoreceptors in the outer retina are shown in black, while cones are indicated by red, green, and blue. (**B**) Degenerated IRD retina. The outer nuclear layer is almost completely lost and the outer plexiform layer has essentially disappeared. Curiously, when the retina has lost all functionality, a small number of cone photoreceptors may still be present, possibly for many years beyond the loss of rod photoreceptors. BC = bipolar cell; GC = ganglion cell; MC = Müller glial cell. Note that the retinal structure has been simplified for clarity and that not all retinal cell types are shown.

The IRD group of diseases is characterized by a vast genetic heterogeneity, with disease-causing mutations known in over 270 genes (https://sph.uth.edu/retnet; information retrieved April 2019). This diversity severely hinders both the understanding of degenerative mechanisms and the development of treatments. To complicate matters further, each of these IRD-linked genes may carry many different types of either recessive or dominant mutations, ranging from complete loss-of-function to gain-of-function [3]. At present, a rough estimate will put the total number of disease mutations to amount to at least several tens of thousands. This enormous heterogeneity calls for the development of treatment approaches targeting common mechanisms, that can effectively treat this condition regardless of the underlying genetic causes.

2. cGMP-Signaling in Phototransduction and Degeneration

The physiology of photoreceptors and the phototransduction cascade critically depends on the signaling of the second messenger molecule cGMP [9]. Mutations affecting genes related to the phototransduction cascade often cause a dysregulation of cGMP, triggering a series of down-stream processes, which eventually kill photoreceptors [10,11]. This highlights cGMP-signaling as one principle common to many disease-causing mutations and, hence, as a plausible target for therapeutic interventions.

In the phototransduction cascade, in the dark, high levels of cGMP in photoreceptor outer segments (OS) allow for the sensitization of photoreceptor cells down to the level of single-photon sensitivity [12]. cGMP binds to and opens the prototypic phototransduction target, the cyclic nucleotide-gated channel (CNGC), located in the outer membrane of the photoreceptor OS [13]. The CNGC opening allows for an influx of Na$^+$ and Ca^{2+} into the OS, yet, at the same time K$^+$ and Ca^{2+} ions are constantly extruded via the Na$^+$/Ca^{2+}/K$^+$ exchanger (NCKX). This continuous influx and outflow of ions in the absence of light is referred to as the dark current [14]. The conformational change in the rhodopsin protein brought about by the absorption of a photon of light, leads to the sequential activation of the G-protein transducin and the phosphodiesterase-6 (PDE6). PDE6, which is located to the membranous disks within photoreceptor OS, hydrolyses cGMP, leading to the closure of CNGC and a hyperpolarization of the OS due to continued activity of NCKX. This in turn promotes the generation of an electro-chemical signal that is transmitted to second order neurons [15].

The toxicity of high levels of cGMP for photoreceptors was already established by Deborah Farber and Frank Lolley in the 1970s [10,16]. The discovery of disease-causing mutations in the PDE6 α and β genes [17,18] provided an explanation for excessive photoreceptor cGMP levels. Many more disease mutations are nowadays known to be associated with high cGMP-dependent photoreceptor cell death, including mutations in the genes encoding for CNGC [19], rhodopsin [11], AIPL1 [20], and photoreceptor guanylyl cyclase [21]. However, cGMP elevation was also found in cells with mutations in genes that seem to have no obvious connection to cGMP metabolism. An example for this situation are mutations in the *PRPH2* gene [22], which encodes for an OS structural protein [23].

Overall, high cGMP and cGMP-dependent cell death are likely involved in a significant proportion of IRD patients [24], making it an attractive target for therapeutic interventions, and additionally highlighting it, or its downstream processes, for biomarker development.

3. Targeting cGMP-Signaling

cGMP acts as a second messenger and plays a critical role in the regulation of different processes in many organisms. Cyclic nucleotide research began in the 1960s but the biological role of cGMP was identified only in the 1980s thanks to two important discoveries: the cGMP synthesis stimulation by the atrial natriuretic peptide (ANP) in the heart, and the cGMP synthesis stimulation by nitric oxide (NO) in smooth muscle cells causing vasorelaxation [25]. In the retina, cGMP was identified in the 1970s when the presence of high activities of guanylate cyclase, as well as a protein kinase stimulated by cGMP, were described in the OS of bovine rods [26]. Today, we know that cGMP, when localized to the photoreceptor OS, is an essential component of the phototransduction cascade [9]. However, cGMP also has targets outside the phototransduction cascade, notably protein kinase G (PKG; also referred to as cGMP-dependent protein kinase, cGK), which appears to be highly relevant for photoreceptor cell death [22].

3.1. Regulation of Photoreceptor cGMP Synthesis

The synthesis of cGMP is catalyzed by membrane guanylyl cyclases (GCs), which convert guanosine 5′-triphosphate (GTP) into cGMP. Photoreceptor GCs work differently compared to other membrane GCs: They do not respond to extracellular ligands, but instead are regulated by Ca^{2+}-binding, and GC activating proteins (GCAPs) [27]. GCAPs are proteins containing EF-hand motifs and once these motifs are occupied by Ca^{2+} they inhibit cGMP production. In the darkness, when intracellular Ca^{2+} is relatively high, photoreceptor guanylyl cyclases (RetGC1 and RetGC2) are inhibited by GCAPs and do not synthesize cGMP. Illumination induces rhodopsin conformational changes, which enable the activation of transducin, a GTP-binding protein. Activated transducin disinhibits PDE6, thereby allowing the hydrolysis of cGMP and the closure of CNGC leading to the interruption of Ca^{2+} influx. Since Ca^{2+} is constantly extruded via NCKX, CNGC closure quickly lowers intracellular Ca^{2+} levels. In this situation, Mg^{2+} replaces the Ca^{2+} bound to GCAPs, activates RetGCs, and promotes the synthesis of cGMP [27–29] (Figure 2).

A. Dark

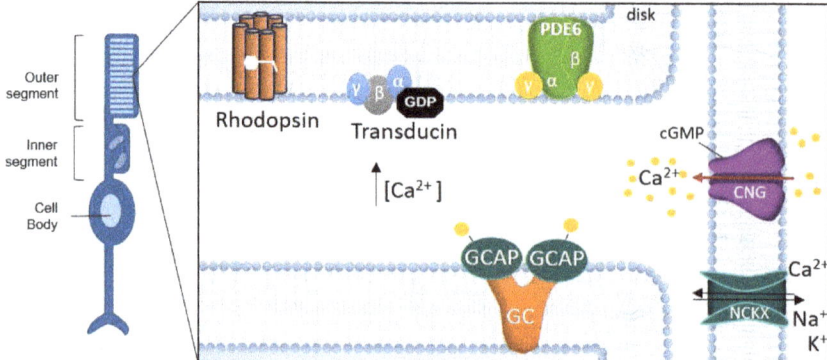

B. Light

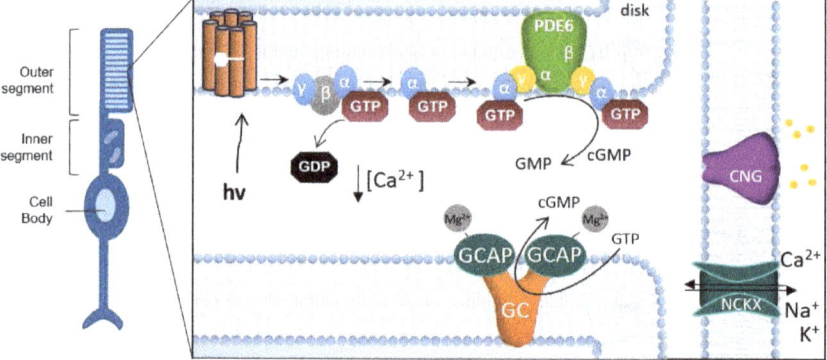

Figure 2. Phototransduction and the photoreceptor cGMP-Ca^{2+} feedback loop. Schematic representation of the interplay between cGMP and Ca^{2+} in the photoreceptor outer segment (OS). (**A**) In darkness, cGMP binds to the cyclic nucleotide-gated channel (CNGC). The opening of CNGC allows for an influx of Na^+ and Ca^{2+} into the photoreceptor OS. At the same time K^+ and Ca^{2+} ions are constantly extruded via $Na^+/Ca^{2+}/K^+$ exchanger (NCKX) creating a continuous influx and outflow of ions called the dark current. Ca^{2+} binds GC activating proteins (GCAPs), which inhibit the synthesis of cGMP by limiting guanylyl cyclase (GC) activity. (**B**) In light, photon (hv) absorption induces conformational changes in the rhodopsin protein. Rhodopsin stimulates the GTP-binding protein transducin to detach from heteromeric G-protein complex, by replacing bound GDP with GTP. The activated transducin α subunit binds to the PDE6 complex, abolishing the inhibitory effect exerted by its γ subunits. Activated phosphodiesterase-6 (PDE6) hydrolyses cGMP to GMP, which in turn limits the CNGC opening and leads to a reduction of Ca^{2+} influx. The closure of the CNGC and a hyperpolarization of the OS, due to continued activity of NCKX, promote the generation of an electro-chemical signal that is transmitted to second order neurons. When OS Ca^{2+} concentration is reduced, Mg^{2+} replaces the Ca^{2+} bound to GCAP, reactivating GCAP and stimulating GC to synthesize cGMP, opening the CNGC again.

In this way, both cGMP and Ca^{2+} concentrations in the photoreceptor are closely linked by a feedback loop that would normally limit the levels of both second messengers to their physiological ranges [30]. The reasons why this feedback loop fails in IRD mutations are not currently known. A major focus of IRD research in the past was on the role of CNGC and the Ca^{2+} influx that it mediates, and a number of studies suggested that excessive activation of CNGC and too high intracellular Ca^{2+} levels would drive photoreceptor degeneration [31–33]. However, other, more recent studies failed to show a clear causal connection between Ca^{2+} and photoreceptor loss in IRD [15,34–36]. Therefore, in the following section, we focus on the role of PKG in photoreceptor degeneration and how this may be exploited for IRD therapy developments.

3.2. The Role of PKG in Normal Physiology

Elevation of cGMP intracellular concentration induces a binding-dependent activation of PKG, a serine/threonine-specific protein kinase that phosphorylates a number of biological targets [37]. Mammals express two different genes for PKG: the *PRKG1* gene encodes for the Iα and Iβ isoforms of PKG I and is located on human chromosome 10, whereas the *PRKG2* gene encodes PKG II and is located on human chromosome 4. PKG is a homodimer of two identical subunits and each PKG subunit consists of an N-terminal regulatory domain, an autoinhibitory sequence, two tandem cGMP binding sites, and a C-terminal catalytic domain [38]. When cGMP binds to PKG it promotes a conformational change, which liberates the catalytic site. In mammals, PKG I mediates many of the effects of NO/cGMP on vasodilation, vascular smooth muscle cell relaxation, proliferation, and apoptosis. PKG II regulates homeostasis of Na$^+$, Cl$^-$, endochondral ossification of bones, and various functions of the nervous system [39]. Not much is known about the role of PKG in retinal photoreceptor cells and its significance for the regulation of phototransduction. Immunohistochemical staining for PKG I and PKG II isoforms revealed a predominant expression of PKG I in photoreceptors ONL [40], while PKG II seems to be expressed in the inner nuclear layer (INL) and the ganglion cell layer (GCL) [41].

Important insight into the physiological functions of PKG isoforms also came from genetic knock-out animals. A full knockout of PKG I (α and β) leads to defects in smooth muscles, intestinal dysfunctions, growth defects, and dwarfism [42]. Interestingly, this effect could be rescued by the reconstitution (knock-in) of the murine PKG (cGK) Iα or Iβ isozymes in smooth muscles [43] allowing normal development. In sensory cells of the inner ear, a knock-out of the murine *Prkg1* gene did not affect hearing function in detectable ways, yet, *Prkg1* knock-out animals were protected against acoustic trauma and resistant against noise induced hearing loss [44]. When *Prkg2* was knocked-out in mice, the animals appeared generally healthy but showed a defect in the entrainment of circadian rhythm, even though retinal morphology and function appeared normal [45]. It remains unclear whether PKG II deficiency leads to changes in the photosensitive retinal ganglion cells. Overall, the results obtained on animals deficient for PKG enzymes [37] suggest that targeted inhibition of PKG would unlikely produce major adverse effects.

The idea that PKG activity plays a role in cell death has been widely established. For instance, activation of PKG has been used for the induction of apoptosis in colon cancer cells and in human breast cancer cells [46,47], and is linked to pro-apoptotic effects in ovarian cancer [48]. Excessive activation of PKG has been shown to cause cell death in certain neuronal cell types [49,50]. Several studies pointed to the importance of the cGMP/PKG-dependent cell death mechanism in photoreceptor degeneration and demonstrated the existence of a non-apoptotic cell death mechanisms involving cGMP-dependent over activation of PKG [11,22,51]. This evidence makes PKG a potential target for neuroprotective strategies.

3.3. Effects of PKG Inhibition

The different physiological functions of PKG in different tissues suggest that its inhibition can lead to various effects. For example, PKG inhibitors DT-2 and DT-3 have been demonstrated to decrease NO-mediated vasodilation in isolated cerebral arteries [52]. Inhibitors of PKG could; therefore, be used to antagonize vasoplegia, a hypotonic condition characteristic of anaphylactic shock [53]. Selective inhibition of PKG Iα mediated by the balanol-derivative N46 reduced thermal hyperalgesia and osteoarthritic pain in rats [54].

PKG inhibition in cancer treatment appears to have an ambiguous role. In some forms of cancer, the effects seem to be very positive. For example, in colorectal carcinoma (CRC) cell lines inhibition of NO/PKG/extracellular-signal-regulated kinases (ERK)-signaling mediated by the PKG-inhibitor

KT5823 reduced migration and invasion in both scratch wound and modified Boyden chamber assays [55]. PKG seems to exert a pro-apoptotic role in breast cancer cell lines [46]. Some of the PKG inhibitors used in the experiments mentioned above may suffer from lack of specificity and potency. For instance, KT5823 is an ATP-binding site inhibitor and works efficiently as a PKG inhibitor in vitro [56]. However, it is also a weak inhibitor of PKC and PKA, both of which may constitute potential competitive binding sites. [56,57]. Another PKG inhibitor, DT-2, a substrate-binding site inhibitor, has been demonstrated to be inefficient in inhibiting PKG activity in several types of cells. Furthermore, in whole-cell homogenates the PKG specificity over PKA for DT-2 appears to be lost [58].

To understand PKG cellular functions as well as the cGMP/PKG-dependent cell death mechanisms, inhibitors or activators with very high selectivity are needed. A possible and valid alternative is the use of cGMP analogues.

3.4. Design of cGMP Analogues to Inhibit PKG

Analogues of cGMP are a class of second messenger compounds able to inhibit or activate both PKG isoforms (Iα, Iβ, and II) [59] and have been used in a multitude of research areas. Over the last ~40 years, the first generation of cGMP analogues have become standard tools for investigations of biochemical and physiological signal transduction pathways [60]. More recently, newly developed PKG activators have been shown to reduce proliferation in colon cancer cell lines [61], as well as in melanoma cells [62]. The use of PKG inhibitors contributed to identify a common non-apoptotic cGMP-dependent degeneration mechanism in different animal models for IRD [22]. In particular, cGMP analogues used as PKG inhibitors carry the common motif of an Rp-configured phosphorothioate. Therein, sulfur replaces one of the exocyclic oxygens of the 3′,5′-cyclic phosphate (equatorial (eq) position in Figure 3), while the prefix "Rp" defines the configuration of this moiety according to Cahn–Ingold–Prelog rules for chiral atoms. These compounds, further referred to as Rp-cGMPS analogues, are able to bind to the cGMP-binding domains of PKGs, but do not evoke the conformational changes of the enzyme required for activation of the catalytically active C-subunit [63]. This leads to a competitive and reversible inhibition of the various PKG isoforms. Furthermore, Rp-cGMPS analogues were shown to be resistant against hydrolysis by mammalian 3′,5′-cyclic phosphodiesterases (PDEs) [64], the enzyme superfamily that metabolizes cGMP to 5′-GMP in vivo. Due to the sulfur in the cyclic phosphate and other substituents, such as bromine, mainly introduced to the guanine nucleobase, corresponding Rp-cGMPS analogues show improved lipophilicity leading to enhanced membrane permeability compared to cGMP [53,60]. Schematic structural motifs of Rp-cGMPS analogues with improved inhibitory potencies for PKGs are illustrated in Figure 3. Taken together, three factors are responsible for the efficacy of sophisticated Rp-cGMPS analogues in biological systems: 1) The improved stability against degradation, 2) the lipophilicity and membrane permeability, and 3) the inhibitory potential for PKG.

As mentioned above, cGMP-signaling is central to phototransduction, but cGMP levels elevated by excessive production or, conversely, by insufficient hydrolysis may trigger photoreceptor degeneration. Between 2012 and 2016, the DRUGSFORD consortium generated over 80 novel cGMP analogues that target and inhibit PKG, and showed that systemic intraperitoneal injections of a selected liposome-formulated Rp-cGMPS analogue can protect photoreceptors from degeneration in different animal models for IRD. This pharmacological treatment significantly preserved rod and—indirectly—cone photoreceptors, ensuring the maintenance of retinal function [65]. This proof of concept study also highlighted the versatility of cGMP(S) analogues, which can be designed and formulated both to study the cellular functions of PKG and as new lead compounds for therapeutic applications in IRD.

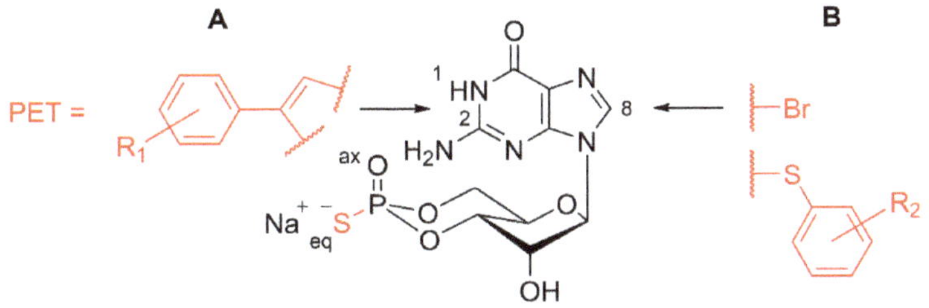

Figure 3. Schematic structure of Rp-cGMPS analogues. Arrows illustrate typical structural positions in Rp-cGMPS used for the introduction of substituents to generate Rp-cGMPS analogues with improved inhibitory potency for cGMP-dependent protein kinase I or II. (**A**) Position 1, N^2: Addition of β-phenyl-1,N^2-etheno-modifications (PET) with varying additional substituents (R_1) to Rp-cGMPS [65,66]. (**B**) Position 8: Addition of halogens (e.g., bromine (Br)) or sulfur-connected aromatic ring systems with varying additional substituents (R_2) [65,67].

4. Pre-Clinical and Clinical Biomarkers for Inherited Retinal Degeneration

Neurodegenerative diseases are often characterized by a slow progression of neuronal cell loss, sometimes over the course of several decades. This implies that disease symptoms may appear only when the damage is advanced and thus the diagnosis is made at a late stage of the disease. The current lack of effective treatment options for most neurodegenerative diseases, including those of the retina, stems in part from a lack of biomarkers to detect neuronal cell death and to study its progression and dynamics. In neurodegenerative diseases biomarkers are needed, not only to aid diagnosis and monitor disease progression, but also, as new medicines are introduced, to detect the patient's response to treatment [68].

4.1. Review of Recent Retinal Biomarker Developments

Over the past decade there has been some progress in the identification and development of biomarkers for retinal cell death, based on the increasing knowledge of the underlying mechanisms behind retinal degeneration. Notably, several attempts have been made to develop molecular probes that target specific degenerative processes [41,69,70].

Perhaps the most straight-forward approach for biomarker development in terms of clinical applicability and patient friendliness would be biomarkers that could be analyzed in blood samples. While to date there are no established biochemical blood markers for retinal degeneration, a study published by Martinez-Fernandez de la Camara et al. [71] showed that in a group of patients affected by retinitis pigmentosa (RP), the serum cGMP levels are increased by approximately 65%, compared to a control group. These results were confirmed in an independent study on a family with autosomal recessive RP due to homozygous mutations in the *PDE6A* gene [72]. The latter study also found cGMP plasma concentration to have a good sensitivity, which means it can detect diseased subjects well, but with a lower specificity, thus carrying the risk that healthy subjects could appear as having the disease. Nevertheless, this example nicely illustrates the potential for the development of blood borne biomarkers. On the other hand, given the high genetic heterogeneity of IRD-type diseases, it is unlikely that a single blood-borne biomarker can be used for all patients. Most likely different mutations, in different genes, will require separate biomarker developments. In the end, this could lead to assays that consider maybe a few dozen different metabolic markers for IRD identification.

Photoreceptors are susceptible to oxidative stress because of their high metabolic rate as well as their exposition to environmental factors, such as ultraviolet radiation or high oxygen tension. Hence, it has been suggested that oxidative stress contributes to the pathogenesis of retinal degeneration [73]. In line with this concept, Martinez-Fernandez de la Camara and colleagues [71] determined the levels of different markers of the antioxidant-oxidant status in aqueous humor and blood from RP patients, and compared them with those in healthy controls to confirm an alteration of this status. The authors found reduced superoxide dismutase (SOD3) activity in aqueous humor as well as reduced SOD3 activity and increased TBARS (thiobarbituric acid reactive substances) formation in peripheral blood. Even though these studies are promising it remains to be seen whether the specificity and sensitivity of these parameters is sufficient for clinical biomarker applications.

Another strategy to assess retinal cell death is to detect and quantify substances released by dying cells in ocular fluids. For instance, neurofilaments (Nf) are essential constituents of the axonal cytoskeleton [74] and, during neuronal cell death and axonal degeneration in the retina, contents of the cytoplasm such as Nf are released into the extracellular fluid [75]. From there, Nf diffuse into the vitreous body and anterior chamber fluid, which are the two compartments adjacent to the retina. Accordingly, in patients who underwent vitrectomy for retinal detachment, epiretinal gliosis, or macular hole surgery, the neurofilament heavy-chain protein could be quantified from the human vitreous body using an ELISA technique [75]. This could make Nf release a potential biomarker for retinal degeneration, provided that vitreous samples can be obtained.

A non-invasive detection of retinal cell death was suggested in a study published by Cordeiro and colleagues [76]. They established a proof-of-principle in reporting the use of fluorescent cell death markers to temporally resolve and quantify the early and late phases of apoptosis and necrosis of single nerve cells in glaucoma and Alzheimer's disease animal models. More specifically, they used Alexa Fluor 488-labelled Annexin V to identify apoptotic cells, as well as propidium iodide to identify necrotic and late apoptotic cells. Fluorescence was visualized using confocal scanning laser ophthalmoscopy. This initial animal study eventually led to a phase 1 clinical trial [69], which established a proof-of-concept demonstrating that retinal cell death can be identified in the human retina with increased levels of activity in glaucomatous neurodegenerative disease.

4.2. Using the cGMP Pathway for Biomarker Development

Cell death in IRD, and in other neurodegenerative diseases, is often thought to be governed by apoptosis, a form of cell death that would display a number of characteristic markers, such as cytochrome c leakage and activation of caspase-type proteases [77]. However, for photoreceptor degeneration in the retina, a growing body of evidence suggests the involvement of non-apoptotic, alternative cell death mechanisms [11,78]. In many cases photoreceptor cell death appears to be driven by cGMP-dependent activation of CNGC [19] and may be even more prominently by PKG [22], also in the absence of functional CNGC expression [79]. A number of cell death-related processes have been discovered down-stream of cGMP-signaling, including excessive activation of histone-deacetylase [80], calpain-type proteases [81], DNA-methyl-transferase [82] and poly-ADP-ribose-polymerase (PARP) [83,84]. Molecular probes targeting these enzymes could be developed and used as biomarkers to detect cell death and study its progression and dynamics in IRD. For instance, an assay previously adapted to resolve PARP activity in photoreceptors ex vivo [41], and which relied on the incorporation of biotin labelled NAD^+ residues as subunits in elongated poly-ADP-ribose chains (Figure 4), could potentially be used to this effect. While the original assay required a two-step detection, using, first, biotinylated NAD^+ and then fluorescently-labelled avidin, in the future it may be possible to develop a single step assay. This might then be used for direct in vivo detection, possibly via fluorescent scanning laser ophthalmoscopy [69].

Similar in vivo biomarkers for the cellular detection of retinal cell death might be developed in the future, using molecular probes targeting cGMP-dependent processes, such as calpain- or caspase-type proteases, histone deacetylases, or DNA-methyl-transferases.

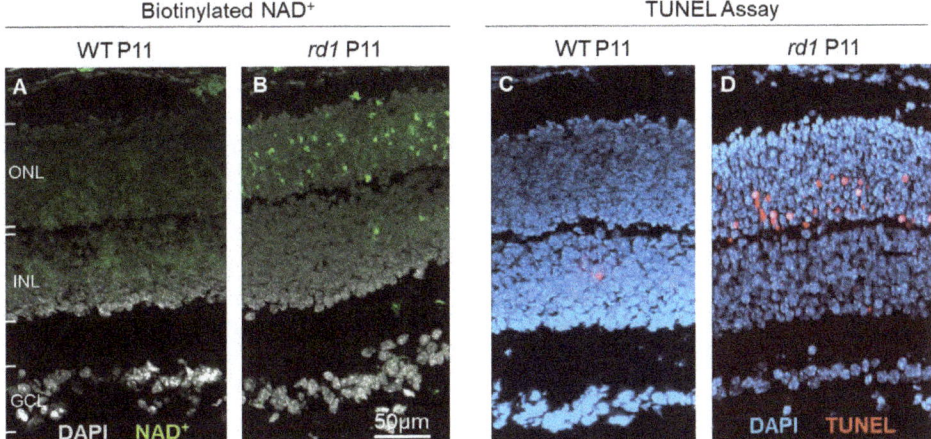

Figure 4. Incorporation of NAD$^+$ as a biomarker for retinal cell death. At post-natal day 11 (P11), when compared to wild-type (WT) retina (**A**), photoreceptors in the *rd1* mouse model (**B**) display marked incorporation of biotinylated NAD$^+$. This is highly correlated with the TUNEL assay for cell death, which at the same age detects only few cells in the WT situation (**C**), while large numbers are detected in the *rd1* outer nuclear layer (ONL; **D**). INL = inner nuclear layer, GCL = ganglion cell layer.

5. Delivery of Compounds to the Retinal Photoreceptors

Compounds targeting photoreceptor cGMP-signaling may have strong therapeutic potential and can, at least in part, address the genetic heterogeneity of IRD-type diseases. Nevertheless, to develop them into successful IRD treatments still requires the delivery of these compounds to the photoreceptor cell, which in most cases will entail formulating the active compound in a suitable drug delivery system (DDS).

5.1. Drug Delivery Systems (DDSs) for the Retina

The retina is protected from detrimental external agents (e.g., toxins, pathogens) by the blood–retinal barrier (BRB), as well as other ocular barriers that prevent therapeutic agents from reaching the photoreceptor cells in the retina [85]. To overcome this obstacle, a variety of different technical approaches have been pursued, using different routes of administration, such as suprachoroidal injection [86], subretinal injection [87], injection into the capsule of Tenon [88], and intravitreal injection [89]. Each of these administration routes may require the use of an adapted DDS such as glutathione conjugated liposomes [65]. Moreover, each of these routes have specific advantages and disadvantages, but which ever administration route is chosen the drug formulation/delivery system used will be critical to successful treatment development.

The use of different application (injection) routes in current clinical practice may be illustrated by two examples: In gene therapy, the most frequently used technique (mostly in clinical trial but also –since 2018–for FDA/EMA approved *RPE65* gene therapy) is subretinal injection of gene constructs delivered in adeno-associated-virus [90,91]. The procedure entails a detachment of the retina from the RPE with the risk for significant and irreversible retinal damage [87]. However, since gene therapy interventions are considered to be needed only once in a lifetime, the overall risk–benefit ratio for subretinal injection is deemed acceptable [90]. For anti-vascular endothelial growth factor (VEGF) medication, commonly used for the treatment of age-related-macular degeneration (AMD) and other retinal diseases, the most frequently used route of administration is intravitreal injection [92]. This form of application is easier to perform than subretinal injection and the risk for damage to the retina is far lower. On the other hand, anti-VEGF drugs require regular re-administration leading to a risk for cumulative damage to the eye, notably intraocular infections [89].

While the last ten years have seen an important development and the appearance of many innovative materials, designs, and technologies for retinal drug delivery, efficient and sustained drug delivery to the photoreceptors remains a major challenge. Importantly, each compound or therapeutic agent may require highly-adapted DDS, which additionally must comply with regulatory requirements from the medicinal drug and product authorities [93]. Therefore, future research into new treatments for IRD should take the retinal delivery problem into consideration as early as possible, and synchronize the compound and delivery system development.

5.2. Retinal Drug Delivery: Local vs. Systemic Administration

Currently, the standard route of administration for retinal drugs, such as anti-VEGF medications, is multiple dosing through intravitreal injection [89,94], while in the case of single-dose, gene therapeutic agents subretinal injection is the preferred technique [95]. Among the advantages of these local administration routes are the limited exposure of the whole body, not the least since the eye is an encapsulated organ. When a treatment does eventually leak out into the systemic circulation, even very high intraocular doses will be diluted about 10.000-fold (volume of the human eye ≈ 6.5 ml; volume of the human body (70 kg) ≈ 66 l; note that this dilution factor will be smaller in children). Therefore, the risk of systemic side-effects of intraocularly applied drugs appears rather small, even though such effects have been reported in some cases after anti-VEGF medication [92].

Among the disadvantages of intraocular application are the patients' discomfort, the need for qualified doctors to perform the injections, and the low (but cumulative) risk for intraocular inflammation [96]. Unfortunately, topical drug application is usually not possible because of the various barriers surrounding the eye and retina, and the alternating lipophilic and hydrophilic nature of these barriers, preventing most drugs from reaching the retina via this route [93].

Systemic drug application might be a more patient-friendly, alternative administration route, yet, for the reasons laid out above, systemic application will require dramatically higher dosing to reach comparable intraocular drug concentration. In addition, cyclic nucleotide analogues are rapidly excreted via the renal system, strongly reducing bioavailability [65,97]. Both problems could potentially be circumvented if a drug intended for the retina was combined with a targeted delivery formulation, such as glutathione (GSH) conjugated liposomes [98]. Such liposomes were recently shown to allow for sufficient drug delivery of PKG inhibitors to the photoreceptors of the retina to obtain a significant morphological and functional rescue in animal models for IRD [65]. Nevertheless, given the potential for systemic adverse effects and the strongly increased consumption of the (often expensive) drug substance, it remains to be seen whether the systemic administration route will be viable in future clinical settings.

6. Conclusions and Outlook

The cGMP-signaling system offers new opportunities for the development of innovative treatments for IRD, as well as for the development of biomarkers that can assess treatment efficacy. Novel small molecule analogues of cGMP allow PKG (and/or CNGC) to be targeted, with high specificity, and have shown to achieve marked photoreceptor protection in different animal models [22,65]. While this was true for inhibitory cGMP analogues in forms of IRD connected to high photoreceptor cGMP levels, it remains to be seen whether activator analogues would have protective capacity in situations where photoreceptor cGMP is too low (e.g., in RetGC loss-of-function mutations [99]).

Nevertheless, translation of new drugs or biomarkers based on cGMP-signaling, and their corresponding DDS, will require substantial development efforts, notably in the areas of ocular pharmacokinetics, GMP manufacturing, safety and tolerability testing, clinical trial design, and suitable clinical endpoints, etc. All these developments require expert knowledge and a broad interdisciplinary oversight, which, unfortunately is rarely found in both basic and clinical researchers. This highlights the need for specific educational programs to train scientists in translational research. Another critical aspect for successful translation into clinical practice is the progression into a viable commercial product that can recoup the development costs and sustain further development and improvements. Additionally, here a specific training and a sensitization of scientists for the requirements of commercialization (e.g., protection of intellectual property, appropriate documentation, regulatory requirements, business models in the rare disease space, etc.) will be important.

Author Contributions: Conceptualization, F.S. and F.P.D.; methodology, S.B., A.R.; writing—original draft preparation, AT, SB, FPD; writing—review and editing, A.T., S.B., A.R., F.S., F.P.D.; visualization, F.P.D., A.T., A.R., S.B.; supervision, F.S. and F.P.D.; funding acquisition, F.P.D.

Funding: This research was funded by grants from the European Union (transMed; H2020-MSCA-765441) and the German research council (DFG; PA1751/7-1, 8-1).

Acknowledgments: We thank Norman Rieger for excellent technical assistance and Michael Power for careful language editing.

Conflicts of Interest: The authors declare no conflicts of interest.

References

1. Hoon, M.; Okawa, H.; Della Santina, L.; Wong, R.O. Functional architecture of the retina: Development and disease. *Prog. Retin. Eye Res.* **2014**, *42*, 44–84. [CrossRef] [PubMed]
2. Verbakel, S.K.; van Huet, R.A.C.; Boon, C.J.F.; den Hollander, A.I.; Collin, R.W.J.; Klaver, C.C.W.; Hoyng, C.B.; Roepman, R.; Klevering, B.J. Non-syndromic retinitis pigmentosa. *Prog. Retin. Eye Res.* **2018**, *66*, 157–186. [CrossRef] [PubMed]
3. Chizzolini, M.; Galan, A.; Milan, E.; Sebastiani, A.; Costagliola, C.; Parmeggiani, F. Good epidemiologic practice in retinitis pigmentosa: From phenotyping to biobanking. *Curr. Genom.* **2011**, *12*, 260–266. [CrossRef]
4. Kennan, A.; Aherne, A.; Humphries, P. Light in retinitis pigmentosa. *Trends Genet.* **2005**, *21*, 103–110. [CrossRef] [PubMed]
5. Hamel, C.P. Cone rod dystrophies. *Orphanet. J. Rare. Dis.* **2007**, *2*, 7. [CrossRef] [PubMed]
6. Trifunovic, D.; Sahaboglu, A.; Kaur, J.; Mencl, S.; Zrenner, E.; Ueffing, M.; Arango-Gonzalez, B.; Paquet-Durand, F. Neuroprotective Strategies for the Treatment of Inherited Photoreceptor Degeneration. *Curr. Mol. Med.* **2012**, *12*, 598–612. [CrossRef] [PubMed]
7. Gargini, C.; Terzibasi, E.; Mazzoni, F.; Strettoi, E. Retinal organization in the retinal degeneration 10 (rd10) mutant mouse: A morphological and ERG study. *J. Comp. Neurol.* **2007**, *500*, 222–238. [CrossRef] [PubMed]
8. Carter-Dawson, L.D.; LaVail, M.M.; Sidman, R.L. Differential effect of the rd mutation on rods and cones in the mouse retina. *Investig. Ophthalmol. Vis. Sci.* **1978**, *17*, 489–498.
9. Stryer, L. Cyclic GMP cascade of vision. *Annu. Rev. Neurosci.* **1986**, *9*, 87–119. [CrossRef]
10. Farber, D.B.; Lolley, R.N. Cyclic guanosine monophosphate: Elevation in degenerating photoreceptor cells of the C3H mouse retina. *Science* **1974**, *186*, 449–451. [CrossRef]
11. Arango-Gonzalez, B.; Trifunovic, D.; Sahaboglu, A.; Kranz, K.; Michalakis, S.; Farinelli, P.; Koch, S.; Koch, F.; Cottet, S.; Janssen Bienhold, U.; et al. Identification of a common non-apoptotic cell death mechanism in hereditary retinal degeneration. *PLoS ONE* **2014**, *9*, e112142. [CrossRef] [PubMed]
12. Field, G.D.; Uzzell, V.; Chichilnisky, E.J.; Rieke, F. Temporal resolution of single-photon responses in primate rod photoreceptors and limits imposed by cellular noise. *J. Neurophysiol.* **2019**, *121*, 255–268. [CrossRef] [PubMed]
13. Michalakis, S.; Becirovic, E.; Biel, M. Retinal Cyclic Nucleotide-Gated Channels: From Pathophysiology to Therapy. *Int. J. Mol. Sci.* **2018**, *19*, 749. [CrossRef] [PubMed]
14. Vinberg, F.; Chen, J.; Kefalov, V.J. Regulation of calcium homeostasis in the outer segments of rod and cone photoreceptors. *Prog. Retin. Eye Res.* **2018**, *67*, 87–101. [CrossRef]
15. Kulkarni, M.; Trifunovic, D.; Schubert, T.; Euler, T.; Paquet-Durand, F. Calcium dynamics change in degenerating cone photoreceptors. *Hum. Mol. Genet.* **2016**, ddw219. [CrossRef] [PubMed]
16. Lolley, R.N.; Farber, D.B.; Rayborn, M.E.; Hollyfield, J.G. Cyclic GMP accumulation causes degeneration of photoreceptor cells: Simulation of an inherited disease. *Science* **1977**, *196*, 664–666. [CrossRef] [PubMed]

17. McLaughlin, M.E.; Sandberg, M.A.; Berson, E.L.; Dryja, T.P. Recessive mutations in the gene encoding the beta-subunit of rod phosphodiesterase in patients with retinitis pigmentosa. *Nat. Genet.* **1993**, *4*, 130–134. [CrossRef]
18. Huang, S.H.; Pittler, S.J.; Huang, X.; Oliveira, L.; Berson, E.L.; Dryja, T.P. Autosomal recessive retinitis pigmentosa caused by mutations in the alpha subunit of rod cGMP phosphodiesterase. *Nat. Genet.* **1995**, *11*, 468–471. [CrossRef] [PubMed]
19. Paquet-Durand, F.; Beck, S.; Michalakis, S.; Goldmann, T.; Huber, G.; Muhlfriedel, R.; Trifunovic, D.; Fischer, M.D.; Fahl, E.; Duetsch, G.; et al. A key role for cyclic nucleotide gated (CNG) channels in cGMP-related retinitis pigmentosa. *Hum. Mol. Genet.* **2011**, *20*, 941–947. [CrossRef]
20. Ramamurthy, V.; Niemi, G.A.; Reh, T.A.; Hurley, J.B. Leber congenital amaurosis linked to AIPL1: A mouse model reveals destabilization of cGMP phosphodiesterase. *Proc. Natl. Acad. Sci. USA* **2004**, *101*, 13897–13902. [CrossRef]
21. Sato, S.; Peshenko, I.V.; Olshevskaya, E.V.; Kefalov, V.J.; Dizhoor, A.M. GUCY2D Cone-Rod Dystrophy-6 Is a "Phototransduction Disease" Triggered by Abnormal Calcium Feedback on Retinal Membrane Guanylyl Cyclase 1. *J. Neurosci.* **2018**, *38*, 2990–3000. [CrossRef] [PubMed]
22. Paquet-Durand, F.; Hauck, S.M.; van Veen, T.; Ueffing, M.; Ekstrom, P. PKG activity causes photoreceptor cell death in two retinitis pigmentosa models. *J. Neurochem.* **2009**, *108*, 796–810. [CrossRef] [PubMed]
23. Goldberg, A.F.; Moritz, O.L.; Williams, D.S. Molecular basis for photoreceptor outer segment architecture. *Prog. Retin. Eye Res.* **2016**, *55*, 52–81. [CrossRef] [PubMed]
24. Marigo, V.; Ekström, P.; Schwede, F.; Rentsch, A.; Paquet-Durand, F. Modulation of cGMP-signaling to prevent retinal degeneration. In *Therapies for Retinal Degeneration: Targeting Common Processes*; De la Rosa, E.J., Cotter, T.G., Eds.; Royal Society of Chemistry: Cambridge, UK, 2019; p. 88.
25. Feil, R.; Kemp-Harper, B. cGMP signaling: From bench to bedside. Conference on cGMP generators, effectors and therapeutic implications. *EMBO Rep.* **2006**, *7*, 149–153. [CrossRef] [PubMed]
26. Pannbacker, R.G.; Fleischman, D.E.; Reed, D.W. Cyclic nucleotide phosphodiesterase: High activity in a mammalian photoreceptor. *Science* **1972**, *175*, 757–758. [CrossRef] [PubMed]
27. Lim, S.; Roseman, G.; Peshenko, I.; Manchala, G.; Cudia, D.; Dizhoor, A.M.; Millhauser, G.; Ames, J.B. Retinal guanylyl cyclase activating protein 1 forms a functional dimer. *PLoS ONE* **2018**, *13*, e0193947. [CrossRef]
28. Dizhoor, A.M.; Olshevskaya, E.V.; Peshenko, I.V. The R838S Mutation in Retinal Guanylyl Cyclase 1 (RetGC1) Alters Calcium Sensitivity of cGMP Synthesis in the Retina and Causes Blindness in Transgenic Mice. *J. Biol. Chem.* **2016**, *291*, 24504–24516. [CrossRef]
29. Makino, C.L.; Wen, X.H.; Olshevskaya, E.V.; Peshenko, I.V.; Savchenko, A.B.; Dizhoor, A.M. Enzymatic relay mechanism stimulates cyclic GMP synthesis in rod photoresponse: Biochemical and physiological study in guanylyl cyclase activating protein 1 knockout mice. *PLoS ONE* **2012**, *7*, e47637. [CrossRef]
30. Olshevskaya, E.V.; Ermilov, A.N.; Dizhoor, A.M. Factors that affect regulation of cGMP synthesis in vertebrate photoreceptors and their genetic link to human retinal degeneration. *Mol. Cell. Biochem.* **2002**, *230*, 139–147. [CrossRef]
31. Fox, D.A.; Poblenz, A.T.; He, L. Calcium overload triggers rod photoreceptor apoptotic cell death in chemical-induced and inherited retinal degenerations. *Ann. N. Y. Acad. Sci.* **1999**, *893*, 282–285. [CrossRef]
32. Frasson, M.; Sahel, J.A.; Fabre, M.; Simonutti, M.; Dreyfus, H.; Picaud, S. Retinitis pigmentosa: Rod photoreceptor rescue by a calcium-channel blocker in the rd mouse. *Nat. Med.* **1999**, *5*, 1183–1187. [CrossRef] [PubMed]
33. Takeuchi, K.; Nakazawa, M.; Mizukoshi, S. Systemic administration of nilvadipine delays photoreceptor degeneration of heterozygous retinal degeneration slow (rds) mouse. *Exp. Eye Res.* **2008**, *86*, 60–69. [CrossRef]
34. Pearce-Kelling, S.E.; Aleman, T.S.; Nickle, A.; Laties, A.M.; Aguirre, G.D.; Jacobson, S.G.; Acland, G.M. Calcium channel blocker D-cis-diltiazem does not slow retinal degeneration in the PDE6B mutant rcd1 canine model of retinitis pigmentosa. *Mol. Vis.* **2001**, *7*, 42–47.
35. Pawlyk, B.S.; Li, T.; Scimeca, M.S.; Sandberg, M.A.; Berson, E.L. Absence of photoreceptor rescue with D-cis-diltiazem in the rd mouse. *Investig. Ophthalmol. Vis. Sci.* **2002**, *43*, 1912–1915.
36. Barabas, P.; Cutler, P.C.; Krizaj, D. Do calcium channel blockers rescue dying photoreceptors in the Pde6b (rd1) mouse? *Adv. Exp. Med. Biol.* **2010**, *664*, 491–499. [CrossRef]
37. Hofmann, F.; Feil, R.; Kleppisch, T.; Schlossmann, J. Function of cGMP-dependent protein kinases as revealed by gene deletion. *Physiol. Rev.* **2006**, *86*, 1–23. [CrossRef]

38. Hofmann, F.; Bernhard, D.; Lukowski, R.; Weinmeister, P. cGMP regulated protein kinases (cGK). *Handb. Exp. Pharmacol.* **2009**, 137–162.
39. Piwkowska, A.; Rogacka, D.; Audzeyenka, I.; Kasztan, M.; Angielski, S.; Jankowski, M. Intracellular calcium signaling regulates glomerular filtration barrier permeability: The role of the PKGIalpha-dependent pathway. *FEBS Lett.* **2016**, *590*, 1739–1748. [CrossRef] [PubMed]
40. Feil, S.; Zimmermann, P.; Knorn, A.; Brummer, S.; Schlossmann, J.; Hofmann, F.; Feil, R. Distribution of cGMP-dependent protein kinase type I and its isoforms in the mouse brain and retina. *Neuroscience* **2005**, *135*, 863–868. [CrossRef]
41. Ekstrom, P.A.; Ueffing, M.; Zrenner, E.; Paquet-Durand, F. Novel in situ activity assays for the quantitative molecular analysis of neurodegenerative processes in the retina. *Curr. Med. Chem.* **2014**, *21*, 3478–3493. [CrossRef]
42. Pfeifer, A.; Klatt, P.; Massberg, S.; Ny, L.; Sausbier, M.; Hirneiss, C.; Wang, G.X.; Korth, M.; Aszodi, A.; Andersson, K.E.; et al. Defective smooth muscle regulation in cGMP kinase I-deficient mice. *EMBO J.* **1998**, *17*, 3045–3051. [CrossRef] [PubMed]
43. Weber, S.; Bernhard, D.; Lukowski, R.; Weinmeister, P.; Worner, R.; Wegener, J.W.; Valtcheva, N.; Feil, S.; Schlossmann, J.; Hofmann, F.; et al. Rescue of cGMP kinase I knockout mice by smooth muscle specific expression of either isozyme. *Circ. Res.* **2007**, *101*, 1096–1103. [CrossRef] [PubMed]
44. Jaumann, M.; Dettling, J.; Gubelt, M.; Zimmermann, U.; Gerling, A.; Paquet-Durand, F.; Feil, S.; Wolpert, S.; Franz, C.; Varakina, K.; et al. cGMP-Prkg1 signaling and Pde5 inhibition shelter cochlear hair cells and hearing function. *Nat. Med.* **2012**, *18*, 252–259. [CrossRef] [PubMed]
45. Oster, H.; Werner, C.; Magnone, M.C.; Mayser, H.; Feil, R.; Seeliger, M.W.; Hofmann, F.; Albrecht, U. cGMP-dependent protein kinase II modulates mPer1 and mPer2 gene induction and influences phase shifts of the circadian clock. *Curr. Biol.* **2003**, *13*, 725–733. [CrossRef]
46. Fallahian, F.; Karami-Tehrani, F.; Salami, S.; Aghaei, M. Cyclic GMP induced apoptosis via protein kinase G in oestrogen receptor-positive and -negative breast cancer cell lines. *FEBS J.* **2011**, *278*, 3360–3369. [CrossRef] [PubMed]
47. Browning, D.D. Protein kinase G as a therapeutic target for the treatment of metastatic colorectal cancer. *Expert Opin. Ther. Targets* **2008**, *12*, 367–376. [CrossRef] [PubMed]
48. Leung, E.L.; Wong, J.C.; Johlfs, M.G.; Tsang, B.K.; Fiscus, R.R. Protein kinase G type Ialpha activity in human ovarian cancer cells significantly contributes to enhanced Src activation and DNA synthesis/cell proliferation. *Mol. Cancer Res.* **2010**, *8*, 578–591. [CrossRef]
49. Canals, S.; Casarejos, M.J.; de, B.S.; Rodriguez-Martin, E.; Mena, M.A. Nitric oxide triggers the toxicity due to glutathione depletion in midbrain cultures through 12-lipoxygenase. *J. Biol. Chem.* **2003**, *278*, 21542–21549. [CrossRef]
50. Canzoniero, L.M.; Adornetto, A.; Secondo, A.; Magi, S.; Dell'aversano, C.; Scorziello, A.; Amoroso, S.; Di, R.G. Involvement of the nitric oxide/protein kinase G pathway in polychlorinated biphenyl-induced cell death in SH-SY 5Y neuroblastoma cells. *J. Neurosci. Res.* **2006**, *84*, 692–697. [CrossRef]
51. Wang, T.; Tsang, S.H.; Chen, J. Two pathways of rod photoreceptor cell death induced by elevated cGMP. *Hum. Mol. Genet.* **2017**, *26*, 2299–2306. [CrossRef]
52. Dostmann, W.R.; Taylor, M.S.; Nickl, C.K.; Brayden, J.E.; Frank, R.; Tegge, W.J. Highly specific, membrane-permeant peptide blockers of cGMP-dependent protein kinase Ialpha inhibit NO-induced cerebral dilation. *Proc. Natl. Acad. Sci. USA* **2000**, *97*, 14772–14777. [CrossRef] [PubMed]
53. Wolfertstetter, S.; Huettner, J.P.; Schlossmann, J. cGMP-Dependent Protein Kinase Inhibitors in Health and Disease. *Pharmaceuticals (Basel)* **2013**, *6*, 269–286. [CrossRef] [PubMed]
54. Falk, J.; Drinjakovic, J.; Leung, K.M.; Dwivedy, A.; Regan, A.G.; Piper, M.; Holt, C.E. Electroporation of cDNA/Morpholinos to targeted areas of embryonic CNS in Xenopus. *BMC. Dev. Biol.* **2007**, *7*, 107. [CrossRef] [PubMed]
55. Babykutty, S.; Suboj, P.; Srinivas, P.; Nair, A.S.; Chandramohan, K.; Gopala, S. Insidious role of nitric oxide in migration/invasion of colon cancer cells by upregulating MMP-2/9 via activation of cGMP-PKG-ERK signaling pathways. *Clin. Exp. Metastasis* **2012**, *29*, 471–492. [CrossRef] [PubMed]
56. Burkhardt, M.; Glazova, M.; Gambaryan, S.; Vollkommer, T.; Butt, E.; Bader, B.; Heermeier, K.; Lincoln, T.M.; Walter, U.; Palmetshofer, A. KT5823 inhibits cGMP-dependent protein kinase activity in vitro but not in intact human platelets and rat mesangial cells. *J. Biol. Chem.* **2000**, *275*, 33536–33541. [CrossRef] [PubMed]

57. Hidaka, H.; Kobayashi, R. Pharmacology of protein kinase inhibitors. *Annu. Rev. Pharmacol. Toxicol.* **1992**, *32*, 377–397. [CrossRef] [PubMed]
58. Gambaryan, S.; Butt, E.; Kobsar, A.; Geiger, J.; Rukoyatkina, N.; Parnova, R.; Nikolaev, V.O.; Walter, U. The oligopeptide DT-2 is a specific PKG I inhibitor only in vitro, not in living cells. *Br. J. Pharmacol.* **2012**, *167*, 826–838. [CrossRef] [PubMed]
59. Lohmann, S.M.; Vaandrager, A.B.; Smolenski, A.; Walter, U.; De Jonge, H.R. Distinct and specific functions of cGMP-dependent protein kinases. *Trends Biochem. Sci.* **1997**, *22*, 307–312. [CrossRef]
60. Schwede, F.; Maronde, E.; Genieser, H.; Jastorff, B. Cyclic nucleotide analogs as biochemical tools and prospective drugs. *Pharmacol. Ther.* **2000**, *87*, 199–226. [CrossRef]
61. Hoffmann, D.; Rentsch, A.; Vighi, E.; Bertolotti, E.; Comitato, A.; Schwede, F.; Genieser, H.G.; Marigo, V. New dimeric cGMP analogues reduce proliferation in three colon cancer cell lines. *Eur. J. Med. Chem.* **2017**, *141*, 61–72. [CrossRef]
62. Vighi, E.; Rentsch, A.; Henning, P.; Comitato, A.; Hoffmann, D.; Bertinetti, D.; Bertolotti, E.; Schwede, F.; Herberg, F.W.; Genieser, H.G.; et al. New cGMP analogues restrain proliferation and migration of melanoma cells. *Oncotarget* **2018**, *9*, 5301–5320. [CrossRef]
63. Zhao, J.; Trewhella, J.; Corbin, J.; Francis, S.; Mitchell, R.; Brushia, R.; Walsh, D. Progressive cyclic nucleotide-induced conformational changes in the cGMP-dependent protein kinase studied by small angle X-ray scattering in solution. *J. Biol. Chem.* **1997**, *272*, 31929–31936. [CrossRef]
64. Zimmerman, A.L.; Yamanaka, G.; Eckstein, F.; Baylor, D.A.; Stryer, L. Interaction of hydrolysis-resistant analogs of cyclic GMP with the phosphodiesterase and light-sensitive channel of retinal rod outer segments. *Proc. Natl. Acad. Sci. USA* **1985**, *82*, 8813–8817. [CrossRef] [PubMed]
65. Vighi, E.; Trifunovic, D.; Veiga-Crespo, P.; Rentsch, A.; Hoffmann, D.; Sahaboglu, A.; Strasser, T.; Kulkarni, M.; Bertolotti, E.; van den Heuvel, A.; et al. Combination of cGMP analogue and drug delivery system provides functional protection in hereditary retinal degeneration. *Proc. Natl. Acad. Sci. USA* **2018**, *115*, E2997–E3006. [CrossRef] [PubMed]
66. Butt, E.; Pohler, D.; Genieser, H.G.; Huggins, J.P.; Bucher, B. Inhibition of cyclic GMP-dependent protein kinase-mediated effects by (Rp)-8-bromo-PET-cyclic GMPS. *Br. J. Pharmacol.* **1995**, *116*, 3110–3116. [CrossRef] [PubMed]
67. Butt, E.; Eigenthaler, M.; Genieser, H.G. (Rp)-8-pCPT-cGMPS, a novel cGMP-dependent protein kinase inhibitor. *Eur. J. Pharmacol.* **1994**, *269*, 265–268. [CrossRef]
68. Nguyen, C.T.O.; Hui, F.; Charng, J.; Velaedan, S.; van Koeverden, A.K.; Lim, J.K.H.; He, Z.; Wong, V.H.Y.; Vingrys, A.J.; Bui, B.V.; et al. Retinal biomarkers provide "insight" into cortical pharmacology and disease. *Pharmacol. Ther.* **2017**, *175*, 151–177. [CrossRef] [PubMed]
69. Cordeiro, M.F.; Normando, E.M.; Cardoso, M.J.; Miodragovic, S.; Jeylani, S.; Davis, B.M.; Guo, L.; Ourselin, S.; A'Hern, R.; Bloom, P.A. Real-time imaging of single neuronal cell apoptosis in patients with glaucoma. *Brain* **2017**, *140*, 1757–1767. [CrossRef]
70. Smith, B.A.; Smith, B.D. Biomarkers and molecular probes for cell death imaging and targeted therapeutics. *Bioconjug. Chem.* **2012**, *23*, 1989–2006. [CrossRef]
71. Camara, M.-F.d.l.; Salom, D.; Sequedo, M.D.; Hervas, D.; Marin-Lambies, C.; Aller, E.; Jaijo, T.; Diaz-Llopis, M.; Millan, J.M.; Rodrigo, R. Altered antioxidant-oxidant status in the aqueous humor and peripheral blood of patients with retinitis pigmentosa. *PLoS ONE* **2013**, *8*, e74223. [CrossRef]
72. Kjellstrom, U.; Veiga-Crespo, P.; Andreasson, S.; Ekstrom, P. Increased Plasma cGMP in a Family With Autosomal Recessive Retinitis Pigmentosa Due to Homozygous Mutations in the PDE6A Gene. *Investig. Ophthalmol. Vis. Sci.* **2016**, *57*, 6048–6057. [CrossRef] [PubMed]
73. Yu, D.Y.; Cringle, S.J. Retinal degeneration and local oxygen metabolism. *Exp. Eye Res.* **2005**, *80*, 745–751. [CrossRef] [PubMed]
74. Lee, M.K.; Cleveland, D.W. Neuronal intermediate filaments. *Annu. Rev. Neurosci.* **1996**, *19*, 187–217. [CrossRef]
75. Petzold, A.; Junemann, A.; Rejdak, K.; Zarnowski, T.; Thaler, S.; Grieb, P.; Kruse, F.E.; Zrenner, E.; Rejdak, R. A novel biomarker for retinal degeneration: Vitreous body neurofilament proteins. *J. Neural. Transm. (Vienna)* **2009**, *116*, 1601–1606. [CrossRef] [PubMed]
76. Cordeiro, M.F.; Guo, L.; Coxon, K.M.; Duggan, J.; Nizari, S.; Normando, E.M.; Sensi, S.L.; Sillito, A.M.; Fitzke, F.W.; Salt, T.E.; et al. Imaging multiple phases of neurodegeneration: A novel approach to assessing cell death in vivo. *Cell Death. Dis.* **2010**, *1*, e3. [CrossRef]

77. Galluzzi, L.; Vitale, I.; Aaronson, S.A.; Abrams, J.M.; Adam, D.; Agostinis, P.; Alnemri, E.S.; Altucci, L.; Amelio, I.; Andrews, D.W.; et al. Molecular mechanisms of cell death: Recommendations of the Nomenclature Committee on Cell Death 2018. *Cell Death Differ.* **2018**, *25*, 486–541. [CrossRef] [PubMed]
78. Sancho-Pelluz, J.; Arango-Gonzalez, B.; Kustermann, S.; Romero, F.J.; van Veen, T.; Zrenner, E.; Ekstrom, P.; Paquet-Durand, F. Photoreceptor cell death mechanisms in inherited retinal degeneration. *Mol. Neurobiol.* **2008**, *38*, 253–269. [CrossRef]
79. Ma, H.; Butler, M.R.; Thapa, A.; Belcher, J.; Yang, F.; Baehr, W.; Biel, M.; Michalakis, S.; Ding, X.Q. cGMP/Protein Kinase G Signaling Suppresses Inositol 1,4,5-Trisphosphate Receptor Phosphorylation and Promotes Endoplasmic Reticulum Stress in Photoreceptors of Cyclic Nucleotide-gated Channel-deficient Mice. *J. Biol. Chem.* **2015**, *290*, 20880–20892. [CrossRef]
80. Sancho-Pelluz, J.; Alavi, M.; Sahaboglu, A.; Kustermann, S.; Farinelli, P.; Azadi, S.; van Veen, T.; Romero, F.J.; Paquet-Durand, F.; Ekstrom, P. Excessive HDAC activation is critical for neurodegeneration in the rd1 mouse. *Cell Death Dis.* **2010**, *1*, 1–9. [CrossRef] [PubMed]
81. Paquet-Durand, F.; Johnson, L.; Ekstrom, P. Calpain activity in retinal degeneration. *J. Neurosci. Res.* **2007**, *85*, 693–702. [CrossRef]
82. Farinelli, P.; Perera, A.; Arango-Gonzalez, B.; Trifunovic, D.; Wagner, M.; Carell, T.; Biel, M.; Zrenner, E.; Michalakis, S.; Paquet-Durand, F.; et al. DNA methylation and differential gene regulation in photoreceptor cell death. *Cell Death Dis.* **2014**, *5*, e1558. [CrossRef] [PubMed]
83. Paquet-Durand, F.; Silva, J.; Talukdar, T.; Johnson, L.E.; Azadi, S.; van Veen, T.; Ueffing, M.; Hauck, S.M.; Ekstrom, P.A. Excessive activation of poly(ADP-ribose) polymerase contributes to inherited photoreceptor degeneration in the retinal degeneration 1 mouse. *J. Neurosci.* **2007**, *27*, 10311–10319. [CrossRef] [PubMed]
84. Sahaboglu, A.; Barth, M.; Secer, E.; Amo, E.M.; Urtti, A.; Arsenijevic, Y.; Zrenner, E.; Paquet-Durand, F. Olaparib significantly delays photoreceptor loss in a model for hereditary retinal degeneration. *Sci. Rep.* **2016**, *6*, 39537. [CrossRef] [PubMed]
85. Campbell, M.; Ozaki, E.; Humphries, P. Systemic delivery of therapeutics to neuronal tissues: A barrier modulation approach. *Expert. Opin. Drug Deliv.* **2010**, *7*, 859–869. [CrossRef] [PubMed]
86. Yeh, S.; Kurup, S.K.; Wang, R.C.; Foster, C.S.; Noronha, G.; Nguyen, Q.D.; Do, D.V.; Team, D.S. Suprachoroidal Injection of Triamcinolone Acetonide, CLS-TA, for macular edema due to noninfectious uveitis: A Randomized, Phase 2 Study (DOGWOOD). *Retina* **2018**. [CrossRef] [PubMed]
87. Ochakovski, G.A.; Peters, T.; Michalakis, S.; Wilhelm, B.; Wissinger, B.; Biel, M.; Bartz-Schmidt, K.U.; Fischer, M.D.; Consortium, R.-C. Subretinal Injection for Gene Therapy Does Not Cause Clinically Significant Outer Nuclear Layer Thinning in Normal Primate Foveae. *Invest. Ophthalmol. Vis. Sci.* **2017**, *58*, 4155–4160. [CrossRef] [PubMed]
88. Ohira, A.; Hara, K.; Johannesson, G.; Tanito, M.; Asgrimsdottir, G.M.; Lund, S.H.; Loftsson, T.; Stefansson, E. Topical dexamethasone gamma-cyclodextrin nanoparticle eye drops increase visual acuity and decrease macular thickness in diabetic macular oedema. *Acta Ophthalmol.* **2015**, *93*, 610–615. [CrossRef] [PubMed]
89. Meyer, C.H.; Krohne, T.U.; Charbel, I.P.; Liu, Z.; Holz, F.G. Routes for Drug Delivery to the Eye and Retina: Intravitreal Injections. *Dev. Ophthalmol.* **2016**, *55*, 63–70. [CrossRef] [PubMed]
90. MacLaren, R.E.; Groppe, M.; Barnard, A.R.; Cottriall, C.L.; Tolmachova, T.; Seymour, L.; Clark, K.R.; During, M.J.; Cremers, F.P.; Black, G.C.; et al. Retinal gene therapy in patients with choroideremia: Initial findings from a phase 1/2 clinical trial. *Lancet* **2014**, *383*, 1129–1137. [CrossRef]
91. Apte, R.S. Gene Therapy for Retinal Degeneration. *Cell* **2018**, *173*, 5. [CrossRef]
92. Solomon, S.D.; Lindsley, K.; Vedula, S.S.; Krzystolik, M.G.; Hawkins, B.S. Anti-vascular endothelial growth factor for neovascular age-related macular degeneration. *Cochrane Database Syst. Rev.* **2019**, *3*, CD005139. [CrossRef] [PubMed]
93. Himawan, E.; Ekström, P.; Buzgo, M.; Gaillard, P.; Stefansson, E.; Marigo, V.; Loftsson, T.; Paquet-Durand, F. Drug delivery to retinal photoreceptors. *Drug Discov. Today* **2019**, in press. [CrossRef] [PubMed]
94. Del Amo, E.M.; Rimpela, A.K.; Heikkinen, E.; Kari, O.K.; Ramsay, E.; Lajunen, T.; Schmitt, M.; Pelkonen, L.; Bhattacharya, M.; Richardson, D.; et al. Pharmacokinetic aspects of retinal drug delivery. *Prog. Retin. Eye Res.* **2017**, *57*, 134–185. [CrossRef] [PubMed]
95. Reichel, F.F.; Peters, T.; Wilhelm, B.; Biel, M.; Ueffing, M.; Wissinger, B.; Bartz-Schmidt, K.U.; Klein, R.; Michalakis, S.; Fischer, M.D.; et al. Humoral Immune Response After Intravitreal But Not After Subretinal AAV8 in Primates and Patients. *Investig. Ophthalmol. Vis. Sci.* **2018**, *59*, 1910–1915. [CrossRef] [PubMed]

96. Rayess, N.; Rahimy, E.; Shah, C.P.; Wolfe, J.D.; Chen, E.; DeCroos, F.C.; Storey, P.; Garg, S.J.; Hsu, J. Incidence and clinical features of post-injection endophthalmitis according to diagnosis. *Br. J. Ophthalmol.* **2015**, *100*, 1058–1061. [CrossRef]
97. Coulson, R.; Baraniak, J.; Stec, W.J.; Jastorff, B. Transport and metabolism of N6- and C8-substituted analogs of adenosine 3',5'-cyclic monophosphate and adenosine 3'5'-cyclic phosphorothioate by the isolated perfused rat kidney. *Life Sci.* **1983**, *32*, 1489–1498. [CrossRef]
98. Maussang, D.; Rip, J.; van Kregten, J.; van den Heuvel, A.; van der Pol, S.; van der Boom, B.; Reijerkerk, A.; Chen, L.; de Boer, M.; Gaillard, P.; et al. Glutathione conjugation dose-dependently increases brain-specific liposomal drug delivery in vitro and in vivo. *Drug Discov. Today Technol.* **2016**, *20*, 59–69. [CrossRef]
99. Williams, M.L.; Coleman, J.E.; Haire, S.E.; Aleman, T.S.; Cideciyan, A.V.; Sokal, I.; Palczewski, K.; Jacobson, S.G.; Semple-Rowland, S.L. Lentiviral expression of retinal guanylate cyclase-1 (RetGC1) restores vision in an avian model of childhood blindness. *PLoS Med.* **2006**, *3*, e201. [CrossRef]

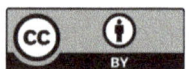

© 2019 by the authors. Licensee MDPI, Basel, Switzerland. This article is an open access article distributed under the terms and conditions of the Creative Commons Attribution (CC BY) license (http://creativecommons.org/licenses/by/4.0/).

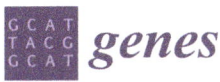

Article

In Vitro Gene Delivery in Retinal Pigment Epithelium Cells by Plasmid DNA-Wrapped Gold Nanoparticles

Sònia Trigueros [1,*], Elena B. Domènech [2,3], Vasileios Toulis [2,3] and Gemma Marfany [2,3,4,*]

1. Department of Zoology, University of Oxford, Oxford OX1 3PS, UK
2. Departament de Genètica, Microbiologia i Estadística, Universitat de Barcelona, 08028 Barcelona, Spain; elenabdomenech@ub.edu (E.B.D.); vtoulis@ub.edu (V.T.)
3. CIBERER, ISCIII, Universitat de Barcelona, 08028 Barcelona, Spain
4. Institute of Biomedicine (IBUB-IRSJD), Universitat de Barcelona, 08028 Barcelona, Spain
* Correspondence: sonia.trigueros@zoo.ox.ac.uk (S.T.); gmarfany@ub.edu (G.M.)

Received: 19 March 2019; Accepted: 8 April 2019; Published: 9 April 2019

Abstract: Many rare diseases course with affectation of neurosensory organs. Among them, the neuroepithelial retina is very vulnerable due to constant light/oxidative stress, but it is also the most accessible and amenable to gene manipulation. Currently, gene addition therapies targeting retinal tissue (either photoreceptors or the retinal pigment epithelium), as a therapy for inherited retinal dystrophies, use adeno-associated virus (AAV)-based approaches. However, efficiency and safety of therapeutic strategies are relevant issues that are not always resolved in virus-based gene delivery and alternative methodologies should be explored. Based on our experience, we are currently assessing the novel physical properties at the nanoscale of inorganic gold nanoparticles for delivering genes to the retinal pigment epithelium (RPE) as a safe and efficient alternative approach. In this work, we present our preliminary results using DNA-wrapped gold nanoparticles (DNA-gold NPs) for successful in vitro gene delivery on human retinal pigment epithelium cell cultures, as a proof-of-principle to assess its feasibility for retina in vivo gene delivery. Our results show faster expression of a reporter gene in cells transfected with DNA-gold NPs compared to DNA-liposome complexes. Furthermore, we show that the DNA-gold NPs follow different uptake, internalization and intracellular vesicle trafficking routes compared to pristine NPs.

Keywords: gene therapy; gold nanoparticles; DNA-wrapped gold nanoparticles; ARPE-19 cells; retinal pigment epithelium; clathrin-coated vesicles; endosomal trafficking

1. Introduction

The dysfunction and death of photoreceptors are the main cause of vision loss in inherited retinal diseases (IRDs), a group of mendelian rare disorders with high genetic and clinical heterogeneity. After more than 30 years of intense clinical and genetic studies to identify IRD genes, around 300 causative genes have been identified that cause the dysfunction of photoreceptors or alter the function of the adjacent retinal pigment epithelium (RPE), thus leading to the progressive attrition of photoreceptors [1,2].

From the clinical side and most relevant to patients, the main challenge is to devise effective treatments to halt the progression of the disease or regain visual capacity. Depending on the gene and type of mutation, different molecular approaches for therapy can be devised; but, at least for autosomal recessive retinal diseases, the most straightforward strategy is the restoration of a fully functional version of the protein via DNA-based gene therapy, even though gene delivery to fully differentiated and mature cells is not an easy task [3,4]. On the other hand, the eye is an excellent target for gene therapy since it is accessible, amenable to non-invasive examination, possesses a well-defined anatomy and is relatively immune privileged [3–5]. Ocular gene therapy for retinal disorders is starting to be developed and the first commercial gene therapy to treat a severe infantile genetic blindness (Leber congenital amaurosis caused by bi-allelic mutations in the *RPE65* gene) was approved last year. These and other ongoing therapies in different clinical trial phases are based on adeno-associated virus (AAV) vectors [6]. However, viral gene delivery also raises several concerns, such as small size capacity (maximum packaging size for 5 kb), high production costs, probability of immunogenicity and inflammatory responses and their invasive route of administration to the retina (subretinal microinjection), which have fostered basic research on non-viral vectors such as nanoparticles (NPs) for gene delivery.

NPs are highly customizable, and can be designed and optimized for cellular uptake, bypassing the degradative machinery of the cells and improving gene expression in the nucleus [7]. Although a priori NPs might yield lower transgene expression levels compared to viral vectors, they overcome most safety concerns of viral vectors, are cost-effective and easily customizable and, most relevant, have a large DNA capacity, critical for gene delivery of large ocular disease genes [4,8]. All these desirable characteristics make the study of NPs for gene delivery to ocular tissues (cornea, retina and retinal pigment epithelium (RPE)) a research priority in order to explore viable alternatives to viral vectors. Nanoparticles made from different materials that display distinct properties, such as inorganic NPs, liposomes, solid lipids and polymeric NPs, have potential use in retinal cells [3,4,9,10]. Some successful attempts using compact DNA polycationic nanoparticles for gene delivery into the retina of pre-clinical animal models have also been reported [11,12].

However, more basic research is still needed to provide a full toolbox of NPs for different uses in the retina, including gene therapy. For instance, liposomal-based NPs, particularly those with positive charges, show cytotoxicity at the large quantities required for efficient gene delivery [13]. The use of polyethilenimine (PEI)-coated NPs increases cellular uptake but PEI is also cytotoxic [3,9]. Gold NPs are mostly non-toxic, but cellular uptake strongly depends on their size and diameter. Several reports indicate that gold NPs ranging between 20 and 50 nm are non-toxic [10]. Indeed, NPs display different physicochemical properties depending on the size, shape, surface charge and hydrophilicity, and these parameters directly impact cellular uptake by different types of vesicular and non-vesicular entry pathways, thereby determining the endocytic route and the final destination of NPs. In gene delivery, the internalization of NPs through the endosomes and eventual fusion of late endosomes with lysosomes should be avoided since it involves the destruction of nucleic acids by lysosomal hydrolases before the genetic material reaches the nucleus [7,14]. Moreover, it has been shown that the lysosomal accumulation of inorganic NPs, elicited by the acidic conditions of the lysosomal cellular compartment, enhance surface instability and ion release. Intracellular ion release is responsible for the cascading events associated with nanoparticle-induced intracellular toxicity [15] and therefore, accumulation of NPs in lysosomes should be avoided.

In this work, we explored the feasibility of gene delivery in cultured differentiated RPE cells using DNA-wrapped gold NPs (DNA-gold NPs). In particular, we focused on cellular uptake and intracellular endosomal trafficking routes of pristine gold NPs and DNA-gold NPs, showing that a higher proportion of DNA-gold NPs (compared to pristine gold NPs) are internalized through clathrin-independent routes that do not end up in late endosomes, thereby avoiding lysosomal degradation. These uptake routes most probably allow faster gene delivery into the nucleus as measured by an early expression of the green fluorescent protein (GFP) reporter gene.

2. Materials and Methods

2.1. ARPE-19 Cell Culture and Differentiation Conditions

Human ARPE-19 cells, acquired from ATCC (CRL_2302), were cultured in 1:1 Dulbecco's Modified Eagle's Medium (DMEM) (ATCC, Manassas, VA, USA) and Ham's F-12 Nutrient Mix (Life Technologies, Carlsbad, CA, USA) supplemented with 10% foetal bovine serum (FBS) (Life Technologies, Carlsbad, CA, USA) and 1% penicillin-streptomycin (Life Technologies, Carlsbad, CA, USA) in a 5% CO_2 humidified chamber at 37 °C. For immunocytochemistry, human ARPE-19 cells (1.5×10^5 cells/well) were seeded in growth medium without antibiotics onto poly-L-lysine-coated coverslips in 24-well plates. To induce differentiation, ARPE-19 cells were deprived of FBS for 48 h and maintained in a 1:1 media of DMEM and Ham's F-12 Nutrient Mix. Subsequently, 48 h post-differentiation, cells were transfected with either nanoparticles or liposomes. For dynasore treatment, the media was changed at 48 h of differentiation, cells were washed once in PBS 1×, and dynasore was added at 80 µM (final concentration) for 30 min. Cell medium was then changed and cells were immediately nanotransfected.

2.2. Lipofection

After 48 h of differentiation, cells were co-transfected with the pEGFP reporter vector (500 ng/well), using Lipotransfectine (Niborlab, Guillena, Spain) (DNA: Lipotransfectine ratio of 1:3) in differentiation medium without antibiotics. This medium was replaced 5 h post-transfection with differentiation medium with antibiotics. After 16 h or 48 h of transfection, cells were fixed with 4% PFA for 20 min at RT and used for immunocytochemistry.

2.3. Gold NP Production and Nanotransfection

Gold nanoparticles (40 nm) at OD 1, stabilized in sodium citrate, were purchased from Sigma-Aldrich (St. Louis, MO, USA) (S-741981). One hundred microliters of gold nanoparticles at OD1 were spun down and resuspended in 10 µL of Milli-Q water and mixed with 1 µL (0.250 µg/µL) of pEGFP plasmid DNA per well. Plasmid DNA-gold hybrid structures were produced by allowing conditions in which double-stranded DNA (dsDNA) loops wrap over the surface of the nanoparticle. The dsDNA-nanoparticle complexes made by this method have an excellent dispersion in different solutions from water to cell culture medium [16]. DNA-wrapped gold nanoparticles were introduced in each well with seeded cells. Photothermal plasmon resonance of the DNA-gold nanoparticles was activated by white light irradiation [17]. Cells were allowed to grow for either 2 h (for immunocytochemistry), or 16 h/48 h (for EGFP expression). For transfection efficiency studies, cells were allowed to grow for 4 h before medium was changed. The details of the wrapping reaction and cell-transfection are currently subject to a patent and published under standard free patent procedures [18].

2.4. Immunocytochemistry

After 2 h, 16 h or 48 h post-transfection with either pristine gold NPs, DNA-wrapped gold NPs or liposomes, cells were fixed with 4% PFA for 20 min at RT, washed in PBS (3×5 min), permeabilized in 0.2% Triton X-100 (St. Louis, MO, USA) in PBS (20 min at RT), and blocked for 1 h in 4% sheep serum in PBS. Primary antibodies were incubated overnight at 4 °C in a 1:200 dilution in blocking solution (rabbit anti-GFP, rabbit anti-EEA1, mouse anti-RAB7, all from Abcam, Cambridge, UK). After incubation, coverslips with cells were rinsed in PBS 1× (3×5 min), incubated with the corresponding secondary antibodies conjugated to either Alexa Fluor 488, 568 or 647 (Life Technologies, Grand Island, NY, USA) (1:400) at RT (1 h) in blocking solution, nuclei were stained with DAPI (Roche Diagnostics, Indianapolis, IN, USA) (1:1000), washed again in PBS 1× (3×5 min), mounted in Mowiol 4–88 (Merck, Darmstadt, Germany) and analysed by confocal microscopy and optical transmission microscopy (Zeiss LSM 880, Thornwood, NY, USA). To quantify GFP-positive cells, coverslips were visualized in a ZOE™ Fluorescent Cell Imager (Bio-Rad, Hercules, CA, USA).

2.5. Imaging and Statistical Analyses

Image analyses were performed using ImageJ (FIJI) software 1.52i. Stack images from five consecutive planes (0.46 µm of separation each) centred on the subcellular location with maximum vesicle intensity were retrieved, segmented in the different channels (clathrin, EEA1, RAB7 or NP), measured and analysed. In the case that the total concentration of the protein of interest had to be determined, the fluorescence threshold value was manually selected and converted into a binary mask.

Then, the binary mask of each protein was converted to area values. In the case that the area of the nanoparticles had to be determined, the threshold value was restricted to the dark spots produced by the plasmon resonance of the nanoparticles. The binary mask of NPs was superimposed over the image of interest—for example, the mask of the NP field was superimposed over the image of the clathrin-positive vesicles' signal. Then, the intersection area between the two selected channels generated a new image, of which the total intensity was determined. To calculate the percentage of NPs in each type of intracellular vesicles, the area of intersection image (e.g., NPs on clathrin-positive cells) was measured and compared to the total area covered by NPs. For statistical analysis, three independent replicates were performed per condition, and three representative different regions of interest (ROIs) per condition and replicate were quantified. Values, ratios and statistical significance were analysed using GraphPad Prism 7.03 (San Diego, CA, USA).

3. Results

3.1. Comparison of Transfection Efficiency of Standard Liposomes Versus DNA-Wrapped Gold NPs in Differentiated ARPE-19 Cells

Differentiated cells are usually difficult to transfect by standard means even in in vitro cell cultures, since lipofection, electroporation or calcium phosphate-mediated transfection strongly depend on plasma and nuclear membrane composition and physicochemical characteristics, such as lability or stiffness. As a first assay, we attempted to directly compare the transfection efficiency in differentiated retinal pigment epithelium cells using GFP as a reporter gene. Dividing ARPE-19 cells (1.5×10^5 cells) were seeded in 24-well plates. The shift to DMEM minimal medium without supplementation of FBS together with cell confluence promotes differentiation to retinal pigment epithelium cells. Under those conditions, ARPE-19 cells stop dividing and in 48 h produce one cilium per cell, demonstrative of their differentiation state. At that stage, liposome-DNA complexes obtained following manufacturer's conditions (Lipotransfectine, 0.500 µg per well) and DNA-wrapped gold NPs (40 nm gold nanoparticles from Sigma-Aldrich (St. Louis, MO, USA), wrapped with pEGFP plasmid DNA following the procedure stated in [18]) (0.250 µg per well) were used to transfect ARPE-19 cells. The plasmon resonance of DNA-gold NPs was activated by white light. After 16 h or 48 h post-transfection, fluorescence images were obtained in a ZOE fluorescent cell imager using the same fluorescence settings (Figure 1A,B and Figure S1). Several images were processed per well and condition and the number of green positive cells was counted manually in a total of 1100–1600 cells.

The number of transfected cells, around 1.4%, was very similar using both methods after 48 h (Figure 1C), even though the amount of DNA used was lower (half) for DNA-gold NP complexes. These results indicated that DNA-gold NPs can be used to transfect differentiated cells with a similar yield than other widely used transfection methods. Remarkably, when using DNA-gold NPs, the same percentage of transfected cells (around 1.2%) was detectable at 16 h and at 48 h, which suggested that the expression of the reporter gene was relatively fast (Figure 1C). Liposome-DNA complexes enter through clathrin-coated vesicles and after trafficking through the endosomal pathway mainly end up fusing to lysosomes (where DNA and lipids are degraded) [19–21]. Our results showing an early reporter gene expression at 16 h indicated that at least a pool of DNA-gold NP complexes might enter the cell through faster routes than clathrin-coated vesicles, thus escaping the endosomal-lysosomal pathway and reaching the nucleus in less time.

3.2. DNA-Gold Nanoparticles Enter RPE Cells by Clathrin-Mediated Vesicles and Other Cellular Uptake Routes

In order to assess whether the cellular uptake of DNA-wrapped gold NPs was clathrin-dependent or independent, we performed colocalization assays of gold NPs and DNA-gold NPs with clathrin-coated vesicles at 2 h post-transfection. Since clathrin internalization is dependent on dynamin activity for closure of the forming vesicles at the membrane, we also treated cells with dynasore for 30 min immediately before transfection. Dynasore is a strong and irreversible inhibitor of dynamin enzymatic activity and therefore, clathrin-coated vesicles can be neither closed up nor internalized. Dynasore also affects the cell membrane stiffness and thus alters lipid raft-mediated processes [22,23].

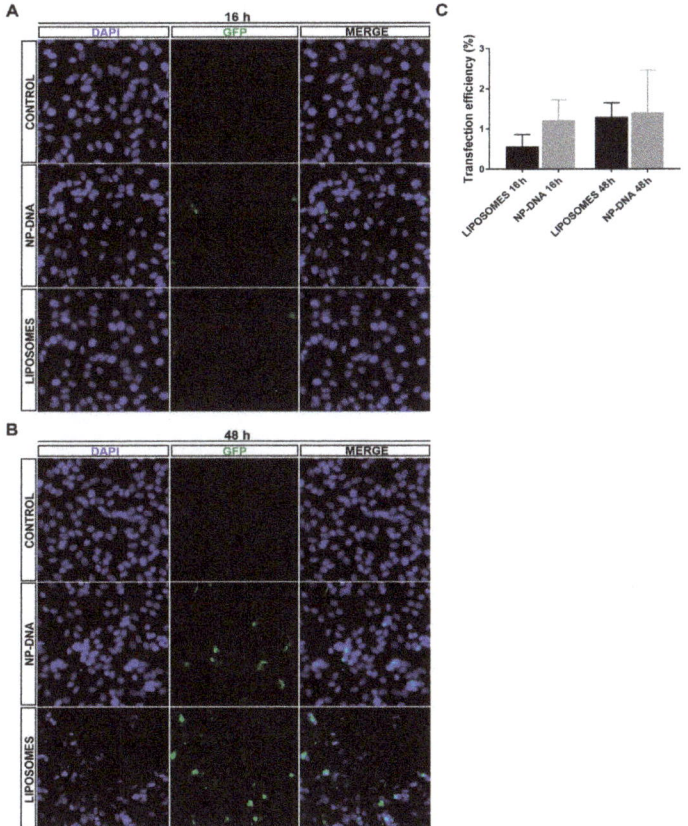

Figure 1. Analysis of transfection efficiency of DNA-wrapped gold nanoparticles (40 nm) compared to liposomes in differentiated ARPE-19 cells. Representative images of differentiated ARPE-19 cells transfected with the pEGFP reporter vector using either liposomes (LIPOTRANSFECTINE) or nanoparticles at (**A**) 16 h and (**B**) 48 h (for wider field images with a lower amplification, see Supplementary Materials, Figure S1). (**C**) Quantification of green fluorescent protein (GFP)-positive cells showed similar levels of transfection efficiency by nanoparticles (1.4% positive cells using 0.25 µg/150,000 cells) compared to standard lipofection (1.31% positive cells using 0.5 µg/150,000 cells) at 48 h. Remarkably, nanoparticles promoted GFP expression in transfected cells at an earlier time after transfection compared to liposomes, since at 16 h, 1.2% cells were GFP-positive in nanoparticle-transfected cells compared to 0.54% in those transfected with liposomes, thus suggesting different cellular uptake and/or intracellular vesicular trafficking routes for the two transfection systems. Quantification on 1100–1600 cells per condition.

Figure 2A shows representative images of the intracellular localization of clathrin vesicles (immunodetected in red) and NPs (detected as black dots in optic tomography field, see zoom panels) in differentiated ARPE-19 cells at 2 h post-transfection. Confocal image stacks were centred in the subcellular localization where clathrin vesicles were more prominent (relatively close to the plasma membrane). Several image masks were used to analyse the localization of NPs in the clathrin-coated vesicles under control (panels at the left) and dynasore treatment (panels at the right) conditions.

Inhibition of dynamin-mediated events by addition of dynasore was effective, since it significantly reduced the number of clathrin-coated vesicles down to 60% in control untransfected cells (Figure 2A,B).

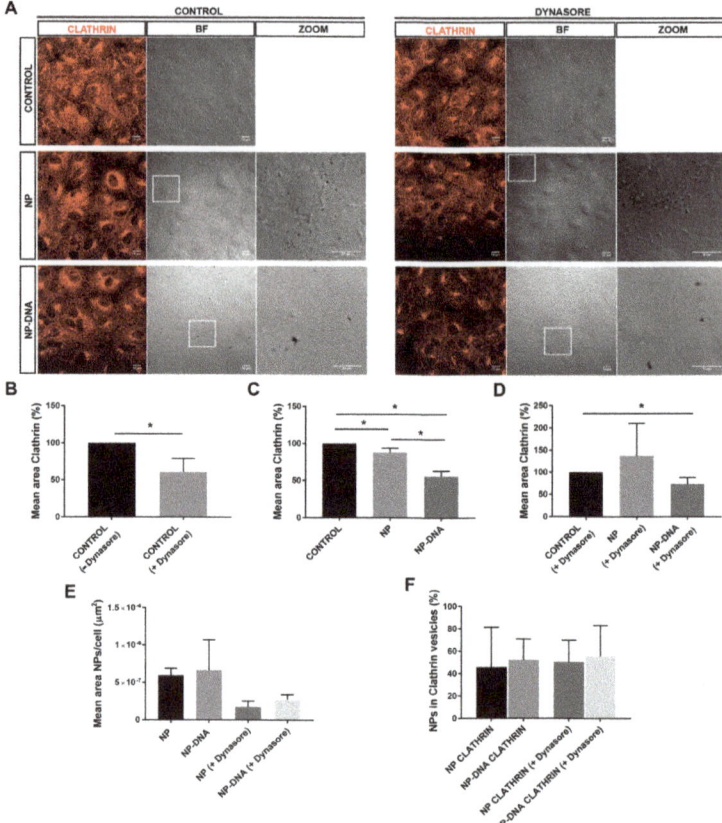

Figure 2. DNA-gold nanoparticles are uptaken by differentiated ARPE-19 cells through different vesicular and/or non-vesicular routes. (**A**) After 2 h post-transfection, between 40 and 60% of pristine gold NPs and DNA-wrapped gold NPs are detected in clathrin-coated vesicles. NPs are visualized as black dots in the optic transmission microscopy channel (BF-bright field, see also zoom panels). DNA nanoparticles appear in clusters compared to pristine 40 nm gold particles. Clathrin-coated vesicles are immunodetected in red. Dynasore treatment inhibited the uptake by dynamin-mediated events. Image analyses of colocalization were performed by using masks over different channels. (**B**) Treatment with dynasore reduced down to 60% the number of clathrin-coated vesicles in untransfected cells, after 2 h. Addition of DNA nanoparticles in either (**C**) control conditions or (**D**) with dynasore treatment significantly reduced down to 55% the number of clathrin-coated particles. (**E**) At 2 h post-transfection, the mean area of NPs/cell uptaken by differentiated RPE is reduced two-fold in dynasore-treated cells, reflecting that at least half of the nanoparticles are internalized by dynamin-mediated events; remarkably, the mean area of internal NPs is higher in cells transfected by DNA-wrapped NPs compared to pristine NPs. (**F**) Percentage of NPs/cell in clathrin-coated vesicles is highly similar in all conditions, ranging between 40 and 50%, indicating that a large pool of NPs was not uptaken by RPE cells using this route. Representative images from three independent replicates (three images per replicate and condition) were quantified. Statistical significance was analysed by the non-parametric Mann–Whitney test (* indicates $p < 0.05$).

Notably, the addition of pristine gold NPs, but particularly of DNA-gold NPs, also significantly reduced the area of clathrin vesicles down to 55% compared to control untransfected cells, which were considered the control reference (Figure 2A panels at the left, and Figure 2C), in a reduction effect similar to that caused by dynasore treatment. This reduction in the area of clathrin vesicles in cells transfected with DNA-gold NPs was also observed after treatment with dynasore (Figure 2A panels at the right, and Figure 2D). This consistent reduction in clathrin area (in all cases after correction per number of cells in each image) may reflect that at the cell–NP interface, surface properties of the DNA-gold NPs, which also differ from those of pristine gold NPs, can alter the formation in number and/or size of clathrin vesicles at the cell membrane of ARPE-19 cells.

Cell uptake of either pristine gold NPs or DNA-gold NPs (measured by the mean area covered by black dots in each image corrected per cell) was reduced, but not abrogated, after dynamin-inhibition in both cases (Figure 2E). However, the percentage of NPs colocalizing within clathrin-coated vesicles was maintained in all conditions and for both types of NPs, with no statistically significant differences (Figure 2F). Therefore, although dynasore treatment reduced the number of clathrin vesicles as well as the total amount of internalized NPs per cell, the percentage of NP uptake via clathrin by ARPE-19 cells was maintained close to 50%.

Overall, these results showed that the presence of DNA-gold NPs (40 nm diameter) altered the dynamics of the differentiated ARPE-19 plasma membrane since the area of clathrin-coated vesicles was diminished at 2 h post-transfection. The percentage of gold NPs in clathrin-coated vesicles was around 50% in all tested conditions, irrespective of the presence of the DNA wrapping and despite inhibition of dynamin activity. Therefore, at least 50% of gold NPs (40 nm), with or without DNA, could enter differentiating ARPE-19 cells through non-clathrin-mediated means.

3.3. Differences in the Intracellular Endosomal Trafficking of DNA-Wrapped Gold NPs Compared to Pristine Gold NPs in RPE Cells

Once inside the cell, clathrin-coated and other endocytic vesicles (e.g., receptor- or caveolin-mediated) enter into the dynamics of the endosomal pathway. The key internalization proteins (clathrin, receptors, caveolin) are recycled and the vesicles fuse to endosomes. Early endosomes mature into late endosomes, and this maturation process involves shifts in the protein epitopes of the endosomal membranes. Late endosomes usually fuse to lysosomes, which degrade the engulfed particles within. There are some exceptions to this endosomal trafficking pathway that leads to degradation. For instance, caveolin-mediated vesicles fuse to neutral endosomes and particles within can be liberated in the cytoplasm and bypass degradation [7,14]. Therefore, we decided to analyse the colocalization of internalized gold NPs with endosomal markers, to assess whether NPs were localized in early and/or late endosomes. After 2 h post-transfection with either pristine gold NPs or DNA-gold NPs, under control and dynamin inhibition conditions, differentiated ARPE-19 were immunodetected for EEA1 (in red) and RAB7 (in white), which are markers for early and late endosomes (Figure 3A). Confocal image stacks were selected at the internal subcellular region with an optimum detection of early and late endosomes. NPs were visualized as black dots in optic transmission microscopy. Several masks were applied to quantify mean areas of NPs and colocalization of NPs within early or late endosomes.

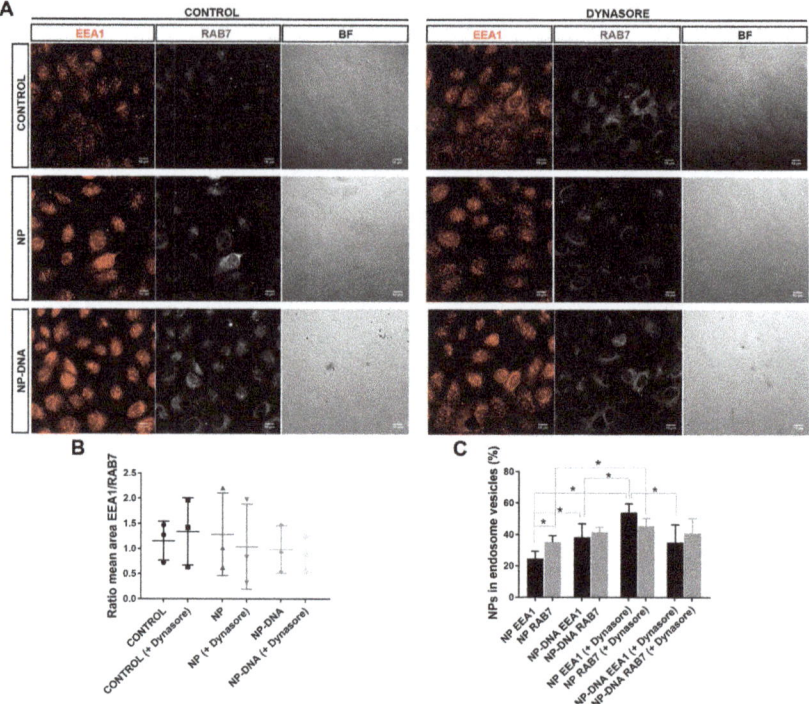

Figure 3. A significant pool of DNA-wrapped gold NPs colocalized in early and late endosomes in differentiated ARPE-19 cells. (**A**) After 2 h post-transfection, a significant pool of NPs colocalized in early endosomes (early endosome marker EEA1, in red) and late endosomes (mature endosome marker RAB7, in white). NPs are visualized as black dots in the optic transmission microscopy channel (BF). Dynasore treatment (panels at the right) was also performed to inhibit dynamin-mediated uptake events. The merge field is not shown since nanoparticles were not distinguishable on the dark background of immunofluorescent images, but image analyses of colocalization were performed by using masks over different channels. (**B**) The number of early and late endosomes was analysed as a ratio (to normalize per cell and condition). After 2 h of transfection with NPs, the ratio EEA1/RAB7 was variable but not significantly different either between cells treated with dynasore compared to controls or between control cells compared to cells transfected with pristine gold NPs or DNA nanoparticles. (**C**) Percentage of pristine NPs and DNA–nanoparticle colocalization with early or late endosomes/cell. At 2 h post-transfection, NPs showed a fluid trafficking between early and late endosomal compartments, as detected by 35% localization in late (35%) versus 25% in early endosomes. Instead, DNA NPs showed a higher localization in the endosomal compartment (close to 100%) but with a similar distribution between early and late endosomes. The addition of dynasore changed the proportion of NPs detected in early and late endosomes when analysing pristine NPs, but not when analysing DNA NPs, indicating that internalization and intracellular trafficking routes differ between pristine gold NPs and DNA NPs. Representative images from three independent replicates (three images per replicate and condition) were quantified. Statistical significance was analysed by the non-parametric Mann–Whitney test (* indicates $p < 0.05$).

First, we assessed that the ratio of early and late endosomes did not vary comparing control cells with cells transfected with either pristine gold NPs or DNA-gold NPs after 2 h post-transfection, in either normal conditions or post-treatment with dynasore (when applicable). No significant differences between the ratio of areas of total early/late endosomes per cell were observed in any tested condition and transfection, including cells treated with dynasore (Figure 3B). However, a more accurate quantification to assess the percentage of NPs within each endosomal compartment, whether in early or in late endosomes, did show statistically significant differences (Figure 3C) when using different NPs and conditions.

Concerning pristine gold NPs, 35% localized in late endosomes and only 25% within the early endosome compartment (Figure 3C). Therefore, the amount of gold NPs that did not localize to the endosomal pathway was close to 40%. In clear contrast, DNA-gold NPs showed an equivalent distribution in both compartments, early and late, summing up to a total of 80% of NPs within the analysed endosomal compartments and 20% outside endosomes. These difference in distribution between pristine and DNA-gold NPs was statistically significant (Figure 3C).

On the other hand, the NPs trafficking through the endosomal pathway after inhibiting dynamin was also divergent between the two types of NPs. After dynasore treatment, pristine gold NPs were mainly found in the endosomal compartments (summing up to 100%), with a significant high increase in the localization within the early endosomes compared to control conditions. Cells transfected with DNA-gold NPs responded differently, since there was no significant variation between NPs localizing at early or late endosomes, rendering similar values to untreated cells, overall indicating that a pool of DNA-gold NPs did not enter through clathrin-coated vesicles. The high number of early endosomes with DNA-wrapped NPs in treated and untreated cells suggest that these particles promote an endocytosis route with a higher number of early endosomes that do not mature into the late compartment. These endosomes might release the cargo into the cytoplasm (in this case, the reporter plasmid pEGFP), which could reach the nucleus and be expressed much faster compared to the early/late endosomal trafficking followed by liposomes, as observed by the early GFP detection at 16 h when using DNA-gold NPs.

4. Discussion

Gene augmentation therapy in recessive mendelian disorders caused by loss of function mutations is, in principle, a plausible option for treatment. Addition of a wild-type copy of the gene should be effective, provided that the gene is delivered and correctly expressed at the target tissue. In IRDs, retinal degeneration is caused by mutations in either genes expressed in photoreceptors or genes expressed in the adjacent RPE, as it is the case with mutations in RPE65, MERTK or LRAT. AAV-based vectors are being used for gene delivery to photoreceptors, but non-viral vectors based on NPs should be concurrently explored for cases in which viral approaches may not be desirable [3,4,8]. Several reports have shown that RPE is particularly amenable for transfection with NPs. This apparent feasibility may be due to the phagocytic nature of RPE cells, which easily engulf and internalize photoreceptor outer segments as well as other exogenous particles [4,9]. Phagocytosis involves the formation of large vesicles, but most small particles enter the cell via pinocytosis, which involve internalization routes mediated by different protein and lipid interactions, for example, clathrin- and caveolae-mediated vesicles as well as clathrin- and caveolae-independent endocytosis [7,14]. The endocytic entry route is key to the final outcome of the internalized particles, since cargo internalized via clathrin vesicles mainly end up being degraded by the lysosome, whereas cargo internalized by caveolin-mediated vesicles or clathrin-independent routes bypass lysosomal degradation. In this context, we have explored the potential use of gold NPs to transfect RPE cells in culture, focusing on the uptake routes and the intracellular endosomal trafficking pathways.

Several authors have reported that in vitro biocompatibility of gold nanoparticles largely depended on their shape and size, and determined that sizes between 5 and 30 nm were more cytotoxic, even though the rate of internalization was higher than that of the less toxic NPs of 50–100 nm (reviewed in [10]). We have used NPs of 40 nm as a compromise between cytotoxicity and internalization. In addition, surface chemical modification of NPs is a critical step that decreases toxicity, increases stability, reduces aggregation and modulates cellular uptake. Most NPs use positive charges at the surface to facilitate the entry at the negatively charged cell membranes, but positively charged NPs induce cell death, whereas negatively charged surfaces induce internalization by clathrin/caveolae-independent endocytosis [7,14].

In this context, we have used plasmid DNA wrapping over gold NPs for two different but relevant reasons: as a means to stabilize gold NPs [8] and favour clathrin-independent cellular uptake, as well as to provide the DNA molecule to be delivered.

In differentiated ARPE-19 cells, at least up to 48 h post-transfection, DNA-wrapped gold NPs did not show any toxicity. DAPI staining did not detect any pyknotic cells, and the transfection efficiency was equivalent for both systems (Figure 1 and Figure S1), even though NPs required half the amount of DNA for the same rate of transfection, thus indicating that this point could be further optimized in the future. Interestingly, in cells transfected with DNA-gold NPs, the same number of cells expressed the reporter GFP gene at 16 h as at 48 h, which suggested that DNA-gold NPs might use a faster uptake/internalization route than cationic liposome-DNA complexes, which are mostly internalized via clathrin vesicles [14,19–21].

Our assays also determined that, in vitro, RPE cells responded differently to pristine gold NPs and DNA-gold NPs, since the area of clathrin vesicles was reduced in the presence of DNA-gold NPs. These differences might be due to changes in the membrane–NP interface. On the one hand, at least 50% of the pool of pristine gold NPs and DNA-gold NPs were internalized via clathrin-coated vesicles, which most probably ended up in the endo-lysosomal degradation pathway (Figure 2). It is likely that this 50% of 40 nm NPs internalized by clathrin-dependent endocytosis corresponded to soluble NPs. On the other hand, the other half of the pool of pristine gold NPs and DNA-gold NPs uses different alternative endocytic routes for internalization, as shown by different localization/trafficking to endosomal compartments. At least 30% of pristine gold NPs are internalized by non-vesicular routes and localized neither in early nor in late endosomes. Since after dynasore treatment this alternative entry route was inhibited and all pristine NPs were detected in the endosomal pathway, the internalization of a significant pool of gold NPs was through lipid rafts or diffusion by destabilization of the cell membrane [22,23]. In contrast, the pool of DNA-gold NPs that was not detected in the endosomal pathway was much lower. A preference for vesicular entry could be explained by the larger size of the DNA-gold NP complexes. Interestingly, DNA-gold NPs are equivalently distributed in early and late endosomes, irrespective of dynasore treatment, thus indicating that a pool of DNA-gold NPs are found in early endosomes that will not mature into late endosome vesicles. These results are in agreement with the earlier expression of the reporter gene detected at 16 h post-transfection, which point to a pool of DNA-gold NPs being internalized by clathrin-independent endocytosis (for instance, via caveolin-mediated vesicles [7,14]) and to cargo escaping lysosomal degradation. Nonetheless, we cannot discard the result that DNA-gold NPs used alternative endosomal trafficking or recycling routes [24].

Our results are but a first step towards the potential use of non-cytotoxic gold NPs for in vivo gene therapy in retinal disorders. Indeed, several basic biological questions should be first addressed, such as the internalization routes and their intracellular endosome trafficking. According to our initial results, DNA-wrapped gold NPs might be considered for gene delivery in retinal tissues. However, before considering this system for in vivo applications, further work is required to fully understand the complexity of cell–NP interaction, which is crucial to increase their transfection efficiency, optimize the cargo delivery by avoiding lysosomal, autophagic or other degradative pathways, and ensure sustained expression of the therapeutic gene.

5. Patents

S.T. declares that the DNA wrapping protocol on NPs is unpublished and currently subject to a patent (S. Trigueros Great Britain Patent GB201201207484A and United States Patent Application 20180318424).

Supplementary Materials: The following are available online at http://www.mdpi.com/2073-4425/10/4/289/s1, Figure S1. Wider field image of Figure 1, showing transfection efficiency of NPs in ARPE-19 cells.

Author Contributions: Conceptualization, S.T. and G.M.; Methodology and Experimental work, E.B.D., V.T. and S.T.; Figures, E.B.D. and V.T.; Result Analysis, all signing authors; Writing Manuscript and Review, all signing authors; Funding Acquisition, S.T. and G.M.

Funding: This research was supported by grants SAF2016-80937-R (Ministerio de Economía y Competitividad/ FEDER), 2017 SGR 738 (Generalitat de Catalunya) and La Marató TV3 (Project Marató 201417-30-31-32) to G.M. E.B.D. is an FI fellow of the Generalitat de Catalunya. V.T. is a fellow of the MINECO (BES-2014-068639, Ministerio de Economía, Industria y Competitividad, Spain). S.T. was supported by EPSRC IAA D4D00620 (UK).

Acknowledgments: Authors acknowledge support from the Oxford Martin School.

Conflicts of Interest: S.T. declares that the DNA wrapping protocol on NPs is unpublished and currently subject to a patent (S. Trigueros Great Britain Patent GB201201207484A and United States Patent Application 20180318424). The rest of the authors declare no conflict of interest.

References

1. RetNet. Retinal Information Network. Available online: https://sph.uth.edu/retnet/ (accessed on 28 February 2019).
2. Farrar, G.J.; Carrigan, M.; Dockery, A.; Millington-Ward, S.; Palfi, A.; Chadderton, N.; Humphries, M.; Kiang, A.S.; Kenna, P.F.; Humphries, P. Toward an elucidation of the molecular genetics of inherited retinal degenerations. *Hum. Mol. Genet.* **2017**, *26*, R2–R11. [CrossRef]
3. Solinís, M.Á.; del Pozo-Rodríguez, A.; Apaolaza, P.S.; Rodríguez-Gascón, A. Treatment of ocular disorders by gene therapy. *Eur. J. Pharm. Biopharm.* **2015**, *95*, 331–342. [CrossRef]
4. Zulliger, R.H.; Conley, S.M.; Naash, M. Non-viral therapeutic approaches to ocular diseases: an overview and future directions. *J. Control. Release* **2015**, *219*, 471–487. [CrossRef] [PubMed]
5. Goureau, O.; Dalkara, D.; Marazova, K. Let There Be Light:Gene and Cell Therapy for Blindness. *Hum. Gene Ther.* **2016**, *27*, 134–147.
6. Bennett, J. Taking Stock of Retinal Gene Therapy:Looking Back and Moving Forward. *Mol. Ther.* **2017**, *25*, 1076–1094.
7. Foroozandeh, P.; Aziz, A.A. Insight into Cellular Uptake and Intracellular Trafficking of Nanoparticles. *Nanoscale Res. Lett.* **2018**, *13*, 339. [CrossRef]
8. Garcia-Guerra, A.; Dunwell, T.L.; Trigueros, S. Nano-Scale Gene Delivery Systems: Current Technology, Obstacles, and Future Directions. *Curr. Med. Chem.* **2018**, *25*, 2448–2464. [CrossRef] [PubMed]
9. Adijanto, J.; Naash, M.I. Nanoparticle-based Technologies for Retinal Gene Therapy. *Eur. J. Pharm. Biopharm.* **2015**, *95*, 353–367. [CrossRef]
10. Masse, F.; Ouellette, M.; Lamoureux, G. Gold nanoparticles in ophthalmology. *Med. Res. Rev.* **2019**, *39*, 302–327. [CrossRef]
11. Han, Z.; Banworth, M.J.; Makkia, R.; Conley, S.C.; Al-Ubaidi, M.R.; Cooper, M.J.; Naash, M.I. Genomic DNA nanoparticles rescue rhodopsin-associated retinitis pigmentosa phenotype. *FASEB J.* **2019**, *29*, 2535–2544. [CrossRef]
12. Kelley, R.A.; Conley, S.M.; Cooper, M.J.; Naash, M.I. DNA nanoparticles are safe and nontoxic in non-human primate eyes. *Int. J. Nanomed.* **2018**, *13*, 1361–1379. [CrossRef] [PubMed]
13. Li, Y.; Cui, X.-L.; Chen, Q.-S.; Yu, J.; Zhang, H.; Gao, J.; Sun, D.X.; Zhang, G.Q. Cationic liposomes induce cytotoxicity in HepG2 via regulation of lipid metabolism based on whole-transcriptome sequencing analysis. *BMC Pharmacol. Toxicol.* **2018**, *19*, 43. [CrossRef] [PubMed]
14. Yameena, B.; Choi, W., II; Vilosa, C.; Swamia, A.; Shia, J.; Farokhzada, O.C. Insight into nanoparticle cellular uptake and intracellular targeting. *J. Control. Release* **2014**, *190*, 485–499. [CrossRef] [PubMed]
15. Sabella, S.; Carney, R.P.; Brunetti, V.; Malvindi, M.A.; Al-Juffali, N.; Vecchio, G.; Janes, S.M.; Bakr, O.M.; Cingolani, R.; Stellacci, F.; et al. A general mechanism for intracellular toxicity of metal-containing nanoparticles. *Nanoscale* **2014**, *12*, 7052–7061. [CrossRef] [PubMed]
16. Civit, S.; Trigueros, S. Analysis of Surface Alignment of SWCNTs–DNA based Nanobiosensors. *Res. Med. Eng. Sci.* **2018**, *5*, 1–7.
17. Lajunen, T.; Viitala, L.; Kontturi, L.-S.; Laaksonen, T.; Liang, H.; Vuorimaa-Laukkanen, E.; Viitalaa, T.; Le Guèvel, X.; Yliperttula, M.; Murtomäki, L.; et al. Light induced cytosolic drug delivery from liposomes with gold nanoparticles. *J. Control. Release* **2015**, *203*, 85–98. [CrossRef] [PubMed]

18. Trigueros, S. Nanostructure Coated with a Twist-Strained Double-Stranded Circular Deoxyribonucleic Acid (DNA), Method for Making and Use. U.S. Patent Application 20180318424, 11 August 2018.
19. Rejman, J.; Conese, M.; Hoekstra, D.J. Gene Transfer by Means of Lipo and Polyplexes:Role of Clathrin and Caveolae-Mediated Endocytosis. *J. Liposome Res.* **2006**, *16*, 237–247. [CrossRef]
20. Soriano, J.; Villanueva, A.; Stockert, J.C.; Cañete, M. Vehiculization determines the endocytic internalization mechanism of Zn(II)-phthalocyanine. *Histochem. Cell. Biol.* **2013**, *139*, 149–160. [CrossRef]
21. Agirre, M.; Ojeda, E.; Zarate, J.; Puras, G.; Grijalvo, S.; Eritja, R.; García del Caño, G.; Barrondo, S.; González-Burguera, I.; López de Jesús, M.; et al. New Insights into Gene Delivery to Human Neuronal Precursor NT2 Cells: A Comparative Study between Lipoplexes, Nioplexes, and Polyplexes. *Mol. Pharm.* **2015**, *12*, 4056–4066. [CrossRef]
22. Girard, E.; Paul, J.L.; Fournier, N.; Beaune, P.; Johannes, L. The Dynamin Chemical Inhibitor Dynasore Impairs Cholesterol Trafficking and Sterol-Sensitive Genes Transcription in Human HeLa Cells and Macrophages. *PLoS ONE* **2011**, *6*, e29042. [CrossRef]
23. Preta, G.; Cronin, J.G.; Sheldon, I.M. Dynasore-not just a dynamin inhibitor. *Cell Commun. Signal.* **2015**, *13*, 24. [CrossRef] [PubMed]
24. Zhang, J.; Chang, D.; Yang, Y.; Zhang, X.; Tao, W. Systematic investigation on the intracellular trafficking network of polymeric nanoparticles. *Nanoscale* **2017**, *9*, 3269–3282. [CrossRef] [PubMed]

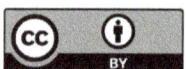

© 2019 by the authors. Licensee MDPI, Basel, Switzerland. This article is an open access article distributed under the terms and conditions of the Creative Commons Attribution (CC BY) license (http://creativecommons.org/licenses/by/4.0/).

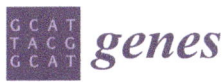

Review

Molecular Therapies for Inherited Retinal Diseases—Current Standing, Opportunities and Challenges

Irene Vázquez-Domínguez, Alejandro Garanto *,† and Rob W. J. Collin *,†

Department of Human Genetics and Donders Institute for Brain, Cognition and Behaviour, Radboud University Medical Center, 6525GA Nijmegen, The Netherlands
* Correspondence: alex.garanto@radboudumc.nl (A.G.); rob.collin@radboudumc.nl (R.W.J.C.); Tel.: +31-24-36-14107 (A.G.); +31-24-36-13750 (R.W.J.C.)
† Both senior authors contributed equally.

Received: 31 July 2019; Accepted: 26 August 2019; Published: 28 August 2019

Abstract: Inherited retinal diseases (IRDs) are both genetically and clinically highly heterogeneous and have long been considered incurable. Following the successful development of a gene augmentation therapy for biallelic *RPE65*-associated IRD, this view has changed. As a result, many different therapeutic approaches are currently being developed, in particular a large variety of molecular therapies. These are depending on the severity of the retinal degeneration, knowledge of the pathophysiological mechanism underlying each subtype of IRD, and the therapeutic target molecule. DNA therapies include approaches such as gene augmentation therapy, genome editing and optogenetics. For some genetic subtypes of IRD, RNA therapies and compound therapies have also shown considerable therapeutic potential. In this review, we summarize the current state-of-the-art of various therapeutic approaches, including the pros and cons of each strategy, and outline the future challenges that lie ahead in the combat against IRDs.

Keywords: inherited retinal diseases; IRD; DNA therapies; RNA therapies; compound therapies; clinical trials

1. Introduction

1.1. Inherited Retinal Diseases (IRDs)

Inherited retinal diseases (IRDs) are a rare and heterogeneous group of neurodegenerative disorders that collectively result in progressive visual impairment. IRDs are estimated to affect around 1 in 2000 people worldwide [1]. Over 250 causative genes have been identified in which mutations can cause one or more of the clinical subtypes of IRD (https://sph.uth.edu/retnet/). IRDs can be familial or sporadic, isolated (non-syndromic) or syndromic and stationary or progressive. In terms of geographic distribution, they could be diffused or localized. Most forms of IRD mainly affect photoreceptors but other forms can also primarily affect the retinal pigment epithelium (RPE) or the inner retina. IRDs can propagate through all modes of inheritance—autosomal dominant (AD), autosomal recessive (AR), X-linked (XL) or mitochondrial, whilst digenic cases or uniparental disomy have also been described occasionally [2].

1.2. Present Treatment of IRD

The eye is an ideal target for molecular therapies, for various reasons. First, the tight junctions of the blood-retina barrier (BRB) define the retina to be a relatively immune-privileged tissue [3]. In other words, the introduction of a foreign antigen (like a viral vector) is generally well tolerated without evoking severe inflammatory responses [4,5]. The risk of widespread dissemination of the locally administered vector is low, preventing unwanted systemic effects. Furthermore, relatively small amounts of the vector are needed to achieve a therapeutic response [6,7]. The eye is easily accessible by surgery [8], which allows intravitreal and subretinal administration of vectors to the affected tissue. As retinal cells are differentiated and non-dividing, there is no loss of the transgene even with the use of non-integrating vectors [9]. Finally, there are many different non-invasive approaches that are able to monitor disease progression [10]. Examples include fundus autofluorescence that provides a topographical map of lipofuscin changes in the RPE cells, spectral domain OCT to assess retinal thickness and photoreceptor layer architecture, as well as other known tests like visual acuity and biomicroscopy [11–13].

Currently, there are various (overlapping) approaches to treat IRDs under development, including molecular therapies but also stem cell-based therapies and retinal prostheses [14–18] (Figure 1). Despite the promising results obtained with some of these approaches, there are still many challenges that must be overcome in order to reach a broad implementation of treatment modalities for IRDs. The great heterogeneity of these diseases [19] hampers the development of a common treatment for a large number of patients [20]. In addition, a significant proportion of genes involved in IRDs has a cDNA size that exceeds the cargo capacity of adeno-associated viral (AAV) vectors, generally considered the most preferred viral vector for retinal delivery of therapeutic molecules [21]. Finally, the costs of developing gene or even mutation-specific approaches are substantial, while often having only a limited number of individuals that could potentially benefit from a given therapeutic molecule.

In this review, we summarize the current state-of-the-art of the therapeutic approaches for IRDs, with a strong emphasis on molecular therapies.

2. Molecular therapies

Due to the severity and heterogeneity of IRDs, avid research is ongoing to identify therapeutic strategies that could ameliorate symptoms and/or disease progression, including many that focus on resolving the consequences of a particular genetic defect [22]. However, a good candidate for molecular therapies requires—(i) a substantial disease burden and a favourable risk/benefit ratio compared to another therapy, if any; (ii) the relevant gene/locus involved in the disease has already been identified and there is ample knowledge of the molecular mechanism of disease and its progression; (iii) the right target cell(s) can be reached, with or without using a therapeutic vehicle; (iv) phenotypic improvement can preferably be achieved with limited expression levels of the therapeutic gene, while its overexpression does not exert any toxic effect [23].

We can subdivide the molecular strategies into different groups—DNA, RNA and compound therapies, as graphically depicted in Figures 1 and 2. Ongoing clinical trials for genetic subtypes of IRDs are summarized in Table 1 (DNA therapies), Table 2 (RNA therapies) and Table 3 (Compound therapies).

2.1. DNA Therapies

2.1.1. Gene Augmentation

In gene augmentation therapy (also known as gene replacement therapy), a normal copy of the mutated gene is inserted into the host cells using therapeutic vectors (for details on the various types of vectors, see Section 3). To enable this, the gene of interest could be delivered as DNA, as messenger RNA (mRNA) or as mRNA analogue. The big advantage of the mRNA platform is that it does not require delivery into the nucleus and the risk of integration into the host genome is reduced [24,25]. Two of the main challenges of mRNA delivery however are immunogenicity and stability of the RNA molecule [24,26]. Thus, since sustained production of the protein of interest is required for continued improvement of visual function, the DNA platform is the preferred strategy for ocular gene augmentation therapy [25]. With this, the gene of interest is introduced to the cell nucleus, where it often remains in an episomal state while promoters and enhancers can facilitate its expression [25,27].

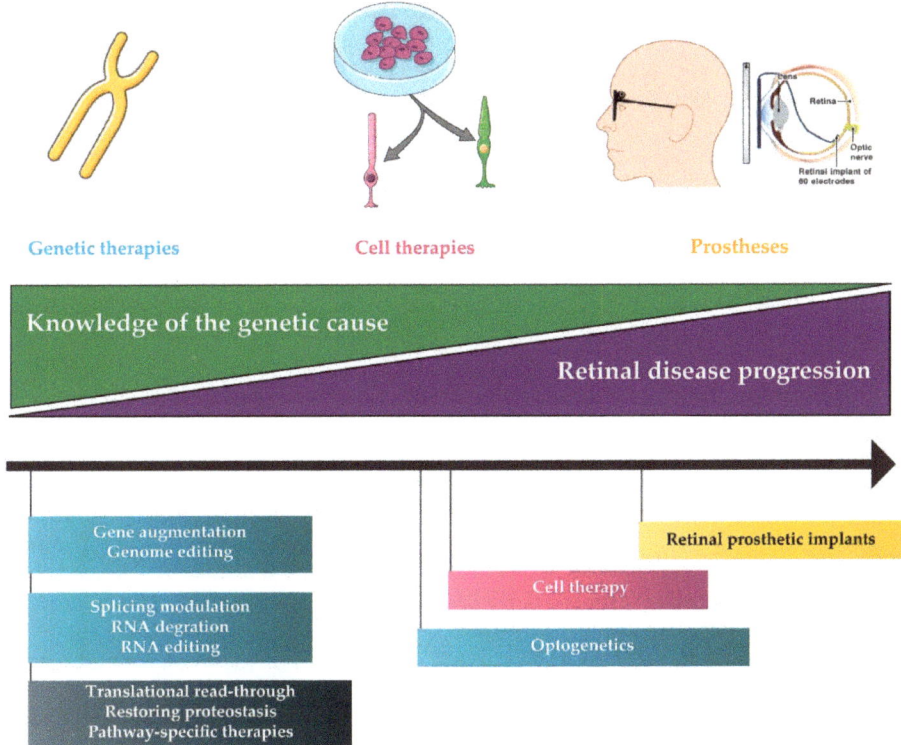

Figure 1. Schematic representation of potential therapeutic approaches according to the retinal disease progression and the knowledge of the genetic cause of the retinal disease. Genetic therapies (blue boxes) are preferred in the first steps of the disease progression (retinal cells are still alive) and when knowledge of the genetic causes of the diseases is present. As the disease progresses and the knowledge of the pathogenesis decreases, other approaches such as cell therapies (pink box) or retinal prosthetic implants (yellow box) can be used. Compound therapies (black box), based on pharmacological treatments, could be used as an alternative approach when the genetic cause of the disease or the pathway involved are either known or unknown. For late-stage diseases, optogenetics or retinal prostheses may be the only option. Image sources—smart.servier.com and Doheny Retina Institute (new.bbc.co.uk/2/hi/science/nature/6368089).

DNA can be delivered using one of several different vectors but in particular for IRDs, adeno-associated viruses (AAVs) have been most commonly used due to their high tropism for certain retinal cells and their low immunogenicity [14]. Other vectors under study are lentiviruses and nanoparticles, which have larger cargo capacities [28].

Advanced stages of retinal degeneration are not compatible with the use of gene augmentation therapy, since this approach requires the target cells to be alive [29]. Moreover, reaching substantial levels of gene expression is crucial for a significant and strong rescue of the phenotype [30]. This requirement can for instance be improved by varying the serotypes of AAVs that are used to deliver the transgene [31–33], by varying the promoter sequence [30] or by producing codon-optimized cDNA versions of a given gene [34,35].

For IRDs, gene augmentation is currently the most advanced therapeutic strategy, with market approval for one gene (*RPE65*, Luxturna^{TM}), several ongoing clinical studies for other genes (Table 1) and preclinical development for a plethora of genes mutated in these diseases [36]. Despite these promising results, gene augmentation strategies may not be the best approach when treating dominant conditions [37], as the mutated allele underlying the disease most often first needs to be inactivated such that it does not interfere with the normal allele [38]. Such an allele-specific inhibition of expression can be achieved either at the DNA level (Section 2.1.2) or at the RNA level (Section 2.2) and, if needed, can be combined with gene augmentation [39]. In addition, the cargo capacity of AAV remains a challenge, since several of the recurrently mutated genes (e.g., *USH2A, EYS,* etc.) are by far exceeding it. Several studies using dual or even triple AAVs [40–43], or microgenes (smaller versions of the gene) [44] are ongoing.

2.1.2. Genome Editing

In addition to gene augmentation, precise editing of genomic DNA has gained an enormous attention over the last five years. Currently, there are two main approaches in genome editing—an in vivo approach, in which the disease-causing mutations are corrected inside the retina and an *ex vivo* approach to first correct the mutation in patient-derived cells, which can be followed by cell transplantation [45]. The editing itself can be achieved by different classes of molecules, as outlined below.

ZFNs and TALENs: Zinc-finger nucleases (ZFNs) and transcription activator like effector nucleases (TALENs) are molecules that pioneered genome editing. Both can induce a wide range of genetic modifications by generating double-strand breaks (DSBs) in the DNA that subsequently stimulate one of the DNA repair pathways of the cell—non-homologous end-joining (NHEJ), homology-directed repair (HDR) or microhomology-mediated end joining [46,47]. To induce DSBs, either nuclease needs to be guided to its target sequence by a DNA-binding protein domain. These approaches are thus depending on the engineering of new proteins for each target, making them laborious and challenging [48]. Nevertheless, ZFNs have been used as a proof-of-concept treatment in IRD. Human embryonic cells carrying the c.68C>A; p.P23H mutation in *RHO* were targeted using ZFNs, which led to an increase in homologous recombination events when the ZFNs were transfected with a homologous donor template, compared to delivery in the absence of this template [49].

TALENs have been used in the correction of the *Crbrd8* allele in C57BL/6N mice. HDR triggered by a combination of TALEN and a single-stranded donor oligonucleotide repair template was observed in 27% of the treated mouse embryos and resulted in an improvement of retinal function [50].

CRISPR/Cas system: The CRISPR/Cas system is considered a more advanced genome editing tool compared to ZFNs and TALENs, as it presents many advantages including the simple design of the target, its higher efficacy and its ability to introduce mutations in multiple genes at the same time by using a combination of guide RNAs (gRNAs) [25]. The CRISPR/Cas system has been improved to a simpler version, CRISPR/Cas9, which nowadays is commonly used for mammalian genome editing [51–53]. The Cas9 endonuclease is delivered into a cell in conjunction with a gRNA, after which it can cut the genome specifically at any desired location [52,54].

As for other genome-editing tools, its major limitation is the possibility of off-target effects [46]. To overcome this aspect, researchers have developed different strategies—(i) using ribonucleoproteins (RNPs) as a form of delivery [55]; (ii) titrating the concentration of gRNA and Cas9 or using two gRNAs flanking the target region [56]; (iii) adding two additional guanine bases at the 5′ end of the gRNA sequence for Cas9 derived from *Streptococcus pyogenes* (SpCas9); interestingly, this modification in the design did not reduce the on-target ratio both in vivo and *in vitro* [57]; (iv) selecting unique DNA target sites with no homology to any other gene sequence [58]; (v) using paired Cas9 nickases, modified Cas9 nucleases that cut only one strand of DNA and thus can produce DSBs with two times more specificity [52,57,59], (vi) employing a high-fidelity version of Cas9 (SpCas9-HF1) [59] or (vii) using the 'enhanced specificity' SpCas9, which is reported to not only decrease the off-target events but also to obtain a higher on-target efficacy [60]. All these strategies have allowed researchers to yield relatively high editing rates *in vitro* but these rates are generally lower in vivo, for instance in treated retinas [52,61–72]. The first challenge is the delivery of the CRISPR system directly into the cells or tissue of interest. As it was previously mentioned, AAV vectors are currently considered the most potent therapeutic vector for retinal delivery. However, its limited cargo capacity hampers an efficient delivery of the complete CRISPR/Cas9 system [73]. One solution for this problem is the delivery of the SpCas9 and gRNA separated into two vectors, with which Hung and colleagues obtained an editing efficacy of 84% in the mouse retina [52]. Other studies using two AAV vectors have also obtained good results over the last years, although it should be mentioned that these in vivo studies only used CRISPR/Cas9 technology to activate NHEJ, resulting in indels and subsequent gene inactivation [55,74–77]. A major concern that remains to be solved is how to increase the efficacy of genome correction in the retina, since photoreceptors are post-mitotic cells that to a large extent lack HDR mechanisms. Suzuki and colleagues developed a strategy coined homology-independent targeted integration which allows for targeted knock-in in non-dividing cells like photoreceptors [45,77]. This appears as a promising approach, as it is based on the NHEJ mechanism, as opposed to HDR, for specific integration of a desired DNA sequence [45,77].

Besides precise editing, the CRISPR/Cas9-system can also be used in other ways, such as the invalidation of mutant alleles that underlie autosomal dominant IRD (reviewed by Diakatou et al.) [78], or the removal of intronic sequences harbouring pathogenic pseudoexons. For the latter, Maeder and colleagues recently developed a CRISPR/Cas9-based approach (EDIT-101) for the splice mutation c.2991+1655A>G in *CEP290*. EDIT-101 promotes the deletion of part of intron 26 where the deep-intronic variant is located. It was tested in a humanized *Cep290* mouse model carrying the c.2991+1655A>G variant [79] and a comparable surrogate non-human primate (NHP) vector also showed efficient editing in photoreceptor and somatic primate cells [80].

Although several hurdles still need to be overcome, the development of the CRISPR/Cas9 system has opened new avenues for the future treatment of various genetic subtypes of IRD.

2.1.3. Optogenetics

Although gene-specific augmentation therapy is a very attractive approach in patients with a known genotype and at a relative early stage of the disease, it is not suitable for patients who present a more advanced stage of the disease in which many of the photoreceptors have been lost (Figure 1).

Optogenetics is a technique used to monitor or control neural activity with light, which can be achieved by the genetic introduction of light-sensitive proteins into retinal cells. This strategy is often used to convert secondary or tertiary neurons into "photoreceptors" or, less often, to restore sensitivity of degenerating photoreceptor cells [81–83]. One advantage of optogenetics is that it may more precisely excite the neural pathway compared to for example, electronic retinal implants [82,84]. In addition, optogenetics can be used independent of the primary genetic defect.

Opsins represent the major optogenetic tool [85]. They function as sensory receptors or light-responsive ion channels. Two types of opsin have been described—microbial opsins (type I) and animal opsins (type II) [81,82]. Type-I opsins (channelrhodopsins, halorhodopsins and archaerhodopsins), following light capture, result in a passive flow of ions across the cell membrane. When they are introduced into non-light sensitive cells, microbial opsins can induce rapid optical control of specific cellular processes. Type-I opsins allow high-speed neural activation and silencing, without requiring any additional chemicals [86]. Type-II opsins (rhodopsin and melanopsin) are part of the large family of naturally occurring light-sensitive G protein-coupled receptors (GPCRs). In contrast to microbial opsins, animal opsins present a much higher light sensitivity, as the light signal is amplified by G-protein-coupled signalling cascades [87]. Both types of opsins are small enough to be encapsidated in AAVs [81,82].

Experiments in animal models (mouse, rat and dog) revealed that expression of type-II opsins resulted in increased light sensitivity, within 1–2 log units of the threshold for normal cone vision, although this sensitivity may come at the cost of slower kinetics [88]. In contrast, the use of type-I opsins is superior in terms of kinetics, yet its sensitivity is lower. Both types however are limited in their operational range of light levels and will likely require modification of the incoming light signal [89]. Moreover, many questions still need to be addressed such as the identification of the best vector and surgical approach for delivery. Although a wide range of ubiquitous, photoreceptor-, bipolar- or ganglion-cell specific promoters have been used, the ideal condition so far remains unclear [82].

Currently, there are two clinical trials ongoing that use optogenetics for vision restoration. One comprises a phase I/II clinical trial (NCT02556736; Table 1) and a second trial is still in a recruiting state (NCT03326336; Table 1), without any results reported yet for both trials.

2.2. RNA Therapies

2.2.1. Splicing Modulation

Antisense oligonucleotides (AONs): Around 15% of all IRD-causing mutations affect the splicing process [90]. Currently, the most widely used genetic therapy to correct aberrant splicing employs antisense oligonucleotides (AONs) [91], small DNA or RNA molecules that bind to their target pre-mRNA in a complementary way [91,92]. Their ability to modulate splicing in fact offers several advantages over gene replacement approaches, especially for IRDs [93]. Initially, AONs were simple antisense RNA molecules but found to be rapidly degraded by nucleases [91]. Therefore, multiple chemical modifications for the backbone or sugar groups were added to improve their target affinity and resistance to nuclease activity [91,94]. These new AONs were classified as first or second generation AONs, depending on their chemical modifications [94]. A third generation class of AONs consists of analogues of nucleic acids. Due to their relatively small size, it has been shown that AONs can be delivered to the eye either as naked molecules or in an AAV using a modified U7-snRNA system [95,96].

The first approved AON-based drug was Formivirsen, also known as Vitravene [97]. Vitravene was used to treat cytomegalovirus retinitis in patients whose immune system was compromised [97,98]. In the last years, the number of IRD-causing mutations that affect pre-mRNA splicing has rapidly increased. An example is a recurrent deep-intronic mutation in *CEP290* (c.2991+1665A>G) underlying congenital blindness [99]. For this mutation, the potential of AON-based therapy was demonstrated first in *in vitro* and in vivo models [96,100–104] and later on, in a phase I/II clinical trial [105]. Promising proof-of-concept studies employing AONs have also been developed for other mutations in *CEP290* [106], and for other genes mutated in IRD such as *OPA1* [107], *CHM* [108], *USH2A* [109] and *ABCA4* [110–113].

Besides the clinical trial for *CEP290* (NCT03140969) there is also an ongoing clinical trial for *USH2A* (Table 2). The results obtained so far indicate that AON-based therapy is a promising therapeutic strategy, albeit only for a selected group of IRD-causing mutations. However, the use of whole genome sequencing or targeted full-gene sequencing will likely identify more mutations amenable for this type of therapy in the near future. Overall, the remaining challenges for AON-based splicing modulation are mainly related to delivery, longevity and potential off-target effects.

U1 spliceosomal RNA: Many exonic splice donor site (SD) mutations have been identified in the last nucleotide of an exon and over 95% of these are predicted to result in aberrant splicing [114]. The splicing process needs the recognition of splice sites and subsequent assembly of the spliceosome. The latter is started by formation of stable complexes consisting of U1 small nuclear RNA (U1 snRNA), pre-mRNA and splice factor proteins. Splice donor sites are recognized directly by the U1 complex and are crucial for a proper splicing of exons. In case nucleotides within the splice donor site of an exon are mutated, an attractive therapeutic approach is to use a modified U1 snRNA. Tanner and colleagues demonstrated that a mutation that induces exon skipping in *RHO* (c.936G>A; p.Q311Q) can be rescued by adapting the U1 snRNA to the mutation [114]. In the last years, this approach has also been successfully employed *in vitro*, to rescue a mutation in exon 5 of the *BBS1* gene that underlies Bardet-Biedl syndrome [115], or a mutation in intron 10 causing *RPGR*-associated X-linked RP [116]. Thus, the U1 snRNA system definitely holds some therapeutic potential for mutations affecting the splice donor site. However, possible off-target effects caused by the delivery of an exogenous modified U1 snRNA are still poorly studied [117,118].

Table 1. Summary of clinical trials for inherited retinal diseases (IRDs) using DNA therapies.

Gene/Condition	Therapeutic Molecule	Clinical Trial Identifier	Status
Gene Augmentation			
ABCA4	SAR422459	NCT01367444	Recruiting
	SAR422459	NCT01736592	Enrolling by invitation
CHM	AAV2-hCHM	NCT02341807	Active, not recruiting
	AAV2-REP1	NCT03496012	Recruiting
	AAV2-REP1	NCT03507686	Recruiting
	AAV2-REP1	NCT02407678	Active, not recruiting
	rAAV2.REP1	NCT02671539	Active, not recruiting
	rAAV2.REP1	NCT02077361	**Completed**
	rAAV2.REP1	NCT01461213	**Completed**
	AAV2-REP1	NCT03584165	Enrolling by invitation
	AAV2-REP1	NCT02553135	**Completed**
CNGA3	AGTC-402	NCT02935517	Recruiting
	AAV2/8-hG1.7p.coCNGA3	NCT03758404	Recruiting
	rAAV.hCNGA3	NCT02610582	Active, not recruiting
CNGB3	rAAV2tYF-PR1.7-hCNGB3	NCT02599922	Recruiting
	AAV2/8-hCARp.hCNGB3	NCT03001310	Recruiting
	AAV-CNGB3	NCT03278873	Recruiting
MERTK	rAAV2-VMD2-hMERTK	NCT01482195	Recruiting
MYO7A	UshStat	NCT02065011	Enrolling by invitation
PDE6B	AAV2/5-hPDE6B	NCT03328130	Recruiting
RPE65	AAV OPTIREP	NCT02946879	Recruiting
	rAAV2-CBSB-hRPE65	NCT00481546	Active, not recruiting
	AAV2-hRPE65v2-	NCT00516477	Active, not recruiting
	AAV2-hRPE65v2	NCT00999609	Active, not recruiting
	AAV2-hRPE65v2	NCT01208389	Active, not recruiting
	AAV2-hRPE65v2	NCT03602820	Active, not recruiting
	tgAAG76 (rAAV 2/2.hRPE65p.hRPE65)	NCT00643747	**Completed**
	rAAV2-CB-hRPE65	NCT00749957	**Completed**
	rAAV2-hRPE65	NCT00821340	**Completed**
	rAAV2/4.hRPE65	NCT01496040	**Completed**
	AAV RPE65	NCT02781480	**Completed**
RLBP1	CPK850	NCT03374657	Recruiting
RPGR	AAV8-RPGR	NCT03116113	Recruiting
	AAV2/5-hRKp.RPGR	NCT03252847	Recruiting
	rAAV2tYF-GRK1-RPGR	NCT03316560	Recruiting
RS1	AAV8-scRS/IRBPhRS	NCT02317887	Recruiting
	rAAV2tYF-CB-hRS1	NCT02416622	Active, not recruiting
Genome editing			
CEP290	EDIT-101 (AGN-151587)	NCT03872479	Recruiting
Optogenetics			
Advanced RP	RST-001	NCT02556736	Recruiting
Non-syndromic RP Retinitis Pigmentosa	GS030-DP	NCT03326336	Recruiting

Black and gray are just used to indicate the different sectiond and can be considered as headers. Gene or disease condition (first column), therapeutic molecule (second column), clinical trial identifier (third column) and the current status of the trial (last column) are indicated. Completed trials are highlighted in bold. Data obtained from https://clinicaltrials.gov/. RP: retinitis pigmentosa.

Trans-splicing: Trans-splicing is a naturally occurring process that results in an alternative processing of the pre-mRNA and was first reported in plants and bacteria [119,120]. Unlike in cis-splicing, trans-splicing takes place between two independent RNA molecules [93,119,120]. In vertebrates, these trans-splicing events occur in some key physiological processes, for example, the regulation of gene expression [121–123]. In humans, trans-splicing has also been reported in some diseases such as cancer [120].

Therapeutic trans-splicing offers an intriguing strategy to remove mutations from the mRNA. Only the introduction of an exogenous RNA molecule can be sufficient to activate the trans-splicing process. This exogenous RNA, also called PTM (pre-mRNA trans-splicing molecule), is constituted by a binding domain that specifically targets the molecule towards a specific region within the endogenous pre-mRNA, an artificial intron sequence harbouring all the elements required for splicing and the sequence that needs to be replaced [93,119]. For a 5′ PTM, the partial coding sequence has to end at the 3′ end of an exon to allow for a 5′ splice site and vice versa for a 3′ splice site [124]. In the last years, trans-splicing has revealed promising results for the correction of mutations in *RHO* and *CEP290*. In the first example, Berger and collaborators were able to correct *RHO* mutations located in exons 2 through 5 by delivering the correct sequence of those exons in an AAV. This led to successful trans-splicing events, both in vivo and *in vitro* [119]. Dooley and colleagues delivered a part of the *CEP290* gene in an AAV and thereby could successfully replace the aforementioned c.2991+1655A>G mutation using the trans-splicing approach [124]. These data support the usefulness of trans-splicing as a therapeutic tool in IRDs.

2.2.2. Post-transcriptional Gene Silencing

iRNA and Ribozymes: Both Hammerhead ribozymes (hhRz) and (short) interference RNA ((s)iRNA) catalyse the sequence-specific cleavage of target mRNAs. iRNA molecules are double-stranded RNAs that are able to inhibit gene expression by binding to specific mRNAs (cellular or viral) [93,125]. Despite their affordability and speed, the effect of iRNA is often incomplete and temporary, with potential off-target effects [126]. In addition, variations between experiments and laboratories often occur. These variations limit the broad application of iRNA technology in many diseases including IRDs [46], although promising results have been obtained in age-related macular degeneration, a multifactorial subtype of retinal disease. Specifically, Ryoo and colleagues used a novel siRNA-based anti-VEGF nanoball that, upon intravitreal administration in mice, showed therapeutic effects for at least two weeks [127].

HhRzs are small RNA molecules causing enzymatic cleavage of polyribonucleotides [128]. The hhRz consists of three helixes surrounding an evolutionary conserved catalytic core. This gives rise to an antisense complementary region that provides the unimolecular RNA the capacity to recognize and subsequently enzymatically cleave its target mRNA [128].

Both types of molecules (iRNA and hhRz) have been successfully used to degrade an incorrect *RHO* transcript responsible for dominant retinitis pigmentosa, a common subtype of IRD [128]. Another alternative is employing microRNAs (miRNAs), which act at the post-transcriptional level to regulate gene expression in the retina. miRNAs generally bind to mRNA and cause a reduction of translated products. Some miRNAs are commonly expressed in all retinal cell types while others are specifically expressed in one or the other [5,129], suggesting that there are possibilities to employ these molecules therapeutically. However, more studies are needed before miRNAs can actually be used [130]. Overall, post-transcriptional gene silencing mediated by iRNA and ribozymes are believed to be a promising strategy for treating dominant-negative mutations.

RNAse H-dependent AONs: Besides redirecting splicing, AONs can also be used to specifically degrade transcripts, even in an allele-specific manner. Some oligonucleotide modifications combine AON segments with conformationally restricted residues that affect cleavage of their intended targets [131]. With this, catalytic activation of RNase H, a ubiquitous enzyme cleaving the RNA part of DNA/RNA hybrid duplexes, can be induced. The big advantage of these hybrid duplexes is that only a low amount of AON is sufficient to induce catalytic turnover. Furthermore, this catalytic turnover provides enough time for AONs to act as a potential drug due to their stability in blood serum, that is, a few days [132]. Murray and colleagues used rodent models genetically modified for *RHO* (p.P23H) to test RNAse H-activating AONs in vivo. They observed that the AON-mediated knockdown of mutant p.P23H rhodopsin expression reduced photoreceptor degradation, thereby preserving the function of photoreceptors in the transgenic rats [133]. Recently, AON-mediated transcript downregulation has also been assessed *in vitro* for a *NR2E3* variant underlying autosomal dominant RP [134], underscoring the usefulness of this approach for some (dominant) mutations.

Cas13: The editing system based on Cas13 can reduce off-target effect rates shown by other systems as explained previously [135]. RNA-guided RNA-targeting CRISPR-Cas effector Cas13 (previously named C2c2) can be engineered to bind and subsequently knockdown mammalian RNA [136]. Abudayyeh and colleagues verified that, for endogenous genes, the knockdown efficiency is transcript-dependent. Despite, the efficacy was comparable to that shown by iRNA, thus the substantially lower off-target ratio makes this approach well-suited for therapeutic applications [137].

2.2.3. RNA Editing (dCas13 and ADAR)

The ADAR (adenosine deaminase acting on RNA) family of proteins can mediate endogenous editing of transcripts via the deamination of adenosine to inosine, a nucleobase that is functionally equivalent to guanosine both in splicing and in translation [135]. Cox and colleagues designed a catalytically inactivated Cas13 (dCas13) that is able to retain its RNA-binding capacity, to direct an ADAR towards the RNA transcript of interest and to perform its adenosine-to-inosine deaminase function [135]. This demonstrated the flexibility of Cas13 to be adapted as a tool for nucleic acid modification. The system that was created is called REPAIRv2 and generates a higher specificity compared to other RNA-editing platforms reported so far [138,139] with high levels of on-target activity. Other advantages include—(i) Cas13 has no targeting sequence constraints and does not present any preferential motif surrounding the target adenosine, allowing any adenosine in the transcriptome to be potentially targeted; (ii) the REPAIRv2 system directly deaminates target adenosines to inosines and does not depend on endogenous repair pathways, thereby enabling RNA editing in post-mitotic cells like neurons and photoreceptors and, (iii) RNA editing, contrary to DNA editing, is transient and thus can be more readily reversed, allowing temporal control over editing events [135]. These features make RNA editing an interesting strategy to be used in future therapeutic studies in IRDs.

Table 2. List of clinical trials for IRDs using RNA therapies.

Gene	Therapeutic Molecule	Clinical Trial Identifier	Status
	QR-110	NCT03140969	Active, not recruiting
CEP290	QR-110	NCT03913130	Recruiting
	QR-110	NCT03913143	Recruiting
USH2A	QR-421a	NCT03780257	Recruiting

Black is just used to indicate the different sectiond and can be considered as headers. Gene (first column), therapeutic molecule (second column), clinical trial identifier (third column) and current status of the trial (last column) are indicated. Data obtained from https://clinicaltrials.gov/.

2.3. Compound Therapies

As happens in other types of diseases, pharmacological development can offer an entirely different approach to the treatment of IRD. However, the great heterogeneity observed in IRDs and the access-limiting BRB present major challenges towards an effective compound therapy [140]. In this section, we focus our attention on some promising drugs for the treatment of IRDs.

2.3.1. Translational Read-Through

Translational read-through (TR) therapy is based on small molecules, also known as TR-inducing drugs (TRIDs), that allow the translation machinery to bypass a premature termination codon (PTC) during translation [141]. In addition, PTCs can induce mRNA degradation through nonsense-mediated decay and thereby also inhibit full-length protein expression [141,142]. The incorporation of an amino acid at the site of the premature stop codon can increase the expression of the full-length protein as well as the reduction of nonsense-mediated decay [142]. Until now, the detailed mechanisms by which TRIDs induce their therapeutic effect are not completely understood. However, it is known that TR efficiency depends on the competition between decoding of the stop codon by a near-cognate tRNA and stop codon recognition by eRF1 [141]. There are two main classes of TRIDs—aminoglycoside and non-aminoglycoside TRIDs. From the first group, gentamicin has been most widely used to analyse TR in different disease models, including those affected with IRD. The efficacy of gentamicin was studied in different rat and mouse models—(i) the S334ter rat model that carries a nonsense mutation (c.1002T>A; p.S334*) in the gene encoding the visual pigment rhodopsin (*Rho*) and (ii) the *rd12* mouse, a model for retinal degeneration caused by a nonsense mutation in *Rpe65*. Systematic gentamicin treatment showed different results between the two models. In S334ter rats, a partial rescue of photoreceptor survival was noticed however, no rescue was observed in *rd12* mice [143]. Studies on genes mutated in Usher syndrome (a syndromic form of IRD accompanied by hearing impairment) demonstrated that aminoglycosides and derivatives thereof can mediate TR of different disease-causing PTCs in the *PCDH15* and *USH1C* genes, in *in vitro* translation assays as well as in cell culture experiments [144–149].

The non-aminoglycoside TRID PTC124 (also known as Ataluren) is used in a wide range of diseases including Duchenne muscular dystrophy and cystic fibrosis [150–153], with several clinical studies having been performed or ongoing. For IRDs, promising results using PTC124 have been reported by the restoration of full-length RP2 protein, the encoding gene of which is mutated in X-linked RP, as well as for the REP1 protein, encoded by the *CHM* gene that is mutated in choroideremia. In X-linked RP, rod photoreceptors mainly suffer from the loss of RP2, although the effect on cone photoreceptors and RPE cells should not be neglected. Schwarz and colleagues used TRIDs (both the aminoglycoside G418 as well as PTC124) to successfully increase full-length RP2 protein levels in the presence of the p.R120ter (c.358C>T; p.R120 *) mutation. In choroideremia, many nonsense mutations in *CHM* have been described. Several studies attempted to use TRIDs, including PTC124 or its analogue PTC-414, to increase REP1 protein levels, either in cellular (human fibroblasts, iPSC-derived RPE) or animal (zebrafish) models [154–156]. The efficacy of read-through was found to be considerably variable, not only depending on the type of nonsense codon and its surrounding sequence but also on the remaining transcript levels that can differ significantly between patients [142]. Another study, based on topical administration of PTC124 to the eye, demonstrated functional restoration of the harmonin protein in a mouse model for Usher syndrome type 1c (USH1C) [141,145].

One of the disadvantages of the systemic use of TRIDs is that for many diseases, drugs need to go through physical barriers (such as the blood-brain barrier or BRB). These barriers can reduce compound availability in the targeted organ after treatment, illustrating the need to increment the dosage administered to the patients or to change the delivery method of TRIDs (commonly intraperitoneal) towards local administration [141]. One strategy to overcome this is the encapsulation of drugs into tissue-specific liposomes [157]. In particular for IRDs, topical applications or intraocular injections should be considered in the future.

2.3.2. Restoring Proteostasis (Protein Therapies)

Photoreceptor cells require a rigorous regulation of proteostasis (maintaining a healthy protein balance) to ensure their correct function and viability. As a result, certain genetic changes in specific genes with an essential function in the photoreceptor cell can have dramatic effects. One example is the dominant-negative effect of mutations in *RHO*, which leads to the disruption of outer segments in the photoreceptor cell [158]. The manipulation of proteostasis mechanisms such as the heat-shock response (HSR) or unfolded protein response could be a good therapeutic target in order to alleviate misfolding diseases (e.g., targeted up-regulation of these pathways to reduce aggregation of proteins such as rhodopsin) [159]. This could be achieved either by the administration of drugs that restore proteostasis (e.g., pharmacological chaperones, kosmotropes, molecular chaperones or autophagy inducers) or by targeting key molecules in the photoreceptor proteostasis network [160,161].

So far, "proteostasis" therapies are mainly focused on rhodopsin, as *RHO* is one of the most frequently mutated genes in autosomal dominant RP. One of the most common mutations in this gene is the p.P23H mutation, which acts in a dominant-negative fashion on wild-type rhodopsin by inducing misfolding [160]. Intriguingly, it was reported that misfolded proteins could be rescued by a ligand that works as a chaperone [161].

Pharmacological chaperones are small, substrate-specific molecules that are able to directly target the protein structure and shift the protein folding equilibrium towards its native state [158,162]. Studies using this kind of chaperones suggested that correction of mutant rhodopsin folding, without improving its stability, could further compromise the outer segments and increase rod cell death. Thus, these data underscore the necessity to ensure opsin stability using parallel treatment strategies [163,164].

Kosmotropes are small, low molecular weight compounds that can enhance the stability of proteins in their native conformation and decrease aggregation. Kosmotropes bind to proteins non-specifically and thus have the potential to be used in a wide range of protein-misfolding diseases [161]. The chemical chaperone tauroursodeoxycholic acid (TUDCA) has been studied in several retinal degeneration models [165–167], although its efficacy was found to vary between different studies, even in the presence of the same IRD-causing mutation, namely p.P23H, in the gene encoding rhodopsin. It has been hypothesized that activation of PERK, one of the receptors responsible for UPR [168] differs between models, thereby explaining the ineffectiveness of TUDCA in some of them [161,165].

Finally, another alternative to restore proteostasis is through the control of the adaptive machinery that is responsible for its maintenance via HSR and UPR [158]. Inhibition of molecular chaperones can activate the HSR by releasing HSF1 and inducing cell stress, which triggers the production of molecular chaperones. The Hsp90 inhibitors and HSR inducers geldanamycin, radicicol and 17-AAG reduced P23H aggregation and cell death *in vitro* [162]. Hsp90 works as a crucial chaperone in the maturation of many proteins. Targeting Hsp90 directly however could affect normal vision, suggesting that an alternative therapeutic approach could include the stimulation of both the HSR and UPR pathways with arimoclomol (a heat shock protein inducer). In rat models carrying the p.P23H rhodopsin mutation, it has been demonstrated that administering arimoclonol via intraperitoneal injection reduced mutant rhodopsin aggregation and ameliorated photoreceptor degeneration [160,161].

2.3.3. Pathway-Specific Therapies

Cyclic guanosine-monophosphate (cGMP) is a crucial molecule for photoreceptor signal transduction and has two main cellular effectors—cyclic nucleotide gated ion channels (CNGCs) and cGMP-dependent protein kinase G (PKG) [169]. It has been reported that over-activation of PKG can be enough to cause photoreceptor cell death and that its activation levels are higher in mutant photoreceptors. Knowing that CNGCs play an important role in driving phototransduction, some interesting observations have been made. The deletion of CNGC beta subunits protects photoreceptors in *rd1* mice that harbour a defect in the *Pde6b* gene, which encodes the phosphodiesterase protein involved in the phototransduction cascade. Therefore, either PKG or CNGCs can be considered as critical disease drivers; consequently, both of them are therapeutic targets for prevention of (further) retinal degeneration [140]. As mentioned above, the BRB can prevent the access of therapeutic agents to the retina. Vighi and colleagues overcame this problem using a liposomal drug delivery method, the liposomal cGMP analogue formulation LP-CN03, and demonstrated improved visual function as well as reduced photoreceptor degeneration in mouse models harbouring mutations in different IRD gene orthologues [140]. Together, these data suggest that cGMP signalling could be a common pathway to target for the treatment of genetically and phenotypically divergent kinds of retinal degeneration [140,169].

Another drug previously tested in clinical trials is an orally delivered synthetic cis-retinoid also known as QLT091001. This drug triggered visual restoration in transgenic and naturally occurring mouse and dog models mutant for *Rpe65* [170]. The results of the clinical trial NCT01014052 (Table 3) showed that QLT091001 did improve visual function in subjects with IRD due to *LRAT* or *RPE65* mutations. Mutations in these genes can cause different subtypes of IRD, usually classified as LCA or RP. Despite this, the exact genetic defect apparently did not affect the drug response in both LCA and RP patients [171]. Upon oral administration of QLT091001, patients showed beneficial effects in the remaining photoreceptors of the retina in both eyes, although it did not stop the progression of photoreceptor degradation completely. The safety profile of this drug showed transient adverse effects such as headaches or nausea [171]. In theory, QLT091001 could be combined with gene augmentation therapy, although the combination of treatments, in particular for orphan diseases, poses additional challenges on drug development.

Table 3. Summary of clinical trials for IRDs using compound therapies.

Gene	Therapeutic Molecule	Clinical Trial Identifier	Status
ABCA4	ALK-001	NCT02402660	Recruiting
	Zimura	NCT03364153	Active, not recruiting
	Emuxustat	NCT03772665	Recruiting
	Emuxustat	NCT03033108	**Completed**
RPE65	QLT091001	NCT01014052	**Completed**
	QLT091001	NCT01521793	**Completed**
	QLT091001	NCT01543906 *	**Completed**
RS1	Dorzolamide 2% TID or brinzolamide 1% TID	NCT02331173	**Completed**

Black is just used to indicate the different sectional and can be considered as headers. Gene (first column), therapeutic molecule (second column), clinical trial identifier (third column) and current status of the trial (last column) are indicated. Completed trials are highlighted in bold. Data obtained from https://clinicaltrials.gov/. * Of note, Trial NCT01543906 describes the use of QLT091001 in patients with a dominant *RPE65* mutation (unlike most *RPE65* mutations inherited in an autosomal recessive manner).

3. Delivery of Therapeutic Molecules

3.1. Methods of Ocular Delivery

Despite its small size, the eye contains several cell and tissue types that can be targeted by therapeutic agents [172]. Local tolerability of vector administration in IRDs has been reported in various studies and no serious systemic problems have been indicated so far [23]. Commonly, we can identify two main potential delivery methods—subretinal and intravitreal injections. Subretinal injections are considered to be more prone towards complications (e.g., retinal detachment), especially in patients with affected retinal integrity, compared to intravitreal injection. Despite, the vector is delivered much closer to its target cells/region, allowing an efficient vector transduction in RPE cells and/or photoreceptors [173]. In contrast, intravitreal injections allow an easier targeting of the optic nerve, lens or inner retina and less often the outer retina or the anterior chamber. It also shows fewer procedure-related complications but the transduction of the viral vector into photoreceptors and RPE cells is less efficient when compared with subretinal injections [23,174]. Apart from these two methods, there is an alternative system—Suprachoroidal delivery. With this, therapeutic agents are delivered directly to the suprachoroidal space located between the sclera and choroid [175,176]. Preclinical animal studies showed that suprachoroidal drug delivery has the same safety profile as intravitreal injections [177–179]. Results from completed clinical trials (e.g., NCT01789320) have also showed encouraging safety profiles [180], although potential spreading of therapeutic vectors into the systemic circulation needs to be considered.

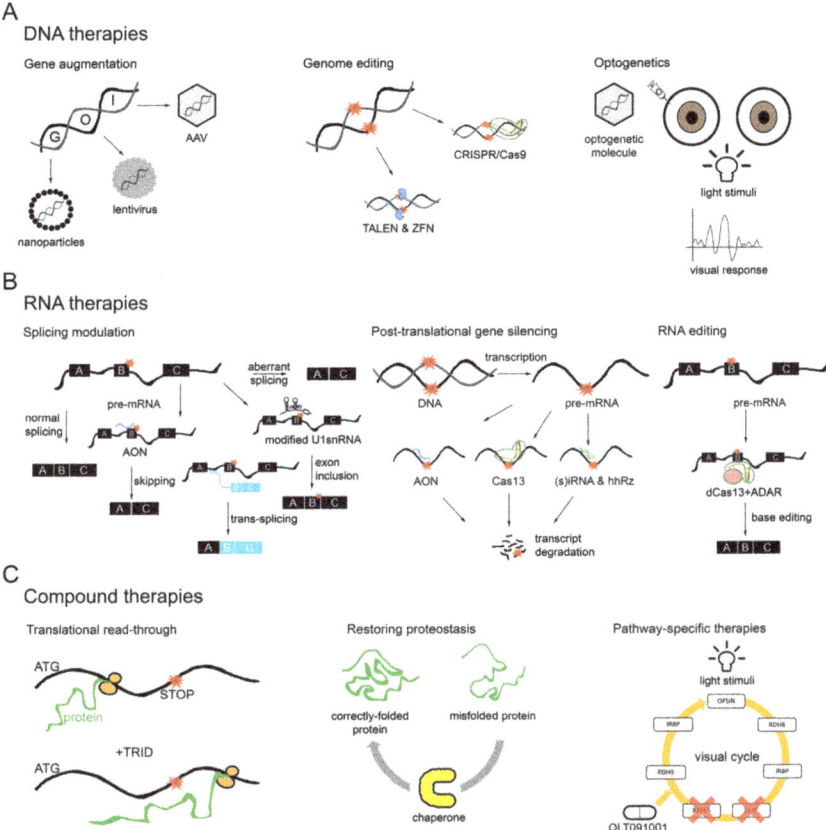

Figure 2. Schematic and simplified representation of the several types of molecular therapies. (**A**) DNA therapies are represented by gene augmentation, genome editing and optogenetics. In gene augmentation, the entire coding sequence of the gene of interest (GOI) is delivered using different vectors. Genome editing employs nucleases able to edit the DNA at a specific position; CRISPR/Cas9 is depicted in green, guide RNA in dark yellow and ZFN and TALEN in blue. Mutations are depicted in red. In optogenetics, a light-sensitive molecule is delivered to the eye to give photosensitive properties to remaining retinal neurons. (**B**) RNA therapies; splicing modulation can be achieved using AONs (in dark blue) for (pseudo)exon skipping or modified U1 snRNA (in black) to favour exon inclusion in cases where mutations (in red) are found in the donor splice site. Trans-splicing occurs between two independent RNA molecules—The original transcript and the exogenous molecule without the mutation. In all cases, splicing is modulated to obtain a transcript with full or residual function. Post-translational gene silencing can be achieved by degrading the RNA transcript using AONs (dark blue), Cas13 (green) with a guide RNA (dark yellow) or (s)iRNA and hhRz (in green). These approaches can be used for dominant-negative mutations by promoting allele-specific degradation. Mutations are indicated in red. With RNA editing using CRISPR/Cas technology, dead Cas13 (in green) is conjugated with an adenosine deaminase (dark yellow) acting at the RNA level (ADAR, in light red). This molecule is guided to the mutation using a guide RNA binding on top of the mutation (in red) to induce a G-to-A transversion. (**C**) Representative examples of compound therapies. Translational read-through allows the ribosome to continue protein synthesis despite a premature stop codon (in red) in the presence of the translational read-through-inducing drugs (TRIDs). Restoring proteostasis can be accomplished by using chaperones to properly fold proteins. QLT091001 is a pathway-specific therapy that acts in the visual cycle and can be used when for example, *RPE65* or *LRAT* are mutated.

Finally, there is the possibility of topical delivery by the use of eye drops. However, this approach can result in lower bioavailability and increased clearance in comparison to the different types of injections. In addition, ocular barriers decrease the bioavailability of topically applied therapeutic agents to less than 5% [181]. Therefore, the effectiveness of this method is less than those reported with the systems previously described.

3.2. Vectors

Besides the routes of administration, a wide range of viral and non-viral gene delivery approaches has been developed over the last twenty years, in order to allow an efficient transfer of therapeutic molecules to the right target cell. Choosing one over another depends on the cell or tissue type to be targeted, the cloning capacity of each of the vectors and safety concerns [23].

3.2.1. Viral Vectors

Adeno-associated viruses (AAVs): Most commonly but not exclusively, therapeutic genes are delivered to their target cells by viral vectors. AAVs are the most common viral vectors used for gene therapy in IRDs, mainly due to their low immunogenicity and toxicity, and allow for long-term transgene expression [182,183].

Recombinant AAV (rAAV) is the most popular viral vector for delivery in IRDs. Its tropism for different types of retinal cells allows efficient transduction of these cells and relatively fast and stable transgene expression [184]. rAAV is available in two forms, single-stranded AAV (ssAAV) and self-complimentary AAV (scAAV). Once a cell is transduced with ssAAV, the single-stranded DNA of the virus needs to be converted into the double-stranded form; this is a rate-limiting step that can be circumvented with scAAVs [25]. The scAAVs are engineered in a way that upon infection two complementary halves will generate a double-stranded DNA, promoting faster and increased transgene expression [185]. However, the main disadvantage of scAAVs is their reduced cargo capacity (2.4 kb), compared to ssAAV (4.8 kb) which limits its transgene selection. scAAV vectors have been demonstrated to transduce retinal ganglion cells, photoreceptors and RPE cells, and can lead to transgene expression within two days after injection in mice while ssAAV requires several weeks [186]; this rapid and increased transgene expression was independent of the AAV serotype tested (i.e. -1, -2 or -5) [25].

Despite its numerous advantages, AAV presents a limited packaging capacity (4.8 kb) [22,25,45]. To overcome this, various strategies have been developed. For instance, with the use of dual AAV vectors, a cDNA can be split in two separate fragments, after which the two parts recombine inside the cells using HDR, trans-splicing or both [41,187]. With this, the capacity can be increased up to 9 kb [41,43,187]. The dual AAV system has been used in preclinical studies to deliver some genes mutated in IRD such as *ABCA4* [188] and *MYO7A* [189], with promising results. However, dual AAVs may still not be sufficient for several other genes mutated in IRD. The use of triple AAV approaches allows to increase the cargo capacity to 14 kb [43,189,190], enabling the development of gene therapies for IRDs caused by mutations in even larger genes. Maddalena and colleagues demonstrated the potential of this system to restore *CDH23* (cDNA size 11.1 kB, mutated in Usher syndrome type 1D) and *ALMS1* (cDNA size 12.9 kb, mutated in Almstrom syndrome) gene expression. Certainly, the enclosed and small subretinal space may facilitate co-infection of the same cell by three independent AAV vectors [43].

To date, up to 12 AAV serotypes and more than 100 variants have been identified in humans and NHPs [25]. From these, AAV2, AAV5 and AAV8 have been most extensively studied, being used as delivery vector in several clinical and preclinical studies for different genes such as *RPE65, CNGB3, RS1* or *PDE6B* (Table 1) [25]. AAV serotypes 2, 5, 7, 8 and 9 are able to transduce photoreceptors, while virtually every AAV serotype is capable of efficiently infecting RPE cells [23]. So far, AAV2 is the only vector described to transduce retinal ganglion cells upon intravitreal delivery [191,192]. However, alternative serotypes of AAV have also been developed. Some examples are the serotypes AAV7m8 [193] and AAV8BP2 [194]. Both of them were designed to alter AAV capsids aiming to improve uptake into the retina and be able to target photoreceptors following intravitreal injection [193,194]. AAV7m8 serotype was generated by in vivo directed evolution in the mouse retina by Dalkara and collaborators [193,195]. They reported that the intravitreal delivery of AAV7m8 resulted in effective pan-retinal photoreceptor and RPE cell transduction in mice. This serotype was also tested in NHP retinas via intravitreal administration. The results indicated a higher transduction rate of foveal and extrafoveal photoreceptors in comparison with the parental serotype AAV2. However, authors also noted toxicity in an NHP injected with a high titre of AAV7m8 [193]. Therefore, a study of safety and efficiency of transduction using lower doses of this serotype is required if this capsid is planned to be used in primates, including humans. The AAV8BP2 serotype was generated in vivo by Cronin and colleagues, it targets ON-bipolar cells and cone photoreceptors efficiently following both intravitreal and subretinal injections in mouse [194]. This research group performed a comparative study between these two novel serotypes. Both vectors showed promising results in mice but in NHPs, either subretinal or intravitreal delivery did not allow to transduce all target cells within the retina. Specifically, AAV7m8 showed some toxicity effects (as previously reported) as well as severe inflammation when using a high titre [195]. For AAV8BP2, a lower transduction of bipolar cells was observed, even at high doses. Taken together, the results of both serotypes indicate that studies in rodents might not provide sufficient information to understand the cellular transduction and pharmacological properties of these engineered AAVs and further studies in for example NHPs are needed before using them in humans. Carvalho and collaborators characterized an *in silico* designed serotype named Anc80 for retinal gene transfer [196]. Three Anc80 variants were evaluated, Anc80L27, Anc80L65 and Anc80L12, in mice and NHP. All of them were capable of efficiently targeting retinal cells following subretinal delivery, although Anc80L65 showed a higher efficiency for targeting retinal cells as well as higher expression levels compared to AAV8. These data support the use of Anc80L65 for gene delivery to the retina. Taken together, all these studies characterizing novel serotypes have illustrated the impact of minimal changes in capsid composition on aspects relevant to experimental and clinical gene transfer applications. This will prove useful for improving delivery to the retina and thus for their use in developing new treatments for IRDs.

Lentiviral vectors: Lentiviruses (LV) are RNA viruses of the retrovirus family. In IRDs, the retroviral variant of human immunodeficiency virus type 1 (HIV-1) or the equine infectious anaemia virus (EIAV) have been tested. LVs have the ability to pass through the cells' intact nuclear membrane and infect both dividing and non-dividing cells [197]. Moreover, LVs efficiently integrate their genome into that of the host-cell, leading to stable expression. LVs are modified to stop replication, so these vectors are not pathogenic after initial gene delivery. LVs present a transgene capacity cargo of ~8–10 kb and, in terms of IRD, are capable of infecting RPE cells and to a lesser extent of differentiated photoreceptors [23,25]. EIAVs have been used for *ABCA4*, as its cDNA size (6.8 kb) outpaced the cargo capacity of AAV but not that of lentiviruses [198]. To assess this strategy in human subjects, a clinical trial (NCT01367444) has been ongoing for several years (Table 1), whilst no clear efficacy data have been reported.

Adenoviruses and helper-dependent adenoviruses: In comparison to the previously mentioned viral vectors, adenoviruses (AdVs) have a cargo capacity of about 8 kb, while its 'gutted' helper-dependent adenovirus (HDAd) has an extremely large capacity of up to 36 kb. It is demonstrated that adenoviral vectors infect RPE cells efficiently but because the coxsackie-AdV receptor is presumed to be absent on the cell membrane of photoreceptors [199,200], these vectors do not efficiently transduce photoreceptor cells [201]. Overall, AdVs have been only sparsely used in the treatment of IRDs [202,203].

3.2.2. Non-Viral Vectors

Although various viral vectors have demonstrated their potential in the treatment of IRDs, there is a continuing need for refinement delivery vectors for the eye. Therefore, research efforts have also been directed towards the development of non-viral delivery systems, such as nanoparticles (NPs), naked DNA or liposomes [174].

Naked DNA is the most elementary form of non-viral gene therapy [204]. As naked DNA does typically not enter into the cells, it is not considered as a suitable therapy for the eye. Different studies have used electroporation or iontophoresis to obtain a significant uptake and expression in the target cells, however both delivery ways presented significant challenges. The side effects of electroporation make it an unlikely method to be clinically feasible, whilst iontophoresis so far presents conflicting information about the real effectiveness of this method [174,204].

In contrast, NPs are well capable of delivering plasmid DNA containing a functional copy of a gene into the retina [205]. The three determinants of the effectiveness of gene delivery using this kind of vectors are cellular uptake, endosomal escape and transfer of the plasmid DNA into the nucleus. All forms of NPs-(metal, lipid or polymers) have some capability to pass through the cell membrane, avoid endosomal trapping and deliver the plasmid DNA into the nucleus. Lipid-based NPs are biocompatible and stable particles; furthermore, there is no inflammatory response to these NPs when injected into the eye. However, there are also some disadvantages, such as lower gene expression when compared to the same transgenes delivered by viral vectors [174]. A new type of delivery system was recently developed by Trigueros and colleagues using gold nanoparticles (DNA-gold NPs), as these are relatively easy to generate and can be adapted to different shapes and sizes [206]. Gold is well-tolerated inside an organism and presents low rates of toxicity. However, they present a low clearance rate, thereby hampering their uptake in specific cells or tissues [207]. Therefore, Trigueros et al. further optimized this system for IRDs. In this study, they compared this new system with DNA-liposome complexes and demonstrated higher expression of a reporter gene. Their results showed that RPE cells responded differently to pristine-gold NPs and DNA-gold NPs, probably because of changes in the membrane-NP interface. Moreover, both types of NPs used different alternative endocytic ways for internalization, as indicated by their detection in different endosomal compartments. DNA-gold NPs were located in early endosomes that later will not mature into late endosome vesicles, resulting in an earlier expression of the reporter gene compared to pristine-gold NPs. This study was the first step to use non-cytotoxic gold NPs for an in vivo gene therapy to treat IRDs. However, some biological questions are still unclear, such as the internalization routes that are used and the exact nature of intracellular endosome trafficking. Furthermore, before using these particles as a delivery method in the retina, it is necessary to understand the complexity of cell–NP interaction, enhance the cargo delivery by avoiding degradative pathways (such as the lysosomal pathway) and ensure a constant expression of the therapeutic gene [206].

Finally, cationic lipids (liposomes) offer an alternative way to deliver DNA into the eye. In addition to the two most common ways of retinal delivery (see above), other delivery methods such as topical or intravenous administration have already reported positive results in eye diseases [174]. Liposomes however also present some limitations such as retinal toxicity and aggregation following administration [208]. Consequently, researchers developed a new type of liposome-PEGylated with perfluoropropane gas-that appears to be safer and more efficient for transfection but, as happened with other lipid-based vectors, presented a drop in gene expression four days after administration [174].

4. Other IRD Treatments

While gene-based therapies may stop or at least delay, the progression of the disease, other promising approaches that are less dependent of the genetic cause of the disease are also gaining momentum. This is for instance the case for stem cell-derived retinal cell transplantation (cell therapy) or the use of prosthetic implants.

4.1. Cell Therapy

Retinal cells, like other cells within the central nervous system, present a low regeneration potential. Therefore, cell therapies could be applied in those IRDs that present an advanced degeneration stage. The use of this type of therapy aims to result in an integration of exogenously delivered cells and subsequent re-activation of visual function [45]. Patient-derived somatic cells could be used to reprogram induced pluripotent stem cells (iPSCs) that subsequently could be differentiated to retinal precursor cells and introduced into the eye to replace either photoreceptors or supporting cells (e.g., RPE) that provide trophic and metabolic maintenance to prevent further degeneration of the remaining photoreceptors [209]. Genome editing tools (such as those described in Section 2.1.2) can be used to repair patient-specific mutations, to eventually transplant the corrected cells back to the patient [210]. The use of embryonic stem cells (ESCs) would not require this genetic modification and it has been demonstrated that these cells also have a high capacity to differentiate into retinal precursors [45,211]. However, the use of ESC is associated with ethical considerations not present with the use of iPSCs generated from the patients. Moreover, the transplantation of iPSC-derived retinal cells would avoid the risk of immune rejection after surgery [45].

Following up on the promising advances that demonstrated that stem cell-derived photoreceptor transplantation can restore rod- and cone-mediated vision [211–214], recent studies showed that these transplanted cells are not able to integrate well into non-degenerative host retinas. Instead, it seems that post-mitotic donor and host photoreceptors can exchange RNA and proteins, including rhodopsin [215,216]. The visual improvements measured after stem cell-derived photoreceptor transplantation could thus also be the result of endogenous photoreceptors that have taken up donor cell-derived proteins. Recently, it was demonstrated that cell integration as well as cytoplasmic transfer can occur but the relative contributions of each depend on the environment within the host retina [45,216].

Some cell therapies that are already tested in the clinic use hESC or hiPSC-derived RPE, for treating diseases such as AMD or Stardgardt disease [217–220]. For the study employing iPSC-derived RPE transplantation, a one-year follow-up analysis indicated that the transplantation did not generate any adverse effect and no immune response was induced, even in the absence of immunosuppression. One of the studies using hESC-derived RPE also reported an improvement of vision in patients with age-related macular degeneration as well as those with Stargardt disease [218]. Nevertheless, more studies are needed to provide reproducible protocols to generate iPSC-derived photoreceptor precursor cells. In addition, if such cells are transplanted after gene mutation repair, stringent quality controls of the iPSCs before and after genome editing are extremely important [45].

4.2. Retinal Prosthetic Implants

Inner retinal neurons largely retain their capability of signal transmission and are still present in advanced stages of retinal degradation. This fact encouraged the use of a stimulation mechanism (prosthetic implants) that is able to restore vision to some extent. Such a device would bypass the degraded photoreceptor layer and directly interact with the still functioning inner retinal neurons [84]. Retinal prostheses work as an integral system that contain an image acquisition device (which is integrated by thousands of light-sensitive microphotodies), an image processor, a stimulator chip and an electrode array [84,221]. In this system, light emanating from visible objects is converted by the microphotodies into little currents of hundreds of microelectrodes, which are directed onto remaining neurons within the neuronal network, the middle and the inner retina [221]. These systems have demonstrated a partial visual restoration, presenting the first evidence of this strategy in the field of vision [222]. To date, several stimulation modalities have been built [84] and four of them have obtained market approval for use in Europe and/or United States (Argus II, IRIS, IMS and AMS) [222]. These devices are classified according to their anatomical placement.

Epiretinal prostheses (Argus II, IRIS and EPI-IRET3) are implanted on the surface of the neurosensory retina, adjacent to nerve fibre and ganglion cell layers. Its location ensures certain advantages such as easy surgical delivery and safe heat dispersion [84,222]. Functionally, the stimulation is directly applied to the retinal ganglion cells, bypassing the residual intraretinal processing system, thereby inhibiting the capacity to mimic the physiological topographic organization. Besides this, as the epiretinal prostheses are close to passing axonal nerve fibres, ectopic visual perceptions from axonal stimulation can occur, thereby decreasing spatial resolution and confusing the intended stimulation pattern. As a note, the epiretinal prostheses have an external camera positioned outside the eye that provides power induction and a data signal that is transmitted to the intraocular simulator [84,221,222]. From these prostheses, Argus II is the most widely-used and it has been implanted in more than 250 patients to date, reporting encouraging results [223].

Subretinal prostheses (ASR, IMS/AMS, PRIMA and BSI) are placed between the degenerated photoreceptor layer and the RPE, such that the intrinsic signal processing capability of the retinal interneurons can be used optimally, generating vision similar to the one that is physiologically generated in the eye [84,222]. Moreover, the device is placed closer to the retina and is therefore favoured over the natural retinal signal amplification, requiring lower stimulation intensities. Unless the system has intrinsic photosensitivity and amplification capacity, it, like the epiretinal devices, requires a power source and a connection serving the delivery of data. Surgically, some studies have indicated that positioning these devices could be technically complicated because of the RPE adhesion caused by the retinal degeneration. Moreover, this surgical approach is less known and practiced outside routine retinal surgery [222]. To date, there are two methods to subretinal stimulation—one that employs a standard electrode array and another that uses a microphotodiode array (MPDA) that is present in all devices with exception of BSI (Boston retinal implant). This last one itself is able to capture light, allowing to avoid the use of cameras, while the visual scene is perceived by the lens on the array [84].

Suprachoroidal prostheses (STS and BVA) are located in the suprachoroidal space. This space is highly vascular and therefore there is a high risk of haemorrhage and fibrosis post-implantation. In comparison with the other two counterparts mentioned above, suprachoroidal devices are relatively far away from the retina. This implies that the design requires greater stimulation power to elicit visual perception [84,222]. Larger numbers are needed to establish solid conclusions about the efficacy of both suprachoroidal and transscleral implants in their present formats; however, results to date suggest greater limitations to these approaches compared to epiretinal or subretinal implants [84].

5. Concluding Remarks

The approval of Luxturna^{TM} as the first approved gene augmentation therapy for an ocular disease has provided an enormous impulse to the development of retinal therapeutics, both in academic centres as well as in industry. As summarized in this review, current developments range from gene augmentation, splice modulation, genome editing, optogenetics and compound therapies to cell replacement strategies and retinal prostheses. Patients with progressive vision loss are in need of treatment, to improve their quality of life by (partially) restoring vision or at least slow down or halt the progression of their diseases. Which strategy has the highest chance of being safe and efficacious depends on many factors, including the person's genetic defect(s) and the stage of disease accompanied by the appearance of the retina. However, therapeutic development also requires appropriate cellular and/or animal models to test the efficacy of a given approach, as well as clinical endpoints to determine whether an improvement of therapeutic intervention can be measured. Only when fundamental and translational scientists, clinicians, funding agencies, patient organizations, industry and regulatory bodies join forces, we can fight these devastating conditions and provide hope and vision, for thousands of visually impaired individuals worldwide.

Author Contributions: I.V.D., A.G. and R.W.J.C. collected data, wrote the manuscript, and performed careful proofreading. All authors approve the final content of the manuscript.

Funding: I.V.D.: A.G. and R.W.J.C. research is supported by Foundation Fighting Blindness USA, grant no. PPA-0517-0717-RAD. In addition, A.G. and R.W.J.C. research is supported by the Algemene Nederlandse Vereniging ter Voorkoming van Blindheid, Stichting Blinden-Penning, Landelijke Stichting voor Blinden en Slechtzienden, Stichting Oogfonds Nederland, Stichting Macula Degeneratie Fonds and Stichting Retina Nederland Fonds (who contributed through UitZicht 2015-31 and 2018-21), together with the Rotterdamse Stichting Blindenbelangen, Stichting Blindenhulp, Stichting tot Verbetering van het Lot der Blinden, Stichting voor Ooglijders and Stichting Dowilvo. A.G. was also supported by an Off Road grant (91215203) from ZonMw. The funding organizations had no role in the design or conduct of this research. They provided unrestricted grants.

Conflicts of Interest: I.V.D. declares no conflict of interest. A.G. and R.W.J.C. are inventors of several patents related to work cited in this review based on splicing modulation for *ABCA4* (P6063546EP, 18184432.5-111, 18210107.1-1111) and R.W.J.C also for splicing modulation of *CEP290* (P6037013PCT).

References

1. Sohocki, M.M.; Daiger, S.P.; Bowne, S.J.; Rodriquez, J.A.; Northrup, H.; Heckenlively, J.R.; Saperstein, D.A. Prevalence of mutations causing retinitis pigmentosa and other inherited retinopathies. *Hum. Mutat.* **2001**, *17*, 42–51. [CrossRef]
2. Khan, M.; Fadaie, Z.; Cornelis, S.S.; Cremers, F.P.; Roosing, S. Identification and Analysis of Genes Associated with Inherited Retinal Diseases. *Methods Mol. Biol.* **2019**, *1834*, 3–27. [PubMed]
3. Kaur, C.; Foulds, W.; Ling, E. Blood–retinal barrier in hypoxic ischaemic conditions: Basic concepts, clinical features and management. *Prog. Retin. Eye Res.* **2008**, *27*, 622–647. [CrossRef] [PubMed]
4. Anand, V.; Duffy, B.; Yang, Z.; Dejneka, N.S.; Maguire, A.M.; Bennett, J. A Deviant Immune Response to Viral Proteins and Transgene Product Is Generated on Subretinal Administration of Adenovirus and Adeno-associated Virus. *Mol. Ther.* **2002**, *5*, 125–132. [CrossRef] [PubMed]
5. Bennett, J. Immune response following intraocular delivery of recombinant viral vectors. *Gene Ther.* **2003**, *10*, 977–982. [CrossRef] [PubMed]
6. Öner, A. Recent Advancements in Gene Therapy for Hereditary Retinal Dystrophies. *Turk. J. Ophthalmol.* **2017**, *47*, 338–343. [CrossRef] [PubMed]
7. Gupta, P.R.; Huckfeldt, R.M. Gene therapy for inherited retinal degenerations: Initial successes and future challenges. *J. Neural Eng.* **2017**, *14*, 051002. [CrossRef]
8. Liang, F.Q.; Anand, V.; Maguire, A.M.; Bennett, J. Intraocular delivery of recombinant virus. *Methods Mol. Med.* **2001**, *47*, 125–139.
9. Ong, T.; Pennesi, M.E.; Birch, D.G.; Lam, B.L.; Tsang, S.H. Adeno-Associated Viral Gene Therapy for Inherited Retinal Disease. *Pharm. Res.* **2019**, *36*, 34. [CrossRef]
10. Sahel, J.-A.; Marazova, K.; Audo, I. Clinical Characteristics and Current Therapies for Inherited Retinal Degenerations. *Cold Spring Harb. Perspect. Med.* **2014**, *5*, a017111. [CrossRef]
11. Robson, A.G. Pattern ERG Correlates of Abnormal Fundus Autofluorescence in Patients with Retinitis Pigmentosa and Normal Visual Acuity. *Investig. Opthalmology Vis. Sci.* **2003**, *44*, 3544–3550. [CrossRef] [PubMed]
12. Koizumi, H.; Spaide, R.F.; Fisher, Y.L.; Freund, K.B.; Klancnik, J.M.; Yannuzzi, L.A. Three-Dimensional Evaluation of Vitreomacular Traction and Epiretinal Membrane Using Spectral-Domain Optical Coherence Tomography. *Am. J. Ophthalmol.* **2008**, *145*, 509–517. [CrossRef] [PubMed]
13. Hagiwara, A.; Yamamoto, S.; Ogata, K.; Sugawara, T.; Hiramatsu, A.; Shibata, M.; Mitamura, Y. Macular abnormalities in patients with retinitis pigmentosa: Prevalence on OCT examination and outcomes of vitreoretinal surgery. *Acta Ophthalmol.* **2011**, *89*, e122–e125. [CrossRef] [PubMed]
14. Lewin, A.S.; Rossmiller, B.; Mao, H. Gene Augmentation for adRP Mutations in RHO. *Cold Spring Harb. Perspect. Med.* **2014**, *4*, a017400. [CrossRef] [PubMed]
15. Salsman, J.; Dellaire, G. Precision genome editing in the CRISPR era. *Biochem. Cell Boil.* **2017**, *95*, 187–201. [CrossRef] [PubMed]
16. Kaczmarek, J.C.; Kowalski, P.S.; Anderson, D.G. Advances in the delivery of RNA therapeutics: From concept to clinical reality. *Genome Med.* **2017**, *9*, 60. [CrossRef] [PubMed]
17. Mead, B.; Berry, M.; Logan, A.; Scott, R.A.; Leadbeater, W.; Scheven, B.A. Stem cell treatment of degenerative eye disease. *Stem Cell Res.* **2015**, *14*, 243–257. [CrossRef] [PubMed]
18. Weiland, J.D.; Humayun, M.S. Retinal prosthesis. *IEEE Trans. Biomed. Eng.* **2014**, *61*, 1412–1424. [CrossRef] [PubMed]
19. Berger, W.; Kloeckener-Gruissem, B.; Neidhardt, J. The molecular basis of human retinal and vitreoretinal diseases. *Prog. Retin. Eye Res.* **2010**, *29*, 335–375. [CrossRef]
20. Smith, J.; Ward, D.; Michaelides, M.; Moore, A.T.; Simpson, S. New and emerging technologies for the treatment of inherited retinal diseases: A horizon scanning review. *Eye* **2015**, *29*, 1131–1140. [CrossRef]
21. Schön, C.; Biel, M.; Michalakis, S. Retinal gene delivery by adeno-associated virus (AAV) vectors: Strategies and applications. *Eur. J. Pharm. Biopharm.* **2015**, *95*, 343–352. [CrossRef] [PubMed]

22. Bennett, J. Taking Stock of Retinal Gene Therapy: Looking Back and Moving Forward. *Mol. Ther.* **2017**, *25*, 1076–1094. [CrossRef] [PubMed]
23. Moore, N.A.; Morral, N.; Ciulla, T.A.; Bracha, P. Gene therapy for inherited retinal and optic nerve degenerations. *Expert Opin. Biol. Ther.* **2018**, *18*, 37–49. [CrossRef] [PubMed]
24. Zuris, J.A.; Thompson, D.B.; Shu, Y.; Guilinger, J.P.; Bessen, J.L.; Hu, J.H.; Liu, D.R. Cationic lipid-mediated delivery of proteins enables efficient protein-based genome editing in vitro and in vivo. *Nat. Biotechnol.* **2015**, *33*, 73–80. [CrossRef] [PubMed]
25. Arbabi, A.; Liu, A.; Ameri, H. Gene Therapy for Inherited Retinal Degeneration. *J. Ocul. Pharmacol. Ther.* **2019**, *35*, 79–97. [CrossRef] [PubMed]
26. Zangi, L.; Lui, K.O.; Von Gise, A.; Ma, Q.; Ebina, W.; Ptaszek, L.M.; Später, D.; Xu, H.; Tabebordbar, M.; Gorbatov, R.; et al. Modified mRNA directs the fate of heart progenitor cells and induces vascular regeneration after myocardial infarction. *Nat. Biotechnol.* **2013**, *31*, 898–907. [CrossRef] [PubMed]
27. Ameri, H. Prospect of retinal gene therapy following commercialization of voretigene neparvovec-rzyl for retinal dystrophy mediated by RPE65 mutation. *J. Curr. Ophthalmol.* **2018**, *30*, 1–2. [CrossRef] [PubMed]
28. Rowe-Rendleman, C.L.; Durazo, S.A.; Kompella, U.B.; Rittenhouse, K.D.; Di Polo, A.; Weiner, A.L.; Grossniklaus, H.E.; Naash, M.I.; Lewin, A.S.; Horsager, A.; et al. Drug and Gene Delivery to the Back of the Eye: From Bench to Bedside. *Investig. Opthalmol. Vis. Sci.* **2014**, *55*, 2714–2730. [CrossRef] [PubMed]
29. Soofiyani, S.R.; Baradaran, B.; Lotfipour, F.; Kazemi, T.; Mohammadnejad, L. Gene Therapy, Early Promises, Subsequent Problems, and Recent Breakthroughs. *Adv. Pharm. Bull.* **2013**, *3*, 249–255.
30. Jacobson, S.G.; Cideciyan, A.V.; Roman, A.J.; Sumaroka, A.; Schwartz, S.B.; Héon, E.; Hauswirth, W.W. Improvement and Decline in Vision with Gene Therapy in Childhood Blindness. *N. Engl. J. Med.* **2015**, *372*, 1920–1926. [CrossRef]
31. Gao, G.; Vandenberghe, L.H.; Wilson, J.M. New recombinant serotypes of AAV vectors. *Curr. Gene Ther.* **2005**, *5*, 285–297. [CrossRef] [PubMed]
32. Vandenberghe, L.H.; Wilson, J.M.; Gao, G. Tailoring the AAV vector capsid for gene therapy. *Gene Ther.* **2009**, *16*, 311–319. [CrossRef] [PubMed]
33. Le Meur, G.; Stieger, K.; Smith, A.J.; Weber, M.; Deschamps, J.Y.; Nivard, D.; Ali, R.R. Restoration of vision in RPE65-deficient Briard dogs using an AAV serotype 4 vector that specifically targets the retinal pigmented epithelium. *Gene Ther.* **2007**, *14*, 292–303. [CrossRef] [PubMed]
34. Fischer, M.D.; McClements, M.E.; De La Camara, C.M.-F.; Bellingrath, J.-S.; Dauletbekov, D.; Ramsden, S.C.; Hickey, D.G.; Barnard, A.R.; MacLaren, R.E. Codon-Optimized RPGR Improves Stability and Efficacy of AAV8 Gene Therapy in Two Mouse Models of X-Linked Retinitis Pigmentosa. *Mol. Ther.* **2017**, *25*, 1854–1865. [CrossRef] [PubMed]
35. Georgiadis, A.; Duran, Y.; Ribeiro, J.; Abelleira-Hervas, L.; Robbie, S.J.; Sünkel-Laing, B.; Fourali, S.; Cordero, A.G.; Cristante, E.; Michaelides, M.; et al. Development of an optimized AAV2/5 gene therapy vector for Leber congenital amaurosis owing to defects in RPE65. *Gene Ther.* **2016**, *23*, 857–862. [CrossRef] [PubMed]
36. McClements, M.E.; MacLaren, R.E. Gene therapy for retinal disease. *Transl. Res.* **2013**, *161*, 241–254. [CrossRef] [PubMed]
37. Wilson, J.H.; Wensel, T.G. The Nature of Dominant Mutations of Rhodopsin and Implications for Gene Therapy. *Mol. Neurobiol.* **2003**, *28*, 149–158. [CrossRef]
38. Farrar, G.J.; Millington-Ward, S.; Chadderton, N.; Humphries, P.; Kenna, P.F. Gene-based therapies for dominantly inherited retinopathies. *Gene Ther.* **2012**, *19*, 137–144. [CrossRef]
39. O'Reilly, M.; Palfi, A.; Chadderton, N.; Millington-Ward, S.; Ader, M.; Cronin, T.; Tuohy, T.; Auricchio, A.; Hildinger, M.; Tivnan, A.; et al. RNA Interference–Mediated Suppression and Replacement of Human Rhodopsin In Vivo. *Am. J. Hum. Genet.* **2007**, *81*, 127–135. [CrossRef]
40. Dyka, F.M.; Boye, S.L.; Chiodo, V.A.; Hauswirth, W.W.; Boye, S.E. Dual adeno-associated virus vectors result in efficient in vitro and in vivo expression of an oversized gene, MYO7A. *Hum. Gene Ther. Methods* **2014**, *25*, 166–177. [CrossRef]
41. Trapani, I.; Colella, P.; Sommella, A.; Iodice, C.; Cesi, G.; de Simone, S.; Farrar, G.J. Effective delivery of large genes to the retina by dual AAV vectors. *EMBO Mol. Med.* **2014**, *6*, 194–211. [CrossRef] [PubMed]

42. Colella, P.; Trapani, I.; Cesi, G.; Sommella, A.; Manfredi, A.; Puppo, A.; Iodice, C.; Rossi, S.; Simonelli, F.; Giunti, M.; et al. Efficient gene delivery to the cone-enriched pig retina by dual AAV vectors. *Gene Ther.* **2014**, *21*, 450–456. [CrossRef] [PubMed]
43. Maddalena, A.; Tornabene, P.; Tiberi, P.; Minopoli, R.; Manfredi, A.; Mutarelli, M.; Auricchio, A. Triple Vectors Expand AAV Transfer Capacity in the Retina. *Mol. Ther.* **2018**, *26*, 524–541. [CrossRef] [PubMed]
44. Baye, L.M.; Patrinostro, X.; Swaminathan, S.; Beck, J.S.; Zhang, Y.; Stone, E.M.; Sheffield, V.C.; Slusarski, D.C. The N-terminal region of centrosomal protein 290 (CEP290) restores vision in a zebrafish model of human blindness. *Hum. Mol. Genet.* **2011**, *20*, 1467–1477. [CrossRef] [PubMed]
45. Sanjurjo-Soriano, C.; Kalatzis, V. Guiding Lights in Genome Editing for Inherited Retinal Disorders: Implications for Gene and Cell Therapy. *Neural Plast.* **2018**, *2018*, 1–15. [CrossRef] [PubMed]
46. Gaj, T.; Gersbach, C.A.; Barbas, C.F., III. ZFN, TALEN and CRISPR/Cas-based methods for genome engineering. *Trends Biotechnol.* **2013**, *31*, 397–405. [CrossRef] [PubMed]
47. Yao, X.; Wang, X.; Hu, X.; Liu, Z.; Liu, J.; Zhou, H.; Shen, X.; Wei, Y.; Huang, Z.; Ying, W.; et al. Homology-mediated end joining-based targeted integration using CRISPR/Cas9. *Cell Res.* **2017**, *27*, 801–814. [CrossRef] [PubMed]
48. Schierling, B.; Dannemann, N.; Gabsalilow, L.; Wende, W.; Cathomen, T.; Pingoud, A. A novel zinc-finger nuclease platform with a sequence-specific cleavage module. *Nucleic Acids Res.* **2012**, *40*, 2623–2638. [CrossRef] [PubMed]
49. Greenwald, D.L.; Cashman, S.M.; Kumar-Singh, R. Engineered Zinc Finger Nuclease–Mediated Homologous Recombination of the Human Rhodopsin Gene. *Investig. Opthalmol. Vis. Sci.* **2010**, *51*, 6374–6380. [CrossRef] [PubMed]
50. Low, B.E.; Krebs, M.P.; Joung, J.K.; Tsai, S.Q.; Nishina, P.M.; Wiles, M.V. Correction of the Crb1rd8 Allele and Retinal Phenotype in C57BL/6N Mice Via TALEN-Mediated Homology-Directed Repair. *Investig. Opthalmol. Vis. Sci.* **2014**, *55*, 387–395. [CrossRef] [PubMed]
51. Nelson, C.E.; Hakim, C.H.; Ousterout, D.G.; Thakore, P.I.; Moreb, E.A.; Rivera RM, C.; Asokan, A. In vivo genome editing improves muscle function in a mouse model of Duchenne muscular dystrophy. *Science* **2016**, *351*, 403–407. [CrossRef] [PubMed]
52. Hung, S.S.C.; Chrysostomou, V.; Li, F.; Lim, J.K.H.; Wang, J.-H.; Powell, J.E.; Tu, L.; Daniszewski, M.; Lo, C.; Wong, R.C.; et al. AAV-Mediated CRISPR/Cas Gene Editing of Retinal Cells In Vivo. *Investig. Opthalmol. Vis. Sci.* **2016**, *57*, 3470. [CrossRef] [PubMed]
53. Tabebordbar, M.; Zhu, K.; Cheng, J.K.; Chew, W.L.; Widrick, J.J.; Yan, W.X.; Cong, L. In vivo gene editing in dystrophic mouse muscle and muscle stem cells. *Science* **2016**, *351*, 407–411. [CrossRef] [PubMed]
54. Long, C.; Amoasii, L.; Mireault, A.A.; McAnally, J.R.; Li, H.; Sanchez-Ortiz, E.; Olson, E.N. Postnatal genome editing partially restores dystrophin expression in a mouse model of muscular dystrophy. *Science* **2016**, *351*, 400–403. [CrossRef] [PubMed]
55. Kim, S.; Kim, D.; Cho, S.W.; Kim, J.; Kim, J.-S. Highly efficient RNA-guided genome editing in human cells via delivery of purified Cas9 ribonucleoproteins. *Genome Res.* **2014**, *24*, 1012–1019. [CrossRef] [PubMed]
56. Hsu, P.D.; Scott, D.A.; Weinstein, J.A.; Ran, F.A.; Konermann, S.; Agarwala, V.; Li, Y.; Fine, E.J.; Wu, X.; Shalem, O.; et al. DNA targeting specificity of RNA-guided Cas9 nucleases. *Nat. Biotechnol.* **2013**, *31*, 827–832. [CrossRef] [PubMed]
57. Cho, S.W.; Kim, S.; Kim, Y.; Kweon, J.; Kim, H.S.; Bae, S.; Kim, J.S. Analysis of off-target effects of CRISPR/Cas-derived RNA-guided endonucleases and nickases. *Genome Res.* **2014**, *24*, 132–141. [CrossRef] [PubMed]
58. Kim, Y.; Kweon, J.; Kim, A.; Chon, J.K.; Yoo, J.Y.; Kim, H.J.; Kim, S.; Lee, C.; Jeong, E.; Chung, E.; et al. A library of TAL effector nucleases spanning the human genome. *Nat. Biotechnol.* **2013**, *31*, 251–258. [CrossRef] [PubMed]
59. Peddle, C.F.; MacLaren, R.E. The Application of CRISPR/Cas9 for the Treatment of Retinal Diseases. *Yale J. Boil. Med.* **2017**, *90*, 533–541.
60. Slaymaker, I.M.; Gao, L.; Zetsche, B.; Scott, D.A.; Yan, W.X.; Zhang, F. Rationally engineered Cas9 nucleases with improved specificity. *Science* **2016**, *351*, 84–88. [CrossRef]
61. Jo, D.H.; Koo, T.; Cho, C.S.; Kim, J.H.; Kim, J.-S.; Kim, J.H. Long-Term Effects of In Vivo Genome Editing in the Mouse Retina Using Campylobacter jejuni Cas9 Expressed via Adeno-Associated Virus. *Mol. Ther.* **2019**, *27*, 130–136. [CrossRef]

62. Li, F.; Hung, S.S.; Khalid, M.K.N.M.; Wang, J.-H.; Chrysostomou, V.; Wong, V.H.; Singh, V.; Wing, K.; Tu, L.; Bender, J.A.; et al. Utility of self-destructing CRISPR/Cas constructs for targeted gene editing in the retina. *Hum. Gene Ther.* **2019**. [CrossRef]
63. Zelinka, C.P.; Sotolongo-Lopez, M.; Fadool, J.M. Targeted disruption of the endogenous zebrafish rhodopsin locus as models of rapid rod photoreceptor degeneration. *Mol. Vis.* **2018**, *24*, 587–602.
64. Xia, C.-H.; Ferguson, I.; Li, M.; Kim, A.; Onishi, A.; Li, L.; Su, B.; Gong, X. Essential function of NHE8 in mouse retina demonstrated by AAV-mediated CRISPR/Cas9 knockdown. *Exp. Eye Res.* **2018**, *176*, 29–39. [CrossRef]
65. Moreno, A.M.; Fu, X.; Zhu, J.; Katrekar, D.; Shih, Y.-R.V.; Marlett, J.; Cabotaje, J.; Tat, J.; Naughton, J.; Lisowski, L.; et al. In Situ Gene Therapy via AAV-CRISPR-Cas9-Mediated Targeted Gene Regulation. *Mol. Ther.* **2018**, *26*, 1818–1827. [CrossRef]
66. Giannelli, S.G.; Luoni, M.; Castoldi, V.; Massimino, L.; Cabassi, T.; Angeloni, D.; Broccoli, V. Cas9/sgRNA selective targeting of the P23H Rhodopsin mutant allele for treating retinitis pigmentosa by intravitreal AAV9.PHP.B-based delivery. *Hum. Mol. Genet.* **2018**, *27*, 761–779. [CrossRef]
67. Burnight, E.R.; Gupta, M.; Wiley, L.A.; Anfinson, K.R.; Tran, A.; Triboulet, R.; Hoffmann, J.M.; Klaahsen, D.L.; Andorf, J.L.; Jiao, C.; et al. Using CRISPR-Cas9 to Generate Gene-Corrected Autologous iPSCs for the Treatment of Inherited Retinal Degeneration. *Mol. Ther.* **2017**, *25*, 1999–2013. [CrossRef]
68. Kim, E.; Koo, T.; Park, S.W.; Kim, D.; Kim, K.; Cho, H.-Y.; Song, D.W.; Lee, K.J.; Jung, M.H.; Kim, S.; et al. In vivo genome editing with a small Cas9 orthologue derived from Campylobacter jejuni. *Nat. Commun.* **2017**, *8*, 14500. [CrossRef]
69. Latella, M.C.; Di Salvo, M.T.; Cocchiarella, F.; Benati, D.; Grisendi, G.; Comitato, A.; Marigo, V.; Recchia, A. In vivo Editing of the Human Mutant Rhodopsin Gene by Electroporation of Plasmid-based CRISPR/Cas9 in the Mouse Retina. *Mol. Ther. Nucleic Acids* **2016**, *5*, e389. [CrossRef]
70. Bassuk, A.G.; Zheng, A.; Li, Y.; Tsang, S.H.; Mahajan, V.B. Precision Medicine: Genetic Repair of Retinitis Pigmentosa in Patient-Derived Stem Cells. *Sci. Rep.* **2016**, *6*, 19969. [CrossRef]
71. Wu, W.-H.; Tsai, Y.-T.; Justus, S.; Lee, T.-T.; Zhang, L.; Lin, C.-S.; Bassuk, A.G.; Mahajan, V.B.; Tsang, S.H. CRISPR Repair Reveals Causative Mutation in a Preclinical Model of Retinitis Pigmentosa. *Mol. Ther.* **2016**, *24*, 1388–1394. [CrossRef]
72. Zhong, H.; Chen, Y.; Li, Y.; Chen, R.; Mardon, G. CRISPR-engineered mosaicism rapidly reveals that loss of Kcnj13 function in mice mimics human disease phenotypes. *Sci. Rep.* **2015**, *5*, 8366. [CrossRef]
73. Swiech, L.; Heidenreich, M.; Banerjee, A.; Habib, N.; Li, Y.; Trombetta, J.; Zhang, F. In vivo interrogation of gene function in the mammalian brain using CRISPR-Cas9. *Nat. Biotechnol.* **2015**, *33*, 102–106. [CrossRef]
74. Wang, D.; Mou, H.; Li, S.; Li, Y.; Hough, S.; Tran, K.; Li, J.; Yin, H.; Anderson, D.G.; Sontheimer, E.J.; et al. Adenovirus-Mediated Somatic Genome Editing of Pten by CRISPR/Cas9 in Mouse Liver in Spite of Cas9-Specific Immune Responses. *Hum. Gene Ther.* **2015**, *26*, 432–442. [CrossRef]
75. Lin, S.; Staahl, B.T.; Alla, R.K.; Doudna, J.A. Enhanced homology-directed human genome engineering by controlled timing of CRISPR/Cas9 delivery. *eLife* **2014**, *3*, 04766. [CrossRef]
76. Kim, K.; Park, S.W.; Kim, J.H.; Lee, S.H.; Kim, D.; Koo, T.; Kim, K.-E.; Kim, J.H.; Kim, J.-S. Genome surgery using Cas9 ribonucleoproteins for the treatment of age-related macular degeneration. *Genome Res.* **2017**, *27*, 419–426. [CrossRef]
77. Suzuki, K.; Tsunekawa, Y.; Hernandez-Benitez, R.; Wu, J.; Zhu, J.; Kim, E.J.; Hatanaka, F.; Yamamoto, M.; Araoka, T.; Li, Z.; et al. In vivo genome editing via CRISPR/Cas9 mediated homology-independent targeted integration. *Nature* **2016**, *540*, 144–149. [CrossRef]
78. Diakatou, M.; Manes, G.; Bocquet, B.; Meunier, I.; Kalatzis, V. Genome Editing as a Treatment for the Most Prevalent Causative Genes of Autosomal Dominant Retinitis Pigmentosa. *Int. J. Mol. Sci.* **2019**, *20*, 2542. [CrossRef]
79. Garanto, A.; Van Beersum, S.E.C.; Peters, T.A.; Roepman, R.; Cremers, F.P.M.; Collin, R.W.J. Unexpected CEP290 mRNA Splicing in a Humanized Knock-In Mouse Model for Leber Congenital Amaurosis. *PLoS ONE* **2013**, *8*, e79369. [CrossRef]
80. Maeder, M.L.; Stefanidakis, M.; Wilson, C.J.; Baral, R.; Barrera, L.A.; Bounoutas, G.S.; Bumcrot, D.; Chao, H.; Ciulla, D.M.; DaSilva, J.A.; et al. Development of a gene-editing approach to restore vision loss in Leber congenital amaurosis type 10. *Nat. Med.* **2019**, *25*, 229–233. [CrossRef]
81. Duebel, J.; Marazova, K.; Sahel, J.A. Optogenetics. *Curr. Opin. Ophthalmol.* **2015**, *26*, 226–232. [CrossRef]

82. Simunovic, M.; Shen, W.; Lin, J.; Protti, D.; Lisowski, L.; Gillies, M. Optogenetic approaches to vision restoration. *Exp. Eye Res.* **2019**, *178*, 15–26. [CrossRef]
83. Deisseroth, K.; Feng, G.; Majewska, A.K.; Miesenböck, G.; Ting, A.; Schnitzer, M.J. Next-Generation Optical Technologies for Illuminating Genetically Targeted Brain Circuits. *J. Neurosci.* **2006**, *26*, 10380–10386. [CrossRef]
84. Yue, L.; Weiland, J.D.; Roska, B.; Humayun, M.S. Retinal stimulation strategies to restore vision: Fundamentals and systems. *Prog. Retin. Eye Res.* **2016**, *53*, 21–47. [CrossRef]
85. Zhang, F.; Vierock, J.; Yizhar, O.; Fenno, L.E.; Tsunoda, S.; Kianianmomeni, A.; Prigge, M.; Berndt, A.; Cushman, J.; Polle, J.; et al. The Microbial Opsin Family of Optogenetic Tools. *Cell* **2011**, *147*, 1446–1457. [CrossRef]
86. Bernstein, J.G.; Boyden, E.S. Optogenetic tools for analyzing the neural circuits of behavior. *Trends Cogn. Sci.* **2011**, *15*, 592–600. [CrossRef]
87. Ahnelt, P.K.; Kolb, H. The mammalian photoreceptor mosaic-adaptive design. *Prog. Retin. Eye Res.* **2000**, *19*, 711–777. [CrossRef]
88. Gaub, B.M.; Berry, M.H.; Holt, A.E.; Isacoff, E.Y.; Flannery, J.G. Optogenetic Vision Restoration Using Rhodopsin for Enhanced Sensitivity. *Mol. Ther.* **2015**, *23*, 1562–1571. [CrossRef]
89. Sengupta, A.; Chaffiol, A.; Macé, E.; Caplette, R.; Desrosiers, M.; Lampič, M.; Forster, V.; Marre, O.; Lin, J.Y.; Sahel, J.; et al. Red-shifted channelrhodopsin stimulation restores light responses in blind mice, macaque retina, and human retina. *EMBO Mol. Med.* **2016**, *8*, 1248–1264. [CrossRef]
90. Liu, M.M.; Zack, D.J. Alternative splicing and retinal degeneration. *Clin. Genet.* **2013**, *84*, 142–149. [CrossRef]
91. Hammond, S.M.; Wood, M.J. Genetic therapies for RNA mis-splicing diseases. *Trends Genet.* **2011**, *27*, 196–205. [CrossRef]
92. Garanto, A.; Collin, R.W.J. Applications of antisense oligonucleotides for the treatment of inherited retinal diseases. *Curr. Opin. Ophthalmol.* **2017**, *28*, 1–266.
93. Bacchi, N.; Casarosa, S.; Denti, M.A. Splicing-Correcting Therapeutic Approaches for Retinal Dystrophies: Where Endogenous Gene Regulation and Specificity Matter. *Investig. Opthalmol. Vis. Sci.* **2014**, *55*, 3285–3294. [CrossRef]
94. Chan, J.H.; Lim, S.; Wong, W.F. Antisense oligonucleotides: from design to therapeutic application. *Clin. Exp. Pharmacol. Physiol.* **2006**, *33*, 533–540. [CrossRef]
95. Goyenvalle, A.; Vulin, A.; Fougerousse, F.; Leturcq, F.; Kaplan, J.-C.; García, L.; Danos, O. Rescue of Dystrophic Muscle Through U7 snRNA-Mediated Exon Skipping. *Science* **2004**, *306*, 1796–1799. [CrossRef]
96. Garanto, A.; Chung, D.C.; Duijkers, L.; Corral-Serrano, J.C.; Messchaert, M.; Xiao, R.; Bennett, J.; Vandenberghe, L.H.; Collin, R.W. In vitro and in vivo rescue of aberrant splicing in CEP290-associated LCA by antisense oligonucleotide delivery. *Hum. Mol. Genet.* **2016**, *25*, 2552–2563.
97. Vitravene Study Group. Safety of intravitreous fomivirsen for treatment of cytomegalovirus retinitis in patients with AIDS. *Am. J. Ophthalmol.* **2002**, *133*, 484–498.
98. Vitravene Study Group. Randomized dose-comparison studies of intravitreous fomivirsen for treatment of cytomegalovirus retinitis that has reactivated or is persistently active despite other therapies in patients with AIDS. *Am. J. Ophthalmol.* **2002**, *133*, 475–483.
99. Den Hollander, A.I.; Koenekoop, R.K.; Yzer, S.; Lopez, I.; Arends, M.L.; Voesenek, K.E.J.; Zonneveld, M.N.; Strom, T.M.; Meitinger, T.; Brunner, H.G.; et al. Mutations in the CEP290 (NPHP6) Gene Are a Frequent Cause of Leber Congenital Amaurosis. *Am. J. Hum. Genet.* **2006**, *79*, 556–561. [CrossRef]
100. Collin, R.W.; Hollander, A.I.D.; Van Der Velde-Visser, S.D.; Bennicelli, J.; Bennett, J.; Cremers, F.P. Antisense Oligonucleotide (AON)-based Therapy for Leber Congenital Amaurosis Caused by a Frequent Mutation in CEP290. *Mol. Ther. Nucleic Acids* **2012**, *1*, e14. [CrossRef]
101. Gerard, X.; Perrault, I.; Hanein, S.; Silva, E.; Bigot, K.; Defoort-Delhemmes, S.; Rio, M.; Munnich, A.; Scherman, D.; Kaplan, J.; et al. AON-mediated Exon Skipping Restores Ciliation in Fibroblasts Harboring the Common Leber Congenital Amaurosis CEP290 Mutation. *Mol. Ther. Nucleic Acids* **2012**, *1*, e29. [CrossRef]
102. Parfitt, D.A.; Lane, A.; Ramsden, C.M.; Carr, A.-J.F.; Munro, P.M.; Jovanovic, K.; Schwarz, N.; Kanuga, N.; Muthiah, M.N.; Hull, S.; et al. Identification and Correction of Mechanisms Underlying Inherited Blindness in Human iPSC-Derived Optic Cups. *Cell Stem Cell* **2016**, *18*, 769–781. [CrossRef]

103. Duijkers, L.; van den Born, L.; Neidhardt, J.; Bax, N.; Pierrache, L.; Klevering, B.; Garanto, A. Antisense Oligonucleotide-Based Splicing Correction in Individuals with Leber Congenital Amaurosis due to Compound Heterozygosity for the c.2991+1655A>G Mutation in CEP290. *Int. J. Mol. Sci.* **2018**, *19*, 753. [CrossRef]
104. Dulla, K.; Aguila, M.; Lane, A.; Jovanovic, K.; Parfitt, D.A.; Schulkens, I.; Collin, R.W. Splice-Modulating Oligonucleotide QR-110 Restores CEP290 mRNA and Function in Human c.2991+1655A>G LCA10 Models. *Mol. Ther. Nucleic Acids* **2018**, *12*, 730–740. [CrossRef]
105. Cideciyan, A.V.; Jacobson, S.G.; Drack, A.V.; Ho, A.C.; Charng, J.; Garafalo, A.V.; Pfeifer, W.L. Effect of an intravitreal antisense oligonucleotide on vision in Leber congenital amaurosis due to a photoreceptor cilium defect. *Nat. Med.* **2019**, *25*, 225–228. [CrossRef]
106. Barny, I.; Perrault, I.; Michel, C.; Goudin, N.; Defoort-Dhellemmes, S.; Ghazi, I.; Kaplan, J.; Rozet, J.-M.; Gerard, X. AON-Mediated Exon Skipping to Bypass Protein Truncation in Retinal Dystrophies Due to the Recurrent CEP290 c.4723A > T Mutation. Fact or Fiction? *Genes* **2019**, *10*, 368. [CrossRef]
107. Bonifert, T.; Menendez, I.G.; Battke, F.; Theurer, Y.; Synofzik, M.; Schöls, L.; Wissinger, B. Antisense Oligonucleotide Mediated Splice Correction of a Deep Intronic Mutation in OPA1. *Mol. Ther. Nucleic Acids* **2016**, *5*, e390. [CrossRef]
108. Garanto, A.; Van Der Velde-Visser, S.D.; Cremers, F.P.M.; Collin, R.W.J. Antisense Oligonucleotide-Based Splice Correction of a Deep-Intronic Mutation in CHM Underlying Choroideremia. In *Results and Problems in Cell Differentiation*; Springer: Cham, Switzerland, 2018; pp. 83–89.
109. Slijkerman, R.W.; Vaché, C.; Dona, M.; García-García, G.; Claustres, M.; Hetterschijt, L.; Peters, T.A.; Hartel, B.P.; Pennings, R.J.; Millan, J.M.; et al. Antisense Oligonucleotide-based Splice Correction for USH2A-associated Retinal Degeneration Caused by a Frequent Deep-intronic Mutation. *Mol. Ther. Nucleic Acids* **2016**, *5*, e381. [CrossRef]
110. Albert, S.; Garanto, A.; Sangermano, R.; Khan, M.; Bax, N.M.; Hoyng, C.B.; Zernant, J.; Lee, W.; Allikmets, R.; Collin, R.W.; et al. Identification and Rescue of Splice Defects Caused by Two Neighboring Deep-Intronic ABCA4 Mutations Underlying Stargardt Disease. *Am. J. Hum. Genet.* **2018**, *102*, 517–527. [CrossRef]
111. Sangermano, R.; Garanto, A.; Khan, M.; Runhart, E.H.; Bauwens, M.; Bax, N.M.; Born, L.I.V.D.; Khan, M.I.; Cornelis, S.S.; Verheij, J.B.G.M.; et al. Deep-intronic ABCA4 variants explain missing heritability in Stargardt disease and allow correction of splice defects by antisense oligonucleotides. *Genet. Med.* **2019**, *21*, 1751–1760. [CrossRef]
112. Bauwens, M.; Garanto, A.; Sangermano, R.; Naessens, S.; Weisschuh, N.; De Zaeytijd, J.; Khan, M.; Sadler, F.; Balikova, I.; Van Cauwenbergh, C.; et al. ABCA4-associated disease as a model for missing heritability in autosomal recessive disorders: Novel noncoding splice, cis-regulatory, structural, and recurrent hypomorphic variants. *Genet. Med.* **2019**, *21*, 1761–1771. [CrossRef] [PubMed]
113. Garanto, A.; Duijkers, L.; Tomkiewicz, T.Z.; Collin, R.W. Antisense Oligonucleotide Screening to Optimize the Rescue of the Splicing Defect Caused by the Recurrent Deep-Intronic ABCA4 Variant c.4539+2001G>A in Stargardt Disease. *Genes* **2019**, *10*, 452. [CrossRef] [PubMed]
114. Tanner, G.; Glaus, E.; Barthelmes, D.; Ader, M.; Fleischhauer, J.; Pagani, F.; Berger, W.; Neidhardt, J. Therapeutic strategy to rescue mutation-induced exon skipping in rhodopsin by adaptation of U1 snRNA. *Hum. Mutat.* **2009**, *30*, 255–263. [CrossRef] [PubMed]
115. Schmid, F.; Glaus, E.; Barthelmes, D.; Fliegauf, M.; Gaspar, H.; Nürnberg, G.; Nürnberg, P.; Omran, H.; Berger, W.; Neidhardt, J. U1 snRNA-mediated gene therapeutic correction of splice defects caused by an exceptionally mild BBS mutation. *Hum. Mutat.* **2011**, *32*, 815–824. [CrossRef] [PubMed]
116. Glaus, E.; Schmid, F.; Da Costa, R.; Berger, W.; Neidhardt, J. Gene Therapeutic Approach Using Mutation-adapted U1 snRNA to Correct a RPGR Splice Defect in Patient-derived Cells. *Mol. Ther.* **2011**, *19*, 936–941. [CrossRef]
117. Schmid, F.; Hiller, T.; Korner, G.; Glaus, E.; Berger, W.; Neidhardt, J. A Gene Therapeutic Approach to Correct Splice Defects with Modified U1 and U6 snRNPs. *Hum. Gene Ther.* **2013**, *24*, 97–104. [CrossRef] [PubMed]
118. Abad, X.; Vera, M.; Jung, S.P.; Oswald, E.; Romero, I.; Amin, V.; Fortes, P.; Gunderson, S.I. Requirements for gene silencing mediated by U1 snRNA binding to a target sequence. *Nucleic Acids Res.* **2008**, *36*, 2338–2352. [CrossRef]

119. Berger, A.; Lorain, S.; Joséphine, C.; Desrosiers, M.; Peccate, C.; Voit, T.; Garcia, L.; Sahel, J.-A.; Bemelmans, A.-P. Repair of Rhodopsin mRNA by Spliceosome-Mediated RNA Trans. -Splicing: A New Approach for Autosomal Dominant Retinitis Pigmentosa. *Mol. Ther.* **2015**, *23*, 918–930. [CrossRef]
120. Lei, Q.; Li, C.; Zuo, Z.; Huang, C.; Cheng, H.; Zhou, R. Evolutionary Insights into RNA trans-Splicing in Vertebrates. *Genome Boil. Evol.* **2016**, *8*, 562–577. [CrossRef]
121. Li, N.; Zheng, J.; Li, H.; Deng, J.; Hu, M.; Wu, H.; Li, W.; Li, F.; Lan, X.; Lu, J.; et al. Identification of chimeric TSNAX–DISC1 resulting from intergenic splicing in endometrial carcinoma through high-throughput RNA sequencing. *Carcinogenesis* **2014**, *35*, 2687–2697. [CrossRef]
122. Guerra, E.; Trerotola, M.; Arciprete, R.D.; Bonasera, V.; Palombo, B.; El-Sewedy, T.; Ciccimarra, T.; Crescenzi, C.; Lorenzini, F.; Rossi, C.; et al. A Bicistronic CYCLIN D1-TROP2 mRNA Chimera Demonstrates a Novel Oncogenic Mechanism in Human Cancer. *Cancer Res.* **2008**, *68*, 8113–8121. [CrossRef] [PubMed]
123. Hirano, M.; Noda, T. Genomic organization of the mouse Msh4 gene producing bicistronic, chimeric and antisense mRNA. *Gene* **2004**, *342*, 165–177. [CrossRef] [PubMed]
124. Dooley, S.J.; McDougald, D.S.; Fisher, K.J.; Bennicelli, J.L.; Mitchell, L.G.; Bennett, J. Spliceosome-Mediated Pre-mRNA trans-Splicing Can Repair CEP290 mRNA. *Mol. Ther. Nucleic Acids* **2018**, *12*, 294–308. [CrossRef] [PubMed]
125. Saurabh, S.; Vidyarthi, A.S.; Prasad, D. RNA interference: Concept to reality in crop improvement. *Planta* **2014**, *239*, 543–564. [CrossRef] [PubMed]
126. Qiu, S.; Adema, C.M.; Lane, T. A computational study of off-target effects of RNA interference. *Nucleic Acids Res.* **2005**, *33*, 1834–1847. [CrossRef] [PubMed]
127. Ryoo, N.-K.; Lee, J.; Lee, H.; Hong, H.K.; Kim, H.; Lee, J.B.; Woo, S.J.; Park, K.H.; Kim, H. Therapeutic effects of a novel siRNA-based anti-VEGF (siVEGF) nanoball for the treatment of choroidal neovascularization. *Nanoscale* **2017**, *9*, 15461–15469. [CrossRef] [PubMed]
128. Yau, E.H.; Butler, M.C.; Sullivan, J.M. A Cellular High-Throughput Screening Approach for Therapeutic trans-Cleaving Ribozymes and RNAi against Arbitrary mRNA Disease Targets. *Exp. Eye Res.* **2016**, *151*, 236–255. [CrossRef] [PubMed]
129. Lagos-Quintana, M.; Rauhut, R.; Meyer, J.; Borkhardt, A.; Tuschl, T. New microRNAs from mouse and human. *RNA* **2003**, *9*, 175–179. [CrossRef]
130. Zuzic, M.; Arias, J.E.R.; Wohl, S.G.; Busskamp, V. Retinal miRNA Functions in Health and Disease. *Genes* **2019**, *10*, 377. [CrossRef]
131. Mangos, M.M.; Min, K.-L.; Viazovkina, E.; Galarneau, A.; Elzagheid, M.I.; Parniak, M.A.; Damha, M.J. Efficient RNase H-Directed Cleavage of RNA Promoted by Antisense DNA or 2′F-ANA Constructs Containing Acyclic Nucleotide Inserts. *J. Am. Chem. Soc.* **2003**, *125*, 654–661. [CrossRef]
132. Honcharenko, D.; Barman, J.; Varghese, O.P. Comparison of the RNase H Cleavage Kinetics and Blood Serum Stability of theNorth-Conformationally Constrained and 2′-Alkoxy Modified Oligonucleotides†. *Biochemistry* **2007**, *46*, 5635–5646. [CrossRef] [PubMed]
133. Murray, S.F.; Jazayeri, A.; Matthes, M.T.; Yasumura, D.; Yang, H.; Peralta, R.; Watt, A.; Freier, S.; Hung, G.; Adamson, P.S.; et al. Allele-Specific Inhibition of Rhodopsin With an Antisense Oligonucleotide Slows Photoreceptor Cell Degeneration. *Investig. Opthalmol. Vis. Sci.* **2015**, *56*, 6362–6375. [CrossRef] [PubMed]
134. Naessens, S.; Ruysschaert, L.; Lefever, S.; Coppieters, F.; De Baere, E. Antisense Oligonucleotide-Based Downregulation of the G56R Pathogenic Variant Causing NR2E3-Associated Autosomal Dominant Retinitis Pigmentosa. *Genes* **2019**, *10*, 363. [CrossRef] [PubMed]
135. Cox, D.B.; Gootenberg, J.S.; Abudayyeh, O.O.; Franklin, B.; Kellner, M.J.; Joung, J.; Zhang, F. RNA editing with CRISPR-Cas13. *Science* **2017**, *358*, 1019–1027. [CrossRef] [PubMed]
136. Shmakov, S.; Smargon, A.; Scott, D.; Cox, D.; Pyzocha, N.; Yan, W.; Abudayyeh, O.O.; Gootenberg, J.S.; Makarova, K.S.; Wolf, Y.I.; et al. Diversity and evolution of class 2 CRISPR–Cas systems. *Nat. Rev. Genet.* **2017**, *15*, 169–182. [CrossRef] [PubMed]
137. Abudayyeh, O.O.; Gootenberg, J.S.; Essletzbichler, P.; Han, S.; Joung, J.; Belanto, J.J.; Lander, E.S. RNA targeting with CRISPR-Cas13. *Nature* **2017**, *550*, 280–284. [CrossRef]
138. Stafforst, T.; Schneider, M.F. An RNA-Deaminase Conjugate Selectively Repairs Point Mutations. *Angew. Chem. Int. Ed.* **2012**, *51*, 11166–11169. [CrossRef] [PubMed]
139. Wettengel, J.; Reautschnig, P.; Geisler, S.; Kahle, P.J.; Stafforst, T. Harnessing human ADAR2 for RNA repair - Recoding a PINK1 mutation rescues mitophagy. *Nucleic Acids Res.* **2017**, *45*, 2797–2808. [CrossRef]

140. Vighi, E.; Trifunović, D.; Veiga-Crespo, P.; Rentsch, A.; Hoffmann, D.; Sahaboglu, A.; Strasser, T.; Kulkarni, M.; Bertolotti, E.; Heuvel, A.V.D.; et al. Combination of cGMP analogue and drug delivery system provides functional protection in hereditary retinal degeneration. *Proc. Natl. Acad. Sci. USA* **2018**, *115*, E2997–E3006. [CrossRef]
141. Nagel-Wolfrum, K.; Möller, F.; Penner, I.; Baasov, T.; Wolfrum, U. Targeting Nonsense Mutations in Diseases with Translational Read-Through-Inducing Drugs (TRIDs). *BioDrugs* **2016**, *30*, 49–74. [CrossRef]
142. Schwarz, N.; Carr, A.J.; Lane, A.; Moeller, F.; Chen, L.L.; Aguila, M.; Nagel-Wolfrum, K. Translational read-through of the RP2 Arg120stop mutation in patient iPSC-derived retinal pigment epithelium cells. *Hum. Mol. Genet.* **2015**, *24*, 972–986. [CrossRef] [PubMed]
143. Guérin, K.; Gregory-Evans, C.; Hodges, M.D.J.; Moosajee, M.; Mackay, D.; Gregory-Evans, K.; Flannery, J.G.; Mackay, D. Systemic aminoglycoside treatment in rodent models of retinitis pigmentosa. *Exp. Eye Res.* **2008**, *87*, 197–207. [CrossRef] [PubMed]
144. Goldmann, T.; Overlack, N.; Möller, F.; Belakhov, V.; Van Wyk, M.; Baasov, T.; Wolfrum, U.; Nagel-Wolfrum, K. A comparative evaluation of NB30, NB54 and PTC124 in translational read-through efficacy for treatment of an USH1C nonsense mutation. *EMBO Mol. Med.* **2012**, *4*, 1186–1199. [CrossRef] [PubMed]
145. Goldmann, T.; Rebibo-Sabbah, A.; Overlack, N.; Nudelman, I.; Belakhov, V.; Baasov, T.; Ben-Yosef, T.; Wolfrum, U.; Nagel-Wolfrum, K. Beneficial Read-Through of a USH1C Nonsense Mutation by Designed Aminoglycoside NB30 in the Retina. *Investig. Opthalmol. Vis. Sci.* **2010**, *51*, 6671–6680. [CrossRef] [PubMed]
146. Nudelman, I.; Glikin, D.; Smolkin, B.; Hainrichson, M.; Belakhov, V.; Baasov, T. Repairing faulty genes by aminoglycosides: Development of new derivatives of geneticin (G418) with enhanced suppression of diseases-causing nonsense mutations. *Bioorganic Med. Chem.* **2010**, *18*, 3735–3746. [CrossRef] [PubMed]
147. Nudelman, I.; Rebibo-Sabbah, A.; Cherniavsky, M.; Belakhov, V.; Hainrichson, M.; Chen, F.; Schacht, J.; Pilch, D.S.; Ben-Yosef, T.; Baasov, T. Development of novel aminoglycoside (NB54) with reduced toxicity and enhanced suppression of disease-causing premature stop mutations. *J. Med. Chem.* **2009**, *52*, 2836–2845. [CrossRef] [PubMed]
148. Nudelman, I.; Rebibo-Sabbah, A.; Shallom-Shezifi, D.; Hainrichson, M.; Stahl, I.; Ben-Yosef, T.; Baasov, T. Redesign of aminoglycosides for treatment of human genetic diseases caused by premature stop mutations. *Bioorganic Med. Chem. Lett.* **2006**, *16*, 6310–6315. [CrossRef]
149. Rebibo-Sabbah, A.; Nudelman, I.; Ahmed, Z.M.; Baasov, T.; Ben-Yosef, T. In vitro and ex vivo suppression by aminoglycosides of PCDH15 nonsense mutations underlying type 1 Usher syndrome. *Qual. Life Res.* **2007**, *122*, 373–381. [CrossRef]
150. Welch, E.M.; Barton, E.R.; Zhuo, J.; Tomizawa, Y.; Friesen, W.J.; Trifillis, P.; Paushkin, S.; Patel, M.; Trotta, C.R.; Hwang, S.; et al. PTC124 targets genetic disorders caused by nonsense mutations. *Nature* **2007**, *447*, 87–91. [CrossRef]
151. Shimizu-Motohashi, Y.; Komaki, H.; Motohashi, N.; Takeda, S.; Yokota, T.; Aoki, Y. Restoring Dystrophin Expression in Duchenne Muscular Dystrophy: Current Status of Therapeutic Approaches. *J. Pers. Med.* **2019**, *9*, 1. [CrossRef]
152. Sermet-Gaudelus, I.; De Boeck, K.; Casimir, G.J.; Vermeulen, F.; Leal, T.; Mogenet, A.; Roussel, D.; Fritsch, J.; Hanssens, L.; Hirawat, S.; et al. Ataluren (PTC124) Induces Cystic Fibrosis Transmembrane Conductance Regulator Protein Expression and Activity in Children with Nonsense Mutation Cystic Fibrosis. *Am. J. Respir. Crit. Care Med.* **2010**, *182*, 1262–1272. [CrossRef] [PubMed]
153. Xue, X.; Mutyam, V.; Tang, L.; Biswas, S.; Du, M.; Jackson, L.A.; Dai, Y.; Belakhov, V.; Shalev, M.; Chen, F.; et al. Synthetic Aminoglycosides Efficiently Suppress Cystic Fibrosis Transmembrane Conductance Regulator Nonsense Mutations and Are Enhanced by Ivacaftor. *Am. J. Respir. Cell Mol. Boil.* **2014**, *50*, 805–816. [CrossRef] [PubMed]
154. Moosajee, M.; Tracey-White, D.; Smart, M.; Weetall, M.; Torriano, S.; Kalatzis, V.; Da Cruz, L.; Coffey, P.; Webster, A.R.; Welch, E. Functional rescue of REP1 following treatment with PTC124 and novel derivative PTC-414 in human choroideremia fibroblasts and the nonsense-mediated zebrafish model. *Hum. Mol. Genet.* **2016**, *25*, 3416–3431. [CrossRef] [PubMed]
155. Torriano, S.; Erkilic, N.; Baux, D.; Cereso, N.; De Luca, V.; Meunier, I.; Moosajee, M.; Roux, A.-F.; Hamel, C.P.; Kalatzis, V. The effect of PTC124 on choroideremia fibroblasts and iPSC-derived RPE raises considerations for therapy. *Sci. Rep.* **2018**, *8*, 8234. [CrossRef] [PubMed]

156. Sarkar, H.; Mitsios, A.; Smart, M.; Skinner, J.; Welch, A.A.; Kalatzis, V.; Coffey, P.J.; Dubis, A.M.; Webster, A.R.; Moosajee, M. Nonsense-mediated mRNA decay efficiency varies in choroideremia providing a target to boost small molecule therapeutics. *Hum. Mol. Genet.* **2019**, *28*, 1865–1871. [CrossRef] [PubMed]
157. Madni, A.; Sarfraz, M.; Rehman, M.; Ahmad, M.; Akhtar, N.; Ahmad, S.; Tahir, N.; Ijaz, S.; Al-Kassas, R.; Löbenberg, R.; et al. Liposomal Drug Delivery: A Versatile Platform for Challenging Clinical Applications. *J. Pharm. Pharm. Sci.* **2014**, *17*, 401–426. [CrossRef] [PubMed]
158. Parfitt, D.A.; Cheetham, M.E. Targeting the Proteostasis Network in Rhodopsin Retinitis Pigmentosa. *Adv. Exp. Med. Biol.* **2016**, *854*, 479–484. [PubMed]
159. Faber, S.; Roepman, R. Balancing the Photoreceptor Proteome: Proteostasis Network Therapeutics for Inherited Retinal Disease. *Genes* **2019**, *10*, 557. [CrossRef] [PubMed]
160. Parfitt, D.A.; Aguila, M.; McCulley, C.H.; Bevilacqua, D.; Mendes, H.F.; Athanasiou, D.; Novoselov, S.S.; Kanuga, N.; Munro, P.M.; Coffey, P.J.; et al. The heat-shock response co-inducer arimoclomol protects against retinal degeneration in rhodopsin retinitis pigmentosa. *Cell Death Dis.* **2014**, *5*, e1236. [CrossRef]
161. Athanasiou, D.; Aguila, M.; Bellingham, J.; Li, W.; McCulley, C.; Reeves, P.J.; Cheetham, M.E. The molecular and cellular basis of rhodopsin retinitis pigmentosa reveals potential strategies for therapy. *Prog. Retin Eye Res.* **2018**, *62*, 1–23. [CrossRef]
162. Mendes, H.F.; Cheetham, M.E. Pharmacological manipulation of gain-of-function and dominant-negative mechanisms in rhodopsin retinitis pigmentosa. *Hum. Mol. Genet.* **2008**, *17*, 3043–3054. [CrossRef] [PubMed]
163. Bogéa, T.H.; Wen, R.H.; Moritz, O.L. Light Induces Ultrastructural Changes in Rod Outer and Inner Segments, Including Autophagy, in a Transgenic Xenopus laevis P23H Rhodopsin Model of Retinitis Pigmentosa. *Investig. Opthalmol. Vis. Sci.* **2015**, *56*, 7947–7955. [CrossRef] [PubMed]
164. Sakami, S.; Maeda, T.; Bereta, G.; Okano, K.; Golczak, M.; Sumaroka, A.; Roman, A.J.; Cideciyan, A.V.; Jacobson, S.G.; Palczewski, K. Probing Mechanisms of Photoreceptor Degeneration in a New Mouse Model of the Common Form of Autosomal Dominant Retinitis Pigmentosa due to P23H Opsin Mutations. *J. Boil. Chem.* **2011**, *286*, 10551–10567. [CrossRef] [PubMed]
165. Lax, P.; Pinilla, I.; Cuenca, N.; Fernández-Sánchez, L.; Martín-Nieto, J. Tauroursodeoxycholic Acid Prevents Retinal Degeneration in Transgenic P23H Rats. *Investig. Opthalmol. Vis. Sci.* **2011**, *52*, 4998–5008.
166. Tao, Y.; Dong, X.; Lu, X.; Qu, Y.; Wang, C.; Peng, G.; Zhang, J. Subcutaneous delivery of tauroursodeoxycholic acid rescues the cone photoreceptors in degenerative retina: A promising therapeutic molecule for retinopathy. *Biomed. Pharmacother.* **2019**, *117*, 109021. [CrossRef] [PubMed]
167. Lobysheva, E.; Taylor, C.; Marshall, G.; Kisselev, O. Tauroursodeoxycholic acid binds to the G-protein site on light activated rhodopsin. *Exp. Eye Res.* **2018**, *170*, 51–57. [CrossRef] [PubMed]
168. Remondelli, P.; Renna, M. The Endoplasmic Reticulum Unfolded Protein Response in Neurodegenerative Disorders and Its Potential Therapeutic Significance. *Front. Mol. Neurosci.* **2017**, *10*, 187. [CrossRef]
169. Tolone, A.; Belhadj, S.; Rentsch, A.; Schwede, F.; Paquet-Durand, F. The cGMP Pathway and Inherited Photoreceptor Degeneration: Targets, Compounds, and Biomarkers. *Genes* **2019**, *10*, 453. [CrossRef] [PubMed]
170. Palczewski, K. Retinoids for Treatment of Retinal Diseases. *Trends Pharmacol. Sci.* **2010**, *31*, 284–295. [CrossRef]
171. Scholl, H.P.N.; Moore, A.T.; Koenekoop, R.K.; Wen, Y.; Fishman, G.A.; Born, L.I.V.D.; Bittner, A.; Bowles, K.; Fletcher, E.C.; Collison, F.T.; et al. Safety and Proof-of-Concept Study of Oral QLT091001 in Retinitis Pigmentosa Due to Inherited Deficiencies of Retinal Pigment Epithelial 65 Protein (RPE65) or Lecithin:Retinol Acyltransferase (LRAT). *PLoS ONE* **2015**, *10*, e0143846. [CrossRef]
172. Patel, A.; Cholkar, K.; Agrahari, V.; Mitra, A.K. Ocular drug delivery systems: An overview. *World J. Gastrointest. Pharmacol. Ther.* **2013**, *2*, 47–64. [CrossRef] [PubMed]
173. Bordet, T.; Behar-Cohen, F. Ocular gene therapies in clinical practice: Viral vectors and nonviral alternatives. *Drug Discov. Today* **2019**, *24*, 1685–1693. [CrossRef]
174. Conley, S.M.; Cai, X.; Naash, M.I. Non-Viral Ocular Gene Therapy: Assessment and Future Directions. *Curr. Opin. Mol. Ther.* **2008**, *10*, 456–463. [PubMed]
175. Chiang, B.; Jung, J.H.; Prausnitz, M.R. The suprachoroidal space as a route of administration to the posterior segment of the eye. *Adv. Drug Deliv. Rev.* **2018**, *126*, 58–66. [CrossRef] [PubMed]
176. Rodrigues, G.A.; Shalaev, E.; Karami, T.K.; Cunningham, J.; Slater, N.K.H.; Rivers, H.M. Pharmaceutical Development of AAV-Based Gene Therapy Products for the Eye. *Pharm. Res.* **2018**, *36*, 29. [CrossRef] [PubMed]

177. Olsen, T.W.; Feng, X.; Wabner, K.; Conston, S.R.; Sierra, D.H.; Folden, D.V.; Smith, M.E.; Cameron, J.D. Cannulation of the Suprachoroidal Space: A Novel Drug Delivery Methodology to the Posterior Segment. *Am. J. Ophthalmol.* **2006**, *142*, 777–787.e2. [CrossRef] [PubMed]
178. Einmahl, S.; Savoldelli, M.; D'Hermies, F.; Tabatabay, C.; Gurny, R.; Behar-Cohen, F. Evaluation of a novel biomaterial in the suprachoroidal space of the rabbit eye. *Investig. Ophthalmol. Vis. Sci.* **2002**, *43*, 1533–1539.
179. Mandelcorn, E.D.; Kitchens, J.W.; Fijalkowski, N.; Moshfeghi, D.M. Active Aspiration of Suprachoroidal Hemorrhage Using a Guarded Needle. *Ophthalmic Surg. Lasers Imaging Retin.* **2014**, *45*, 150–152. [CrossRef] [PubMed]
180. Goldstein, D.A.; Do, D.; Noronha, G.; Kissner, J.M.; Srivastava, S.K.; Nguyen, Q.D. Suprachoroidal Corticosteroid Administration: A Novel Route for Local Treatment of Noninfectious Uveitis. *Transl. Vis. Sci. Technol.* **2016**, *5*, 14. [CrossRef] [PubMed]
181. Gote, V.; Sikder, S.; Sicotte, J.; Pal, D. Ocular Drug Delivery: Present Innovations and Future Challenges. *J. Pharmacol. Exp. Ther.* **2019**, *370*, 602–624. [CrossRef] [PubMed]
182. Bennett, J.; Ashtari, M.; Wellman, J.; Marshall, K.A.; Cyckowski, L.L.; Chung, D.C.; McCague, S.; Pierce, E.A.; Chen, Y.; Bennicelli, J.L.; et al. AAV2 Gene Therapy Readministration in Three Adults with Congenital Blindness. *Sci. Transl. Med.* **2012**, *4*, 120ra15. [CrossRef] [PubMed]
183. Trapani, I.; Puppo, A.; Auricchio, A. Vector platforms for gene therapy of inherited retinopathies. *Prog. Retin. Eye Res.* **2014**, *43*, 108–128. [CrossRef] [PubMed]
184. Stieger, K.; Lhériteau, E.; Moullier, P.; Rolling, F. AAV-Mediated Gene Therapy for Retinal Disorders in Large Animal Models. *ILAR J.* **2009**, *50*, 206–224. [CrossRef] [PubMed]
185. Petrs-Silva, H.; Dinculescu, A.; Li, Q.; Deng, W.T.; Pang, J.J.; Min, S.H.; Agbandje-McKenna, M. Novel properties of tyrosine-mutant AAV2 vectors in the mouse retina. *Mol. Ther.* **2011**, *19*, 293–301. [CrossRef] [PubMed]
186. Kong, F.; Li, W.; Li, X.; Zheng, Q.; Dai, X.; Zhou, X.; Boye, S.L.; Hauswirth, W.W.; Qu, J.; Pang, J.-J. Self-complementary AAV5 Vector Facilitates Quicker Transgene Expression in Photoreceptor and Retinal Pigment Epithelial Cells of Normal Mouse. *Exp. Eye Res.* **2010**, *90*, 546–554. [CrossRef] [PubMed]
187. Ghosh, A.; Yue, Y.; Duan, D. Efficient transgene reconstitution with hybrid dual AAV vectors carrying the minimized bridging sequences. *Hum. Gene Ther.* **2011**, *22*, 77–83. [CrossRef] [PubMed]
188. Trapani, I. Dual AAV Vectors for Stargardt Disease. *Methods Mol. Biol.* **2018**, *1715*, 153–175. [PubMed]
189. Trapani, I. Adeno-Associated Viral Vectors as a Tool for Large Gene Delivery to the Retina. *Genes* **2019**, *10*, 287. [CrossRef]
190. Patel, A.; Zhao, J.; Duan, D.; Lai, Y. Design of AAV Vectors for Delivery of Large or Multiple Transgenes. *Adv. Struct. Saf. Stud.* **2019**, *1950*, 19–33.
191. Auricchio, A.; Kobinger, G.; Anand, V.; Hildinger, M.; O'Connor, E.; Maguire, A.M.; Wilson, J.M.; Bennett, J. Exchange of surface proteins impacts on viral vector cellular specificity and transduction characteristics: The retina as a model. *Hum. Mol. Genet.* **2001**, *10*, 3075–3081. [CrossRef]
192. Martin, K.R.; Klein, R.L.; Quigley, H.A. Gene delivery to the eye using adeno-associated viral vectors. *Methods* **2002**, *28*, 267–275. [CrossRef]
193. Dalkara, D.; Byrne, L.C.; Klimczak, R.R.; Visel, M.; Yin, L.; Merigan, W.H.; Flannery, J.G.; Schaffer, D.V. In Vivo-Directed Evolution of a New Adeno-Associated Virus for Therapeutic Outer Retinal Gene Delivery from the Vitreous. *Sci. Transl. Med.* **2013**, *5*, 189ra76. [CrossRef] [PubMed]
194. Cronin, T.; Vandenberghe, L.H.; Hantz, P.; Juttner, J.; Reimann, A.; Kacsó, Á.E.; Huckfeldt, R.M.; Busskamp, V.; Kohler, H.; Lagali, P.S.; et al. Efficient transduction and optogenetic stimulation of retinal bipolar cells by a synthetic adeno-associated virus capsid and promoter. *EMBO Mol. Med.* **2014**, *6*, 1175–1190. [CrossRef] [PubMed]
195. Ramachandran, P.S.; Lee, V.; Wei, Z.; Song, J.Y.; Casal, G.; Cronin, T.; Willett, K.; Huckfeldt, R.; Morgan, J.I.; Aleman, T.S.; et al. Evaluation of Dose and Safety of AAV7m8 and AAV8BP2 in the Non-Human Primate Retina. *Hum. Gene Ther.* **2017**, *28*, 154–167. [CrossRef] [PubMed]
196. Carvalho, L.S.; Xiao, R.; Wassmer, S.J.; Langsdorf, A.; Zinn, E.; Pacouret, S.; Shah, S.; Comander, J.I.; Kim, L.A.; Lim, L.; et al. Synthetic Adeno-Associated Viral Vector Efficiently Targets Mouse and Nonhuman Primate Retina In Vivo. *Hum. Gene Ther.* **2018**, *29*, 771–784. [CrossRef] [PubMed]
197. Greenberg, K.P.; Lee, E.S.; Schaffer, D.V.; Flannery, J.G. Gene delivery to the retina using lentiviral vectors. *Adv. Exp. Med. Biol.* **2006**, *572*, 255–266.

198. Han, Z.; Conley, S.M.; Naash, M.I. Gene Therapy for Stargardt Disease Associated with ABCA4 Gene. *Adv. Exp. Med. Biol.* **2014**, *801*, 719–724.
199. Bergelson, J.M.; Modlin, J.F.; Wieland-Alter, W.; Cunningham, J.A.; Crowell, R.L.; Finberg, R.W. Clinical Coxsackievirus B Isolates Differ from Laboratory Strains in Their Interaction with Two Cell Surface Receptors. *J. Infect. Dis.* **1997**, *175*, 697–700. [CrossRef]
200. Cashman, S.M.; Sadowski, S.L.; Morris, D.J.; Frederick, J.; Kumar-Singh, R. Intercellular Trafficking of Adenovirus-Delivered HSV VP22 from the Retinal Pigment Epithelium to the Photoreceptors—Implications for Gene Therapy. *Mol. Ther.* **2002**, *6*, 813–823. [CrossRef]
201. Mallam, J.N.; Hurwitz, M.Y.; Mahoney, T.; Chévez-Barrios, P.; Hurwitz, R.L. Efficient gene transfer into retinal cells using adenoviral vectors: Dependence on receptor expression. *Investig. Opthalmol. Vis. Sci.* **2004**, *45*, 1680–1687. [CrossRef]
202. Kumar-Singh, R.; Farber, D.B. Encapsidated adenovirus mini-chromosome-mediated delivery of genes to the retina: Application to the rescue of photoreceptor degeneration. *Hum. Mol. Genet.* **1998**, *7*, 1893–1900. [CrossRef] [PubMed]
203. Bergelson, J.M.; Cunningham, J.A.; Droguett, G.; Kurt-Jones, E.A.; Krithivas, A.; Hong, J.S.; Horwitz, M.S.; Crowell, R.L.; Finberg, R.W. Isolation of a Common Receptor for Coxsackie B Viruses and Adenoviruses 2 and 5. *Science* **1997**, *275*, 1320–1323. [CrossRef] [PubMed]
204. Andrieu-Soler, C.; Bejjani, R.-A.; De Bizemont, T.; Normand, N.; Benezra, D.; Behar-Cohen, F. Ocular gene therapy: A review of nonviral strategies. *Mol. Vis.* **2006**, *12*, 1334–1347. [PubMed]
205. Foroozandeh, P.; Aziz, A.A. Insight into Cellular Uptake and Intracellular Trafficking of Nanoparticles. *Nanoscale Res. Lett.* **2018**, *13*, 339. [CrossRef] [PubMed]
206. Trigueros, S.; Domènech, E.B.; Toulis, V.; Marfany, G. In Vitro Gene Delivery in Retinal Pigment Epithelium Cells by Plasmid DNA-Wrapped Gold Nanoparticles. *Genes* **2019**, *10*, 289. [CrossRef] [PubMed]
207. Zhang, X. Gold Nanoparticles: Recent Advances in the Biomedical Applications. *Cell Biophys.* **2015**, *72*, 771–775. [CrossRef]
208. Peeters, L.; Sanders, N.N.; Braeckmans, K.; Boussery, K.; Van De Voorde, J.; De Smedt, S.C.; Demeester, J. Vitreous: A barrier to nonviral ocular gene therapy. *Investig. Opthalmol. Vis. Sci.* **2005**, *46*, 3553–3561. [CrossRef] [PubMed]
209. Chen, F.; McLenachan, S.; Edel, M.; Da Cruz, L.; Coffey, P.; Mackey, D. iPS Cells for Modelling and Treatment of Retinal Diseases. *J. Clin. Med.* **2014**, *3*, 1511–1541. [CrossRef]
210. Takahashi, K.; Tanabe, K.; Ohnuki, M.; Narita, M.; Ichisaka, T.; Tomoda, K.; Yamanaka, S. Induction of Pluripotent Stem Cells from Adult Human Fibroblasts by Defined Factors. *Cell* **2007**, *131*, 861–872. [CrossRef] [PubMed]
211. Lamba, D.A.; Gust, J.; Reh, T.A. Transplantation of human embryonic stem cells derived photoreceptors restores some visual function in Crx deficient mice. *Cell Stem Cell* **2009**, *4*, 73–79. [CrossRef] [PubMed]
212. Pearson, R.A.; Barber, A.C.; Rizzi, M.; Hippert, C.; Xue, T.; West, E.L.; Duran, Y.; Smith, A.J.; Chuang, J.Z.; Azam, S.A.; et al. Restoration of vision after transplantation of photoreceptors. *Nature* **2012**, *485*, 99–103. [CrossRef] [PubMed]
213. West, E.L.; Gonzalez-Cordero, A.; Hippert, C.; Osakada, F.; Martinez-Barbera, J.P.; Pearson, R.A.; Ali, R.R. Defining the integration capacity of embryonic stem cell-derived photoreceptor precursors. *Stem Cells* **2012**, *30*, 1424–1435. [CrossRef] [PubMed]
214. Barber, A.C.; Hippert, C.; Duran, Y.; West, E.L.; Bainbridge, J.W.; Warre-Cornish, K.; Pearson, R.A. Repair of the degenerate retina by photoreceptor transplantation. *Proc. Natl. Acad Sci. USA* **2013**, *110*, 354–359. [CrossRef] [PubMed]
215. Pearson, R.A.; Cordero, A.G.; West, E.L.; Ribeiro, J.R.; Aghaizu, N.; Goh, D.; Sampson, R.D.; Georgiadis, A.; Waldron, P.V.; Duran, Y.; et al. Donor and host photoreceptors engage in material transfer following transplantation of post-mitotic photoreceptor precursors. *Nat. Commun.* **2016**, *7*, 13029. [CrossRef] [PubMed]
216. Santos-Ferreira, T.; Llonch, S.; Börsch, O.; Postel, K.; Haas, J.; Ader, M. Retinal transplantation of photoreceptors results in donor–host cytoplasmic exchange. *Nat. Commun.* **2016**, *7*, 13028. [CrossRef] [PubMed]
217. Liu, Y.; Xu, H.W.; Wang, L.; Li, S.Y.; Zhao, C.J.; Hao, J.; Li, Q.Y.; Zhao, T.T.; Wu, W.; Wang, Y.; et al. Human embryonic stem cell-derived retinal pigment epithelium transplants as a potential treatment for wet age-related macular degeneration. *Cell Discov.* **2018**, *4*, 50. [CrossRef] [PubMed]

218. Schwartz, S.D.; Regillo, C.D.; Lam, B.L.; Eliott, D.; Rosenfeld, P.J.; Gregori, N.Z.; Hubschman, J.-P.; Davis, J.L.; Heilwell, G.; Spirn, M.; et al. Human embryonic stem cell-derived retinal pigment epithelium in patients with age-related macular degeneration and Stargardt's macular dystrophy: Follow-up of two open-label phase 1/2 studies. *Lancet* **2015**, *385*, 509–516. [CrossRef]
219. Song, W.K.; Park, K.-M.; Kim, H.-J.; Lee, J.H.; Choi, J.; Chong, S.Y.; Shim, S.H.; Del Priore, L.V.; Lanza, R. Treatment of Macular Degeneration Using Embryonic Stem Cell-Derived Retinal Pigment Epithelium: Preliminary Results in Asian Patients. *Stem Cell Rep.* **2015**, *4*, 860–872. [CrossRef] [PubMed]
220. Mandai, M.; Watanabe, A.; Kurimoto, Y.; Hirami, Y.; Morinaga, C.; Daimon, T.; Fujihara, M.; Akimaru, H.; Sakai, N.; Shibata, Y.; et al. Autologous Induced Stem-Cell–Derived Retinal Cells for Macular Degeneration. *N. Engl. J. Med.* **2017**, *376*, 1038–1046. [CrossRef] [PubMed]
221. Zrenner, E. Will Retinal Implants Restore Vision? *Science* **2002**, *295*, 1022–1025. [CrossRef] [PubMed]
222. Bloch, E.; Luo, Y.; Da Cruz, L. Advances in retinal prosthesis systems. *Ther. Adv. Ophthalmol.* **2019**, *11*, 2515841418817501. [CrossRef] [PubMed]
223. da Cruz, L.; Dorn, J.D.; Humayun, M.S.; Dagnelie, G.; Handa, J.; Barale, P.O.; Salzmann, J. Five-Year Safety and Performance Results from the Argus II Retinal Prosthesis System Clinical Trial. *Ophthalmology* **2016**, *123*, 2248–2254. [CrossRef] [PubMed]

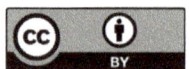

© 2019 by the authors. Licensee MDPI, Basel, Switzerland. This article is an open access article distributed under the terms and conditions of the Creative Commons Attribution (CC BY) license (http://creativecommons.org/licenses/by/4.0/).

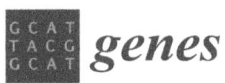

Commentary

The Foundation Fighting Blindness Plays an Essential and Expansive Role in Driving Genetic Research for Inherited Retinal Diseases

Ben Shaberman * and Todd Durham *

Foundation Fighting Blindness, 7168 Columbia Gateway Drive, Suite 100, Columbia, MD 21046, USA
* Correspondence: bshaberman@fightingblindness.org (B.S.); tdurham@fightingblindness.org (T.D.); Tel.: +1-410-423-0634 (B.S. & T.D.)

Received: 20 June 2019; Accepted: 4 July 2019; Published: 6 July 2019

Abstract: The Foundation Fighting Blindness leads a collaborative effort among patients and families, scientists, and the commercial sector to drive the development of preventions, treatments, and cures for inherited retinal diseases (IRDs). When the nonprofit was established in 1971, it sought the knowledge and insights of leaders in the retinal research field to guide its research funding decisions. While the Foundation's early investments focused on gaining a better understanding of the genetic causes of IRDs, its portfolio of projects would come to include some of the most innovative approaches to saving and restoring vision, including gene replacement/augmentation therapies, gene editing, RNA modulation, optogenetics, and gene-based neuroprotection. In recent years, the Foundation invested in resources such as its patient registry, natural history studies, and genetic testing program to bolster clinical development and trials for emerging genetic therapies. Though the number of clinical trials for such therapies has surged over the last decade, the Foundation remains steadfast in its commitment to funding the initiatives that hold the most potential for eradicating the entire spectrum of IRDs.

Keywords: retinitis pigmentosa; Usher syndrome; Stargardt disease; Leber congenital amaurosis; RPE65; nonprofit; patient registry; translational

1. Introduction

The founders of the Foundation Fighting Blindness had no idea how challenging the development of treatments and cures for inherited retinal diseases (IRDs) would be. Little did they know, it would take nearly two decades for Foundation-funded researchers to find the first IRD gene and more than 35 years to advance a gene therapy into a human study.

The nonprofit was established in 1971, when Eliot Berson, MD, brought together Gordon and Lulie Gund and Ben and Beverly Berman to create the first IRD research center: the Berman–Gund Laboratory for the Study of Retinal Degenerations at Massachusetts Eye and Ear Infirmary.

At the time, Dr. Berson had recently diagnosed the Berman's young daughters, Mindy and Joanne, with retinitis pigmentosa (RP). Gordon had recently lost all of his vision to RP after he and Lulie had completed an exhaustive search for something—anything—to save his vision. The Gund's quest for a cure, which included a harrowing journey to a clinic in Russia at the height of the Cold War, came up empty.

It was obvious to the Foundation's founders that virtually nothing was known about the conditions. Furthermore, they understood that no other entity—public or private—would fund research for rare retinal conditions. There was simply no commercial incentive for anyone to do so at the time. Driven by passion and a personal commitment, the small group of families took it upon themselves to get the research off the ground. Their goal was clear and singular: find preventions, treatments, and cures for everyone affected. The Berman–Gund lab was their first step forward, but little did they know how difficult the path forward would be.

"If you put your shoulder to the grindstone, we'd find an answer in five or six years," said Lulie, reflecting on her expectations for conquering RP. "It just never occurred to me it could go on so long."

Today, nearly 50 years later, the Foundation is the world's largest private funding source for research to find preventions, treatments, and cures for the entire spectrum of IRDs. The nonprofit has raised more than $750 million toward its focused mission. Throughout its history, the Foundation has been led by a board and trustees comprised of families and individuals with IRDs. Likewise, it has been largely funded by grassroots donors who are also affected. Its urgent mission has been driven by those who have the greatest stake in its success.

Excitingly, there has been a tremendous surge in human research for treatments over the past 10–15 years. Nearly three dozen clinical trials for IRD therapies are underway. The US Food and Drug Administration's (FDA's) approval of LUXTURNA™ (Voretigene neparvovec)—the first gene therapy for the eye or an inherited condition to receive regulatory marketing approval—was a historical moment for the Foundation, which funded preclinical studies that made the sight-restoring treatment possible. The Foundation's leadership and supporters were ebullient about the advent of the life-changing gene therapy. Finally, something made it across the finish line. Something worked, and it worked well.

However, the Foundation recognized it must optimally leverage the LUXTURNA™ approval and clinical research momentum to save the vision for the millions who still do not have any therapies. The Foundation's funding strategy has therefore evolved from only funding basic lab research to better understand IRDs to also getting treatments across the translational chasm known as "the valley of death"—that is, to the point where biotechnology and pharmaceutical companies would invest in their clinical and commercial development.

A little de-risking from the Foundation has gone a long way. Looking at the current IRD gene therapy and genetic treatment landscape, the Foundation's footprint is virtually everywhere. Most current and emerging genetics-based treatments were made possible by lab, translational, and/or early clinical research funded in part by the Foundation.

In 2018, the Foundation launched its venture philanthropy fund, known as the Retinal Degeneration Fund (RD Fund), with initial capital of $70 million. Its charter is not only to fund translational and early stage clinical projects, but to attract more venture capital into the IRD space and re-invest returns back into research.

"Yes, we are a nonprofit, but that doesn't mean we shouldn't realize and re-invest returns for projects we are funding", said Benjamin Yerxa, PhD, the Foundation's chief executive officer. "The IRD gene therapy business is burgeoning, and we owe it to patients and families to leverage that momentum as much as possible to accelerate and expand therapy development."

While the Foundation has traditionally emphasized research to identify treatment targets and develop therapies for these genetic retinal conditions, its project portfolio has recently expanded to include natural history studies—ProgStar, for people with Stargardt disease, and RUSH2A, for those with *USH2A* mutations—as well as the global patient registry at www.MyRetinaTracker.org. An ancillary study of My Retina Tracker has thus far provided diagnostic genetic testing to approximately 4,000 IRD patients, at no cost to them. The overarching goal for these new initiatives is to gain a better understanding of how these genetic diseases affect vision, share de-identified patient data for disease progression, genetically diagnose more patients, and facilitate recruitment for clinical trials.

Data from both My Retina Tracker and the natural history studies can accelerate clinical development by helping researchers identify more powerful and sensitive clinical endpoints.

2. Patient Perspectives on the Progress of Genetic Research

As mentioned, the FDA's approval of LUXTURNA™ in December 2017 created tremendous excitement and hope for patients and families with IRDs. The success of the gene therapy program provided proof that a genetic treatment could, in fact, save and restore vision and be made commercially available to the people who need it. For the thousands of constituents affiliated with the Foundation—many of whom had been part of the organization for several decades—this was the most important and encouraging advancement in their journey. Also, the advent of additional gene therapy clinical trials in recent years—for several other IRDs, including choroideremia, X-linked RP, Stargardt disease, and Usher syndrome type 1B—boosted optimism for the potential for genetic research to halt and reverse vision loss. The Foundation's constituents are also eager to learn about other genetic therapies, such as clustered regularly interspaced short palindromic repeats/CRISPR-associated protein 9 (CRISPR/Cas9) and antisense oligonucleotides, especially as these approaches begin to move into human studies.

With all the enthusiasm for the current progress in research, those affected are keenly aware that only one treatment has made it through the pipeline thus far. Furthermore, LUXTURNA™ can only help a small fraction of those affected. Much more work needs to be done to address the overall need. Ultimately, sustained hope and excitement about genetic research for each patient is often predicated on the advancement of research directed toward the mutated gene causing their (or a loved one's) IRD.

Jen Walker, a woman with moderate vision loss from RP (*PDE6A* mutations), is excited about the LUXTURNA™ milestone, but recognizes well the unmet need and the urgency to meet it. "Hearing about LUXTURNA™ was life changing. It was astounding to see so many young people with visual impairments regain sight. The feeling of putting away a white cane for good is immeasurable," she said, "but more work needs to be done. This is only one gene, when there are hundreds more. We need a cure quickly, as it's going to be harder to regain sight as we lose more and more photoreceptors. I am hopeful that doctors and researchers are noticing that gene therapy for vision is an up and coming science movement, and I hope everyone gets on board sooner than later."

John Corneille, who has advanced vision loss from RP (*PDE6B* mutations), shares Jen's urgency for answers, but maintains an overall positive outlook. He said, "There are days, for sure, when I get discouraged thinking, at age 59, a treatment will not be found in time to enable me to see the faces of my children and grandchildren again. Most days, however, I remain very optimistic, given how far we have come in the last couple of decades. It was very exciting to learn that a company in France is engaged in a clinical trial for my gene! I try not to think about the complexity of gene studies, replacement, and editing. But it is very reassuring to know that there are countless incredibly talented researchers working hard, each day, to find breakthrough treatments for us."

Though gene-specific therapies are often at the top of patients' minds, more are beginning to appreciate the potential of emerging, cross-cutting genetic treatment approaches, such as optogenetics. "Perhaps most exciting is the diversity of research approaches that seem likely to eventually address any stage of these progressive and devastating diseases," said Martha Steele, who has Usher syndrome type 2A. "As someone with advanced vision loss, I realize that not all treatments under investigation will likely work for me, but some, such as optogenetics, may well be in my future."

Thanks to the advanced power and increasing affordability of gene-sequencing panels, more people are getting genetically tested and having their IRD gene mutation(s) identified. A genetic diagnosis can have a big impact on the patient and their family. Of course, the genetic diagnosis can put people on the path toward a clinical trial or future treatment.

But for many patients, the identification of their gene mutation can also be cathartic. It's a step forward in unravelling the mystery of a disease that has been progressively robbing them of their vision. For parents, the identification of their gene mutation gives them answers about the risk of passing the IRD on to their kids. Depending on the result, the knowledge can be a relief or it can raise new questions and emotions.

For Michelle Glaze, a woman with moderate vision loss from mutations in *RP1*, getting a definitive genetic diagnosis took some time, but the result helped ease her mind about her son's risk of inheriting her IRD. "I had genetic testing done about six years ago. The initial diagnosis helped me to understand what was causing my vision loss. However, there were some missing pieces, which left some things unclear. I was not sure if my son was at risk. Thanks to additional investigation by a genetic counselor,

I learned he was not at risk. Thanks to advances in genetics, and the increased ability to identify pathogenic mutations, I am now able to rest well knowing that my son will not be affected by RP. This was always a fear, always a concern in my mind, until now. As a patient and mother, I am extremely grateful for advances in research, clinical developments, and genetic testing. I have an increased hope that I may be able to see my son's sweet face clearly one day."

Michelle's story underscores how critical a genetic counselor can be to the patient's and family's understanding and journey in managing an IRD, especially when results are inconclusive or additional testing may be advised.

3. In the Beginning: The Foundation's Early Focus on Genetics

When the Foundation began funding research in the early 1970s, one of the few clues scientists had about IRDs was that they ran in families; the conditions were clearly genetic. The nonprofit and its scientific advisors—including prominent visionaries in the retinal research community, such as John Dowling, PhD, Morton Goldberg, MD, and Alan Laties, MD—understood that identifying the genetic causes would be critical to: 1) diagnosing patients, 2) elucidating disease pathways, and 3) the development of therapies.

As a result, throughout its early years and for decades to come, the Foundation aggressively funded (and continues to fund) the leading IRD genetic research labs around the world.

Despite its early and substantial investments in genetic research, it took nearly two decades for Foundation-funded investigators to find the first gene associated with RP (or any IRD). That gene was *RHO*, which was identified in 1989 by a team at Trinity College Dublin [1].

The landmark genetic breakthrough brought momentum to the search for more IRD genes, but the magnitude of the challenge was not well understood. To date, more than 270 genes have been associated with IRDs.

"In the 1980s, we expected there would only be a handful of RP genes. We now know there are more than 80 and still counting. The effort started with a small group of scientists, across the world, working together and sharing ideas, patient samples, and lab reagents," said Stephen Daiger, PhD, a world leader in IRD genetic research at The University of Texas Health Science Center in Houston, who has been funded by the Foundation for genetic research and discovery since 1986. "With the identification of *RHO* in 1989, the field took off. As the Human Genome Project got underway, the first useful byproduct was a much better map of human chromosomes. Because of this improved map, many more RP genes were mapped by 1995."

While most IRD genes have been identified, diagnostic gaps remain. Today, about two out of every three people with an IRD will have their gene mutation(s) identified when they undergo genetic diagnostic testing using a comprehensive gene panel. To address the need to genetically diagnose more patients, the Foundation is funding a five-year, $2.5 million project to find elusive IRD genes and mutations, including those in non-coding regions. The collaborative effort is being led by Dr. Daiger, Dr. Ayyagari, and Kinga Bujakowska, PhD, at Massachusetts Eye and Ear, and will include more than 140 families and an additional 400 individuals.

4. The Trajectory for Gene Therapy Development

With the discovery of the first genes associated with IRDs in the 1990s, the idea of developing gene replacement therapies—using viral vectors to replace mutated copies of an IRD gene with healthy copies—was tantalizingly attractive to the Foundation and its scientific advisors. After all, IRDs were caused by mutations in single genes and the retina was a clear and accessible target for such an approach. So, Foundation funding for IRD gene therapy, and relevant animal models for testing, began in earnest.

However, for Jean Bennett, MD, PhD, and Albert Maguire, MD, the visionaries for what eventually became LUXTURNA™, the idea of gene therapy for a condition like RP came to them in medical school, well before the first IRD gene had been discovered.

"I remember in 1985, my husband, Albert Maguire, asked me if I thought we could do a gene therapy for retinitis pigmentosa. I said, sure. But what I didn't tell him is that we didn't know the genes, we didn't have any animal models, and we didn't know how to deliver DNA to the target cells," recalled Dr. Bennett. "But that planted a seed and I started researching the state of the art. A few years later, I applied for a career development award from what was then the Retinitis Pigmentosa Foundation, now the Foundation Fighting Blindness, and got it. And that launched my whole career developing gene therapy for retinal degenerations."

The Foundation invested approximately $10 million in *RPE65* gene therapy lab studies to enable the launch of the clinical trial in 2007 at the Children's Hospital of Philadelphia (CHOP), which brought to fruition the vision of Drs. Bennett and Maguire. It was the first clinical trial of a gene therapy for an IRD. The company Spark Therapeutics was spun out of CHOP in 2013 to raise the money needed to get the treatment across the regulatory finish line and out to the patients who needed it. In early 2019, Spark was acquired by Roche for nearly $5 billion.

"The Foundation's goal has been, and always will be, to get vision-saving treatments out to the people who need them. LUXTURNA™ was an important first step in achieving that goal, and we will be in business until all inherited retinal diseases are eradicated," said Dr. Yerxa. "We are also delighted that our projects are attracting such large commercial investments, including Roche's potential acquisition of Spark. It affirms we are on the right track with the right science, the right strategies, and the right investments."

Several other clinical trials for IRD gene therapies were made possible by earlier Foundation funding. Take, for example, Nightstar Therapeutics' Phase 3 clinical trial for its choroideremia gene therapy, which has preserved or improved vision for 90 percent of patients in a Phase 1/2 study. That study would not have been possible without earlier lab research by Miguel Seabra, PhD, who received more than $1.5 million from the Foundation for his efforts to characterize the *CHM* gene, develop a rodent model of choroideremia, and evaluate early versions of the *CHM* gene therapy in lab studies. Nightstar was recently acquired by Biogen for approximately $800 million.

Large animal models and related safety and efficacy studies have been invaluable to the advancement of IRD gene therapies, and perhaps no other Foundation-funded lab has been more productive in IRD large animal research than the University of Pennsylvania School of Veterinary Medicine. Its successful studies in canines have led to gene therapy clinical trials for: Leber congenital amaurosis (*RPE65* mutations), X-linked RP (*RPGR* mutations), and achromatopsia (*CNGA3* and *CNGB3* mutations). Human trials resulting from its Best disease and RP (*RHO* mutations) gene therapy canine studies are currently being planned.

5. Beyond Gene Replacement

While momentum for the clinical development of gene replacement therapies for IRDs is strong, the approach has its limitations.

For example, the cargo capacity of the adeno-associated viruses (AAVs) commonly (and successfully) used for gene delivery in LUXTURNA™ and most ongoing clinical trials is limited to about 4.7 kb. Several genes, including *ABCA4* (Stargardt disease), *USH2A* (RP and Usher syndrome), and *CEP290* (LCA) exceed the AAV's capacity.

Also, for autosomal dominant IRDs, such as RP caused by mutations in *RHO*, the delivery of a replacement gene will not be sufficient; a therapy will need to silence the mutated allele encoding the toxic protein or the allele acting in a dominant-negative fashion.

In recent years, the Foundation's research portfolio has expanded to include gene-editing treatment approaches such as CRISPR/Cas9 for autosomal dominant RP caused by mutations in *RHO* (Johns Hopkins and Columbia) and RP1 (Massachusetts Eye and Ear), as well as Usher syndrome type 1B caused by mutations in *MYO7A* (UCLA).

In February 2018, the Foundation Fighting Blindness, through its RD Fund, announced funding of up to $7.5 million for the development of ProQR's QR-421a, an antisense oligonucleotide (AON) designed to block mutations in RNA caused by defects in exon 13 of USH2A. ProQR announced in March 2019 that it had dosed the first patient in its Phase 1/2 clinical trial for QR-421a. Excitingly, the company reported vision improvements for 60 percent of participants in its Phase 1/2 targeting a recurrent mutation in CEP290, which causes LCA10. A Phase 2/3 trial for the LCA10 AON is now underway.

6. Cross-Cutting Gene Therapies

Even before the first gene replacement therapy clinical trial got off the ground (the RPE65 trial at CHOP) in 2007, Foundation-funded scientists were envisioning neuroprotective gene-therapy paradigms that could help people regardless of the mutated gene causing their disease. That is, delivering a gene to express proteins that would slow photoreceptor degeneration.

Neuroprotection became attractive to Foundation leadership and scientific advisors because of the technical and financial infeasibility of developing a gene replacement therapy for the hundreds of mutated genes that cause IRDs. According to RetNet (https://sph.uth.edu/retnet/) there are more than 270 genes associated with IRDs. Furthermore, approximately one third of patients will not have their mutation(s) identified when genetically tested.

In 2005, José Sahel, MD, and Thierry Léveillard, PhD, at the Institut de la Vision, received the Foundation's Board of Director's Award for identifying a protein produced and secreted by rod photoreceptors that prevented cones from degenerating in models of RP. Aptly named the rod-derived cone-viability factor (RdCVF), the protein was an intriguing approach for saving cone-mediated vision in people with RP and related conditions. Perhaps most appealing was that RdCVF had the potential to work independent of the patient's mutated gene—an approach that would be desirable for those whose gene mutation could not be identified, or those for whom gene replacement or editing wasn't technically desirable.

The newly-formed French company SparingVision plans to advance RdCVF into a clinical trial soon, thanks to the culmination of many years of lab funding from the Foundation and its recent commitment of up to €7 million.

The Foundation is also funding optogenetic therapies—the delivery of a gene to retinal ganglion or bipolar cells to express a light-sensitive protein in a retina that has lost all its photoreceptors due to an advanced IRD. In fact, the Foundation funded preclinical research for retinal optogenetic approaches currently in clinical trials—studies sponsored by Allergan and GenSight. The Foundation is also funding John Flannery, PhD, UC Berkeley, who is developing optogenetic alternatives designed to work in more natural lighting conditions.

While still in early clinical trials, optogenetic therapies hold promise for restoring meaningful vision to people who have lost all of their photoreceptors, regardless of the mutated gene causing their blindness.

7. Natural History Studies: Learning about Disease Progression and Genotype–Phenotype Correlations

The successful development of any new therapy requires a thorough understanding of the disease—in the absence of treatment—ideally from the time of diagnosis to its end stages. Understanding this natural history of disease enables clinical researchers to describe the clinical manifestations of disease (the phenotype) and its association with the genotype, estimate how quickly the disease progresses over time, identify patient characteristics that predict slower or faster disease progression, and study which clinical assessments are most appropriate to measure a treatment's benefit. Addressing these objectives is particularly important for IRDs because they are highly variable in their clinical manifestations, they may progress over decades, and because they are rare diseases about which little may be known. Ultimately, the knowledge gained from natural history studies will provide a number of key insights. This fundamental work will inform the designs of clinical trials of new treatments, the patient population most likely to benefit, the length of follow-up required to demonstrate a benefit, and the outcomes that are most sensitive to change [2].

The Foundation funds and conducts natural history studies of IRDs through its Clinical Consortium, a coordinating center and an international group of over 25 leading research centers which are experts in IRDs. The Clinical Consortium's mission is to accelerate the development of treatments for IRDs through collaborative and transparent clinical research. These objectives are met by ensuring the studies are designed, led, and reported by participating investigators and by making the study datasets publicly available for wider use. Because the studies are conducted using industry standards for quality—including good clinical practice (GCP) and site certification for retinal imaging modalities—the Foundation has designed the studies so the data will have broad utility, including, in some situations, to serve as a historical control.

Currently, the Foundation's Clinical Consortium is conducting RUSH2A, a prospective, four-year, natural history study of approximately 100 patients with an IRD associated with mutations in the *USH2A* gene, the most common mutated gene in Usher syndrome type 2 and a frequent cause of non-syndromic RP. The primary objectives of the RUSH2A study are to characterize the progression of the disease with respect to functional outcome measures (e.g., visual acuity and static perimetry) and structural outcome measures (e.g., the area of the ellipsoid zone measured by SD-OCT), to investigate the relationships between structure and function, and to assess whether there are genotypic or phenotypic predictors of progression at four years.

By the end of 2019, the Clinical Consortium plans to initiate a natural history study of retinal dystrophy associated with the *EYS* gene, PRO-EYS. The PRO-EYS study has similar objectives to RUSH2A and will follow approximately 100 patients for four years. A key feature of PRO-EYS is that the patient population will be stratified by the severity of disease at study entry. Thus, the study will provide valuable information that can be used to design trials for treatments at various stages of disease progression.

Natural history studies of IRDs and their associated pathogenic genes will continue to be a major activity of the Foundation's Clinical Consortium. These studies have broad applicability; they therefore represent an ideal partnership opportunity for industry sponsors, who can save time and effort by leveraging the network's existing research infrastructure and access to IRD patients around the world.

8. My Retina Tracker: The Foundation's Global Patient Registry

Patient data for IRDs—both genetic and phenotypic information—is rare. Furthermore, IRD patient data collected by academic research centers is usually not shared widely and often limited to the conditions studied by the institution.

However, the need for comprehensive IRD patient data has become paramount with the surge in clinical trials for emerging therapies. The success of these human studies depends greatly on a sponsor's ability to recruit enough genotypically and phenotypically well-characterized patients.

In 2014, the Foundation launched its secure global patient registry, My Retina Tracker (www.MyRetinaTracker.org), to provide pre-screened researchers and companies with de-identified patient and disease data for relevant studies, including IRD clinical trials and natural history studies.

The registry is patient controlled; the patient uploads and maintains their own record. When a company or researcher searches the registry for potential clinical trial participants, they never receive patient names or personal information. Instead, they are sent an alphanumeric identifier, which Foundation administrators use to identify and notify the patient who matched the search criteria. It is then up to the patient to contact the clinical trial coordinator about possible participation in the trial or study.

As of June 2019, more than 12,260 patients (with an informative profile of their disease) were registered in My Retina Tracker. Approximately 400 new patients register every month.

The Foundation Fighting Blindness has been conducting a genetic testing study for patients registered in My Retina Tracker. Through the study, registrants obtain genetic testing, at no cost to them.

A 266 IRD gene panel (includes copy number variation testing) is being used to screen DNA samples. No cost genetic counseling is provided for those patients who don't receive genetic counseling from their clinic or physician.

"Genetically characterizing IRD patients and making their de-identified molecular and disease information available to the research community is critical for advancing human disease and therapy studies," said Brian Mansfield, PhD, the Foundation's executive vice president research and interim chief scientific officer. "Dozens of therapy developers and investigators from around the world have used data from My Retina Tracker to advance their lab and clinical research. With approximately 200,000 IRD patients in the United States alone, we still have a lot of work to do, but we are building momentum as more patients learn about My Retina Tracker and the genetic testing study."

9. Conclusion: Filling the Gaps to Advance the Field

The Foundation's role in driving genetic research for IRDs has evolved and expanded as a result of advancement in biological sciences, the development of powerful gene sequencing technologies, the mapping of the human genome, and the growth in its own revenues and membership base. Of course, success in gene therapy development—including the regulatory approval of LUXTURNA™ and the impressive results from preclinical research that propelled the *RPE65* gene therapy toward the clinic—has also brought accelerating momentum to clinical development in the field.

However, the Foundation has always maintained (and continues to maintain) a commitment to funding projects that would fill critical gaps in research that were not addressed by commercial or government sectors, especially when doing so advanced the entire IRD field.

Today, the My Retina Tracker patient registry, genetic testing study, and Stargardt disease and *USH2A* natural history studies are all prime examples of significant Foundation investments that are having a wide-reaching impact in the advancement of research, especially when it comes to the clinical development of sight-saving and -restoring therapies. In most cases, these are major investments, each costing several millions of dollars, which other organizations haven't been able or willing to make.

The Foundation's long-standing, guiding imperative—whatever the investment—is to ensure that it is based on good science and it will get more preventions, treatments, and cures for IRDs across the finish line for everyone affected.

Conflicts of Interest: The authors declare no conflict of interest.

References

1. McWilliam, P.; Farrar, G.J.; Kenna, P.; Bradley, D.G.; Humphries, M.M.; Sharp, E.M.; McConnell, D.J.; Lawler, M.; Sheils, D.; Ryan, C.; et al. Autosomal dominant retinitis pigmentosa (ADRP): Localization of an ADRP gene to the long arm of chromosome 3. *Genomics* **1989**, *5*, 619–622. [CrossRef]
2. Food and Drug Administration Center for Drug Evaluation and Research (CDER); Center for Biologics Evaluation and Research (CBER); Office of Orphan Products Development (OOPD). Rare Diseases: Natural History Studies for Drug Development. Guidance for Industry. March 2019. Available online: https://www.fda.gov/media/122425/download (accessed on 1 March 2019).

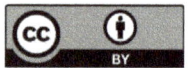

© 2019 by the authors. Licensee MDPI, Basel, Switzerland. This article is an open access article distributed under the terms and conditions of the Creative Commons Attribution (CC BY) license (http://creativecommons.org/licenses/by/4.0/).

MDPI
St. Alban-Anlage 66
4052 Basel
Switzerland
Tel. +41 61 683 77 34
Fax +41 61 302 89 18
www.mdpi.com

Genes Editorial Office
E-mail: genes@mdpi.com
www.mdpi.com/journal/genes